Operating Room Management

Operating Room Management

Ronald A. Gabel, M.D.
Professor and Former Chairman, Department of Anesthesiology, University of Rochester School of Medicine and Dentistry, Rochester, New York; Medical Director, Lattimore Community Surgicenter, Rochester, New York

John C. Kulli, M.D.
Clinical Associate Professor, Department of Anesthesiology, University of Rochester School of Medicine and Dentistry, Rochester, New York; Former Operating Room Director, Strong Memorial Hospital, Rochester, New York

B. Stephen Lee, M.D., M.B.A.
Assistant Professor, Departments of Anesthesiology and Community and Preventive Medicine, University of Rochester School of Medicine and Dentistry, Rochester, New York; Quality Officer, Strong Health System, Rochester, New York

Deborah G. Spratt, R.N., M.P.A., C.N.O.R., C.N.A.A.
Nurse Manager, Operating Room, Strong Memorial Hospital, Rochester, New York; Former Clinical Director, Lattimore Community Surgicenter, Rochester, New York; Former Manager of Surgical Services, Highland Hospital, Rochester, New York

Denham S. Ward, M.D., Ph.D.
Professor and Chairman, Department of Anesthesiology, University of Rochester School of Medicine and Dentistry, Rochester, New York; Professor, Department of Electrical Engineering, University of Rochester, Rochester, New York; Senior Director, Surgical Support Services, Strong Memorial Hospital, Rochester, New York

With a Foreword by
Paul G. Barash, M.D.
Professor, Department of Anesthesiology, Yale University School of Medicine, New Haven, Connecticut; Attending Anesthesiologist, Yale-New Haven Hospital, New Haven

and

Inez E. Tenzer, R.N., M.S., C.N.A.A., C.N.O.R.
Assistant Director, Divisional Nursing, Kaiser Permanente, Pasadena, California; Adjunct Faculty, Department of Nursing, Sonoma State University, Sonoma, California

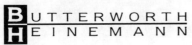

Boston   Oxford   Auckland   Johannesburg   Melbourne   New Delhi

Library of Congress Cataloging-in-Publication Data
Operating room management / Ronald A. Gabel . . . [et al.] ; foreword by
    Paul G. Barash and Inez E. Tenzer.
        p.   cm.
    Includes bibliographical references and index.
    ISBN 0-7506-9911-6
    1. Operating rooms--Administration. 2. Operating room nursing-
-Administration. I. Gabel, Ronald A.
    [DNLM: 1. Operating Rooms--organization & administration.
    2. Surgicenters--organization & administration. WX 200 0605 1999]
    RD63.0625 1999
    617' .917--dc21
    DNLM/DLC
    for Library of Congress   99-20092
                                                                      CIP

British Library Cataloguing-in-Publication Data
A catalogue record for this book is available from the British Library.

The publisher offers special discounts on bulk orders of this book.
For information, please contact:

Manager of Special Sales   For information on all Butterworth–
Butterworth–Heinemann   Heinemann publications available,
225 Wildwood Avenue   contact our World Wide Web home
Woburn, MA 01801-2041   page at: http://www.bh.com
Tel: 781-904-2500
Fax: 781-904-2620

10 9 8 7 6 5 4 3 2 1

Printed in the United States of America

*To Ann T. Mishia, for her abundant contributions to
the preparation of this book and for her long and steadfast
commitment to the Department of Anesthesiology
at the University of Rochester*

Contents

Foreword

As a source of prestige and as a technologic frontier, the operating room (OR) evokes a mystique that is unrivaled in modern medicine. To those who do not work there, the OR is a black box inhabited by demanding, arrogant individuals with enormous egos who require instant gratification. Conversely, those who do work in the OR cannot understand why the "system" does not fully comprehend the enormous benefits of the OR and accommodate to this epicenter of modern health care. The end of the era in which facilities were reimbursed based on how much they spent and physicians were rewarded for the number of procedures performed and the beginning of the economics of managed care have forced a change in attitude. Because it has the potential to spend a significant portion of a facility's budget, the OR must be run with a high degree of efficiency, must be parsimonious in acquiring technology, and must manage logistical support as if the organization is in combat. All of the stakeholders—administrators, physicians, nurses, support staff, and, last but not least, patients—are involved in critical decision making.

Books relating to the OR address various aspects of the perioperative environment from management to clinical preparation. Most are written from the nursing perspective, reflecting the bygone era when a strong head nurse, feared by all, acted as a benevolent dictator for the common good. Currently, individuals from various disciplines—nursing, medicine, and administration—share responsibility for OR management. Until now, no book has analyzed the OR from each of these points of view. *Operating Room Management* offers the unique perspectives of experienced and knowledgeable individuals who present a method for successful administration of the OR that is integrated into the overall goals of the parent facility. The material is presented so that it can be applied to many different practice settings.

At a time when health care is experiencing accelerated change, sometimes verging on chaos, an interdisciplinary approach to coping with the demands of survival and progress is critical. The complexity of the perioperative service requires a leadership team that is knowledgeable about the external and internal environments. This team should know the primary influences on the success of its decisions. For those who have managerial responsibility for the OR, the difference between success and failure is small. We believe that *Operating Room Management* adds considerable value to the reader's armamentarium by reducing the risk of error and enhancing a rational decision-making process.

Paul G. Barash
Inez E. Tenzer

Preface: Why a Book on Operating Room Management?

I keep six honest serving men (They taught me all I knew).
Their names are What and Why and When.
And How and Where and Who.

—Rudyard Kipling (1865–1936)

Health care organizations are increasingly pressured to provide high-quality surgical care at the lowest possible cost. OR suites have historically been considered a substantial source of revenue by senior hospital management. In 1992, a major health care consulting company estimated that the profit from adding just one additional surgical case per day could contribute as much as $500,000 per year to margin. Hence, consultants in the early 1990s advised hospitals to increase the number of ORs to improve profitability. However, the progression of managed care has made this a risky strategy. With mounting constraints on revenues, the need for expert management of expensive hospital resources is increasing. The OR suite is among the most resource-intensive units in a health care organization.

OR suites represent an extremely complex clinical and administrative environment. Various aspects of OR management involve nurses, anesthesiologists, surgeons, health care administrators, and other professionals having specialized knowledge. Because each of these groups has a different perspective and a unique background, it is difficult in one book to provide a unifying, albeit diverse, knowledge base. We have described the OR environment for those unfamiliar with it and included enough detail to make this book a useful reference for hands-on OR managers. We have also kept in mind that senior health care administrators need in-depth knowledge to understand the broad issues behind efficient OR management, including an appreciation of the daily issues that must be dealt with to run an OR suite efficiently. Therefore, this book is descriptive of the OR environment and designed to help managers who are actively engaged in day-to-day OR management or who have broad administrative or fiscal responsibilities for the OR suite.

Besides having dissimilar personal backgrounds and varying responsibilities, readers of this book are likely to work in diverse health care settings. We have taken this into account in the specific examples distributed throughout the book. However, our intent is to focus on broad principles of management that are equally applicable to OR suites in all settings.

Ronald A. Gabel
John C. Kulli
B. Stephen Lee
Deborah G. Spratt
Denham S. Ward

Prologue: Terminology and Scenarios

There are two kinds of people, those who do the work and those who take the credit.
Try to be in the first group; there is less competition there.

—*Indira Gandhi (1917–1984)*

TERMINOLOGY

No universal terminology is available for many of the common roles and items in ORs. In this book, we use the term *operating room* when referring to the specific site in which surgical operations take place and the term *OR suite* when referring to a collection of ORs and their supporting facilities, including a preoperative area and a postanesthesia recovery room, which are usually physically adjacent to the ORs. Because the word *operations* can mean either surgical operations or working systems that support functional areas, we use *surgical operations* when the unqualified term might be ambiguous.

The person in charge of the OR suite is generically referred to as the *operating room manager*. This function is often served by the OR nurse manager, although in larger medical centers a physician sometimes has the title *OR director* or *OR medical director*. We hope that our generic use of the term *OR manager* easily translates to terminology that is already known to readers.

SCENARIOS

Throughout this book, we illustrate typical management problems using hypothetical examples from three settings: a freestanding surgical center, an acute care community hospital, and a university medical center. Each of these settings is fictional, but the problems and settings are quite familiar to

the authors, who have held management and leadership roles in each type of organization. Freestanding Surgical Center (FSC) is a freestanding OR suite, while the OR suites of Community Medical Center (CMC) and University Medical Center (UMC) exist within larger health care organizations.

Although most community hospitals are still nonprofit, we have made CMC part of a growing for-profit health care organization. We have done so partly because this appears to be an evolving trend and partly because the profit status of the parent organization should not influence how the ORs are organized and managed. UMC, like most academic medical centers, is extremely complex and is trying to cope with major changes in health care.

The following descriptions of the three fictional settings are meant primarily to provide background for the examples scattered throughout this book. However, they also give general background for readers who may not be familiar with diverse health care settings. We hope that readers who work in health care organizations find one or more of the fictional settings familiar and realistic.

Freestanding Surgical Center

FSC is a for-profit facility dedicated to performing ambulatory surgery in a medium-sized city. It competes for business with two hospitals and another freestanding ambulatory surgical center (ASC). FSC is owned by a group of physicians (two orthopedic surgeons, a gynecologist, and a gastroenterologist), all of whom use the facility. It is located in an office building for physicians that was built by a developer. FSC has an 8-year lease on its space. The 11,000-square-foot surgical center has four ORs and two treatment rooms. Most of the equipment is less than 5 years old. Last year, FSC purchased an ophthalmologic laser system and several new arthroscopes to accommodate advancing technology.

FSC was conceived approximately 10 years ago as a way to give the surgeons and the gastroenterologist more control over their workplace than was possible in the local hospitals. Surgeons choose to work at the center because it is efficient and provides state-of-the-art equipment. Ophthalmologists, orthopedists, otolaryngologists, general surgeons, and podiatrists are key customers. One treatment room is dedicated to gastroenterologic endoscopies, and minor office procedures are performed in the other treatment room. Approximately 200 operations are performed each month, two-thirds of them surgical and one-third medical procedures, primarily endoscopies.

FSC is governed by a board of directors made up of the owners. The medical director is not an owner, but she is an anesthesiologist and senior partner in the three-member anesthesia group with which FSC contracts. FSC's administrative team is made up of a clinical manager (a registered nurse [RN]) and an administrator. They and the medical director report to the board of directors, currently chaired by one of the orthopedic surgeons.

The professional staff is made up of RNs and OR technicians, all of whom have substantial previous OR experience. Nurses with many years of hospital experience seek employment at FSC because it provides a pleasant working environment and one without night or weekend shifts. FSC is Medicare approved, state certified, and accredited by the Accreditation Association for Ambulatory Health Care, ensuring that, from a quality perspective, many outside observers are monitoring FSC's systems.

Two standing committees advise the board of directors. A multidisciplinary group called the Quality Improvement Committee is composed of representatives from nursing, anesthesiology, surgery, and the business office. The Medical Affairs Committee, made up of the medical director, the chief of surgery, the chief of anesthesiology, the chief of medicine (gastroenterology), and the clinical manager, who is a nonvoting member, conducts credentialing, disciplinary, and policy-making activities. The medical director chairs both of these committees and meets regularly with the board of directors.

Systems set in place to ensure financial viability are focused on improving efficiency. For example, all routine cases have custom packs to help decrease turnover time. All patients receiving anesthesia are screened for medical problems through a telephone call by an RN, using a form jointly developed by the clinical manager and the chief of anesthesiology. Patients with significant medical problems are referred to a preoperative clinic conducted by the anesthesiologists, who handle medical problems in conjunction with primary care physicians. Relatively healthy patients are medically evaluated by an anesthesiologist on the day of surgery.

FSC has a multifunction computer system that (1) schedules by *Current Procedural Terminology* (*CPT*) codes, (2) automatically produces surgeon preference cards, and (3) monitors use of supplies for reordering. The computer software includes a billing function that communicates electronically with most major insurers.

Community Medical Center

CMC is located in a predominantly middle-class, medium-sized suburb of a major metropolitan city. Two large employers, a computer technology firm and an automobile parts manufacturing company, employ about one-half of the working population. Many of the remaining employed population commute to the larger city.

The local community has experienced an economic boom in the last 10 years. The computer technology firm has expanded several times to meet increasing demand for microprocessors and memory chips. The automobile parts company has expanded its numerous contracts with automobile manufacturers. However, recent global competition has forced both firms to focus on increasing productivity and reducing costs.

Employee health care benefits were extremely expensive under traditional indemnity insurance plans. Responding to demands of employee benefit managers for lower-cost health care coverage, health insurers have been implementing stringent utilization review processes for costly procedures and hospital admissions. Insurers are developing health maintenance organizations (HMOs) and other managed care products. Insurance companies are circulating "requests for proposal" to local and regional hospitals for specific high-volume and high-cost medical care, such as obstetric services and cardiac surgery. Requests for proposals for the full continuum of care, including both professional and facility services, are expected soon.

CMC is a 175-bed general hospital with 45 beds allocated to surgical patients. It was built in 1955 to replace an antiquated building that had served the community for the previous 30 years. The hospital was known as Community General Hospital until 1991, when the board of directors, faced with declining revenues and potential losses that could not be sustained by the hospital's meager reserves, reorganized the hospital and merged it with several skilled-nursing facilities and a group of 15 employed family physicians. The new entity was called Community Health Care System (CHCS). The merger was carried out with the assistance of a national for-profit health care chain. The community retains a 50% ownership in the new company through a non-profit community foundation, and the national chain owns the other half. CHCS was reorganized as a for-profit corporation. The community foundation was given a $1-million endowment and receives its share of the profits from CHCS. The foundation supports community health and childhood preventive care in the community. The board of directors is made up of the chief executive officer (CEO) of the hospital, one member of the medical staff, two prominent business people from the community, and four officers of the national chain.

One hundred and twenty-four physicians are on the medical staff, 73 of them on the "active" staff. Most members of the medical staff are primary care physicians, but 19 are surgeons, including three obstetrician/gynecologists, one oral surgeon, and three podiatrists. The three staff anesthesiologists practice as a group and have an exclusive contract with CMC. The group was granted its 3-year exclusive contract 2 years ago after problems with quality of care forced the anesthesiologists previously serving the hospital to leave. The group employs four certified registered nurse anesthetists (CRNAs).

A single suite on the fourth floor of the medical center holds four ORs. The obstetric unit is on the second floor of the hospital, directly below the OR suite. The suite is surrounded by offices and other facilities that would make expansion or renovation difficult. Storage and other support space in the OR suite is inadequate. The suite includes locker rooms and a small staff lounge shared by nurses and doctors. The nurse manager has an office in the suite.

Scheduling is carried out by the clerk at the OR control desk, who works from 7:00 AM to 3:30 PM, Monday through Friday. Surgical operations are scheduled in a loose-leaf notebook kept at the control desk, and the surgical registry and all OR statistics are maintained in handwritten documents; extracting any statistical data for decision making is a labor-intensive job. The new national partners in CHCS are planning to install an electronic information system that includes an OR database (ORDB).

For many years, only two of the four ORs were staffed for elective surgery. A third OR was staffed 2 years ago, however, when four new surgeons were recruited to work exclusively at CMC and a push was made to encourage other surgeons in the region to use the ORs at CMC more heavily. The current anesthesiology group was hired at that time.

The OR has no director position, but the OR nurse manager and the chief of anesthesiology work closely on operational issues.

University Medical Center

UMC, the flagship teaching hospital of a large university in a major metropolitan community, is a 700-bed institution that provides tertiary medical services. The main university campus is at a suburban site approximately 20 miles from the medical center. One other medical school and four other tertiary medical centers are located within the major metropolitan area surrounding UMC. One of the medical centers has recently been acquired by a national for-profit hospital chain.

UMC is a nonprofit institution with an independent board of directors. It was formed 50 years ago in a merger between City Hospital, Doctors' Hospital, and University Clinics. The CEO of UMC was appointed by the board of directors 5 years ago. He has been a faculty member for 20 years and was formerly chief of nephrology in the Internal Medicine Department. The chief operating officer (COO) has been with the medical center for 8 years and has been its COO for 3. He previously held a variety of management positions, mainly at various academic medical centers. The director of nursing has held this position for 15 years. She is a graduate of the University School of Nursing and has been at UMC for her entire career. The OR nurse manager has been a perioperative nurse and supervisor for 15 years, all at UMC, and reports to the director of nursing.

The medical school's dean has held that position for 3 years, having previously been associate dean for education at another medical school after serving for many years as a faculty member in the Department of Family Medicine. As dean, she reports to the president of the university. Each class has about 150 medical students and approximately 200 graduate students in a variety of disciplines. The medical students receive most of their clinical rotations at UMC. Chairs of the academic clinical departments all serve as chiefs of their services at UMC. The dean of the School of Nursing is located on the main university campus, and nursing students receive their clinical education at a variety of community sites, with relatively few rotations at UMC.

The physical plant of the medical center is a conglomeration of buildings, most built after World War II. The oldest buildings are used for various support and medical school research functions. The current UMC hospital was built 20 years ago, and a new ambulatory clinic building was finished 5 years ago. The medical center holds three OR suites: a four-OR ASC in the new ambulatory clinic building, two operative delivery rooms in the obstetric suite on the

second floor, and a 17-OR suite in the basement of the medical center. Approximately 17,000 operative procedures (including cesarean deliveries) are performed yearly in the 23 ORs.

The Department of Surgery is composed of eight divisions: general surgery, plastic surgery, otolaryngology, cardiothoracic surgery, vascular surgery, neurosurgery, transplant surgery, and pediatric surgery. UMC also has departments of orthopedics, obstetrics and gynecology, urology, ophthalmology, dentistry, and oral surgery. The Department of Anesthesiology, which provides all anesthesia services at UMC, has three divisions: cardiothoracic, obstetric, and pediatric anesthesia. All the anesthesiologists and approximately half of the surgeons are full-time faculty members at the university, and the other half of the surgeons are part-time faculty members who have their offices outside the university. The Department of Anesthesiology and all of the surgical specialties have residency programs.

UMC just hired a new OR director. He reports directly to the hospital COO. The ORs were previously managed through the Operating Room Committee, which was composed of the chairs of the surgical and anesthesiology departments, the director of surgical nursing, and the hospital COO. Chairmanship of this committee rotated. The new Operating Room Management Committee, chaired by the OR director, is made up of one anesthesiologist, one surgeon, the nurse manager, and an administrator who works for the OR director.

Operating Room Management

Chapter 1
The Clinical Enterprise

Life is short, the art long, opportunity fleeting, experience treacherous, judgment difficult.

—*Hippocrates (460–359 BC)*

The American system of health care is undergoing a revolutionary change, from a near-total focus on episodic medical care of the acutely ill to a broader view that takes into account the long-term overall health of entire populations. As this shift in clinical emphasis occurs, relationships among health care providers (including physicians and hospitals), health insurers, and the government are rapidly evolving. These changes are largely motivated by an unsustainable rate of growth in national expenditures on health care. Population-based health improvement strategies with emphasis on preventive care may, it is hoped, decrease the need for high-cost intervention after illness has occurred. Similarly, the move to managed care is intended to control costs by bringing the advantages of the competitive marketplace to the business of medicine.

The type of medical care provided in ORs is the antithesis, even the nemesis, of these dual changes in medicine. Surgical care is by definition episodic and by nature costly. Nonetheless, considerable illness remains for which only surgical intervention, extraordinarily expensive as it may be, can improve quality of life, provide palliation, or achieve cure. The conflict between the national goal of health care cost containment and the high cost of surgical operations is a powerful incentive to health care organizations to improve the quality of management of the surgical suite. High-quality OR management not only reduces costs but also improves the satisfaction of the many surgical "customers"—patients, surgeons, anesthesiologists, nurses, technical staff, administrators—and improves the quality of the product. Modern OR management is directed toward the complementary goals of improving quality and increasing productivity, thereby reducing costs.

HISTORY

Although the history of surgery is well documented, the history of the location in which surgery is performed is less well understood. Historical paintings show that the traditional surgical setting—the amphitheater—was primarily used to accommodate an audience. Eighteenth-century ORs were actually lecture auditoriums used to demonstrate dissection of cadavers. Live patients could sometimes be convinced to submit to an operation, which provided spectators with additional instruction. Most surgical procedures were minor, brief, and performed wherever convenient, usually wherever the patient happened to be (e.g., at home).

Because the role of pathogens in causing postoperative infection was not understood, scant consideration was given to this and other aspects of the surgical location. Good lighting was considered no more necessary than architectural embellishments meant to impress spectators or the patient. The introduction of anesthesia in the 1840s did little to influence the location where surgical operations were performed. Not until the late nineteenth century, when Joseph Lister identified the need for antisepsis, did it become necessary to give special consideration to the design of the space in which operations were performed. Lister's antisepsis technique required treatment of everything in contact with the patient with carbolic acid. Because of the caustic nature of the solution, surgeons began to protect their street clothes with aprons and their hands with rubber gloves. The function of the "circulating nurse" was to walk around the operating table spraying a fine mist of carbolic acid into the air to disinfect the dust that rose from the wooden floors. These special requirements ended the use of amphitheaters as ORs.

Gustav Neuber pioneered the use of dedicated ORs in Germany in the late nineteenth century. Like Lister, Neuber met with considerable resistance from the surgical establishment. He went so far as to build a private hospital with ORs designed to limit septic contamination. In Baltimore, Halsted introduced similar aseptic concepts at Johns Hopkins Hospital in the 1890s. By the early twentieth century, most large hospitals had three ORs—one each for general, orthopedic, and gynecologic surgery. This early specialized use of space most likely arose for the convenience of surgeons rather than to accommodate special equipment or staffing needs.

The field of surgery advanced rapidly during and immediately after World War II. Refinement of surgical techniques on the battlefield, coupled with the development of antibiotics, produced an atmosphere in which surgical advances took place almost daily. Changes in anesthesiology kept pace, making it possible for extremely sick patients to survive increasingly complex operations. Although ORs in the 1950s and 1960s were not substantially different from those of the early twentieth century, developing technology required many more pieces of equipment to be used in complex operations.

Surgery on ambulatory (non-hospitalized) patients was performed early in the twentieth century. J. H. Nicoll of Glasgow, Scotland, reported in 1909 to the British Medical Association on his experiences with ambulatory surgery in 8,988 children. Ralph Waters set up an ambulatory surgery clinic for dental procedures and minor surgery in Sioux City, Iowa, in 1916. Ambulatory surgery did not become commonplace, however, until Wallace Reed, a Phoenix anesthesiologist, opened a "Surgicenter"

in 1970. Such centers, initially viewed with some skepticism, proved to offer an equally safe but less expensive alternative to hospital-based surgery. Hospitals responded by developing separate ASCs or by allocating dedicated ambulatory ORs as part of their OR suites.

CHARACTERISTICS OF THE OPERATING ROOM ENVIRONMENT

Surgical teams perform sometimes difficult technical procedures under often unfavorable circumstances. Unavoidable problems inherent in surgery stem from several sources. First, patients and their diseases vary tremendously. Consequently, surgeons can never be certain in advance of what they will find and therefore exactly what operation they will perform. Second, once an operation has begun, turning back is impossible. If an orthopedic surgeon has taken out a native hip, the patient will not walk again until a prosthesis is in place; if the operation cannot be completed and the patient must return another day, the final outcome is usually less favorable than if the operation is completed as planned. Third, help is usually not readily available on short notice. Another surgeon to assist or to give advice is not normally at hand. A trip to the library to try to find the answer to a pressing question is not feasible (although exploring the Internet may become a viable option). Fourth, serious time pressures are present. Surgical operations in expert hands can last several hours. A major surgical misadventure, although not itself disastrous, may prolong surgical and anesthesia time, increase blood loss, and seriously prolong the time a relevant organ is nonfunctional. In cardiac surgery, for example, the length of time in which the heart is not beating during extracorporeal bypass is significantly correlated with outcome. Similarly, in orthopedic surgery a tourniquet may be used to keep the operative field free of blood, but tourniquet time cannot be extended indefinitely. In medical therapy, time for treatment is measured in days, weeks, and months; in surgical therapy, time for treatment is measured in seconds, minutes, and hours. (Of course, time for recovery and healing is another matter.)

Neither surgery nor anesthesia is completely free of risk. Among the risks that should be explained to every patient when obtaining informed consent for anesthesia and surgery is death. Unpredictable events occur, and even the most skilled and careful experts are, in reality, fallible human beings who make mistakes. Consequently, professionals who work in ORs are often demanding perfectionists. They have little tolerance for delay, regardless of the cause. Assistants are held to the highest standards. Given the high stakes, high risks, and difficult circumstances, it should not be surprising that serious interpersonal conflicts sometimes arise. Communication is often blunt and painfully frank, with little thought for the sensitivities of the recipient. Personnel who are unable to tolerate this level of "incivility" usually seek other lines of work.

This behavior style often carries over into nonsurgical situations. Those outside the surgical profession often comment on the rudeness and arrogance of OR personnel. Administrators, who are accustomed to using finesse and compromise in pursuing a goal, may have difficulty dealing with what appears to be an abrupt, confrontational, and sometimes rude style exhibited by a surgeon. In an OR, this style has been thought to foster clear and unambiguous communication and is sometimes intended to be "motivational." Whereas such behavior is a fact of life in many OR suites, mutual respect and common courtesy can also get the job done effectively.

Although cooperation and a shared goal of quality patient care should always be the primary focus, certain conflicts are inherent in the interactions of the three major groups of professionals—surgeons, anesthesiologists, and nurses—who work in the OR. A major role of RNs working in the OR is to be the patient's advocate while the patient is undergoing an operative procedure. While attending to the multiple needs of the surgical patient, the RN is also adhering to and enforcing facility policy and procedure, which may sometimes conflict with the surgeon's intentions or actions. For example, the nurse must ensure that sterile standards are met, which means correcting the doctor who violates a principle of aseptic technique. When this happens, conflict resolution is expected to take place in an atmosphere of professionalism and collegiality, with patient welfare the highest priority.

Anesthesiologists and surgeons may have conflicts as well. A major duty of the anesthesiologist is to ensure that the patient is in satisfactory condition for surgery. In practice, this means that the anesthesiologist must review the adequacy of the surgeon's preoperative evaluation; if it is found inadequate, the surgery is sometimes delayed or canceled. The

selection of anesthesia is a second area of conflict. Some surgeons prefer, or even demand, a particular type of anesthesia for their operations, whereas most anesthesiologists consider it their duty to choose the most appropriate anesthetic based on patient needs and type of operation as well as the surgeon's preference. Finally, contrary to a legal tenet long ago abandoned in the OR, no one is "captain of the ship." Surgeons, anesthesiologists, and nurses have their own realms of competence. Under these circumstances, members of the OR team must be prepared to yield to whomever has the greatest knowledge or skill in the area under contention.

TRENDS IN SURGERY

The rate of growth in surgery currently exceeds population growth, reflecting the increasing health care needs of an aging population. However, the rising rate of surgical operations may also be due to technological advances that allow medical professionals to offer safer surgical therapy to a wider population, as well as to a steady introduction of new surgical treatments for previously untreatable problems. Interaction of technology, managed care, population growth, and aging can be very unpredictable and can result in significant local variations in the rate of growth of surgical therapy. OR managers must be aware of local variations, which are probably larger than national trends, to make correct decisions, especially when they are marketing the services of the OR suite. (See Strategic Management on page 21.)

Growth of Ambulatory Surgery

In 1983, nearly 75% of the surgical operations performed in the United States were on inpatients, whereas only 7 years later, in 1990, more than one-half of operations were performed on ambulatory patients (Figure 1-1). The shift from inpatient to ambulatory surgery has made many aspects of OR management more difficult and good management even more vital.

The growth of freestanding ASCs and of ambulatory surgical cases has been dramatic (Figure 1-2). Surgery in ASCs is at least as safe as in hospital-based surgical facilities, and patient satisfaction may be higher. Many "surgicenters" are providing "23-hour stays" for patients who need overnight care but

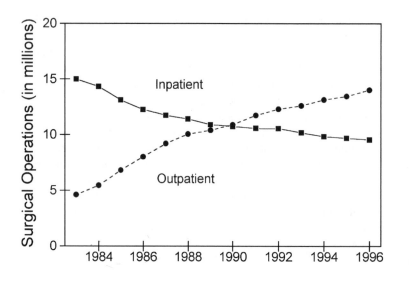

Figure 1-1. Increase in outpatient and decrease in inpatient surgical volume (community hospitals) over 14 years. (Data from American Hospital Association Hospital Statistics, 1986–95 Edition. Chicago: American Hospital Association, 1995; American Hospital Association Hospital Statistics 1998 Edition. Chicago: Healthcare InfoSource Inc., a subsidiary of the American Hospital Association, 1998.)

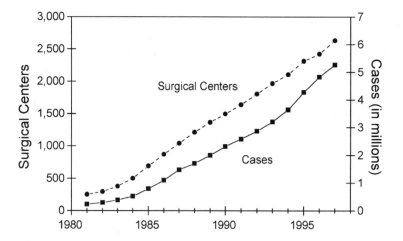

Figure 1-2. Growth in free-standing ambulatory surgical centers and in ambulatory surgical cases from 1981 to 1997. (Data used with permission from SMG Marketing Group Inc., Chicago, IL.)

not the extensive facilities of a hospital. Freestanding surgical centers offer highly competitive services that are attractive to patients and can be profitable at reimbursement levels that would be unfavorable to hospitals. Furthermore, smaller suites of ORs may provide more convenience to surgeons than larger, hospital-based units. On the other hand, many surgeons may wish to mix inpatient and outpatient surgery in a single session rather than having to divide time between facilities. Only hospital-based OR suites are able to provide this option.

Variations in Surgical Rate

The rate at which surgery is performed in different parts of the United States varies widely, even in areas that seem to be demographically similar. Large differences that are observed between apparently comparable venues raise serious questions about whether some surgical procedures are necessary for optimal patient care. The major problem in attempting to answer these questions is to distinguish between appropriate and inappropriate operations.

Back surgery provides a good example of this issue. Figure 1-3 shows the wide variation in the rate of surgical treatment of back pain in Medicare patients. Such surgery is generally an elective procedure for which alternative therapies are available, including watchful waiting and non-medical treatment. Possible causes for observed wide regional variations include differences in rates of disease, in numbers and practice styles of physicians, and in patient income, education, and insurance coverage. However, the "correct" surgical rate is not known. Are some patients denied beneficial operations or others subjected to

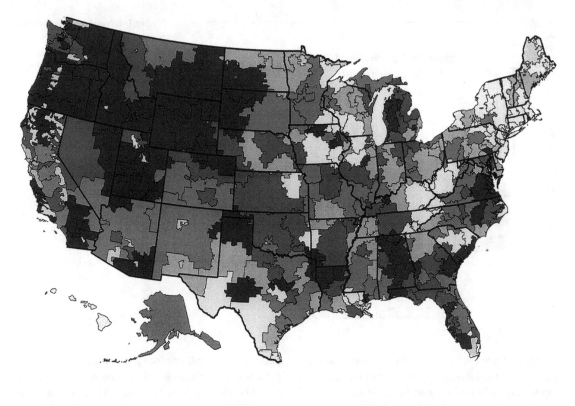

☐ 1.26–2.36 operations per 1,000 enrollees

■ 3.76–7.59 operations per 1,000 enrollees

Figure 1-3. The rate of back surgery among Medicare enrollees in 1995. The rate varied more than sixfold in different regions of the country. (Adapted from JE Wennberg, MM Cooper. The Dartmouth Atlas of Health Care 1998. Chicago: American Hospital Publishing, 1998.)

unnecessary surgery? Why is the rate of back surgery high in the mountain states and low in the northeast?

This issue is not new. Growth in surgical volume and questions about the effectiveness of surgical therapy have been under discussion for decades. The 1974 Moss Subcommittee on Oversight and Investigation of the U.S. House of Representatives claimed to have discovered 12,000 deaths from "unnecessary" surgery.

Effect of Facility Ownership

Most acute-care hospitals have ORs and daily surgical schedules. Ownership of these hospitals includes not-for-profit organizations, investor-owned corporations, and various local, state, and federal government agencies. The number of surgical operations performed in each institution, when normalized by the number of beds, is remarkably similar, at approximately 25 operations per hospital bed per year. Nongovernmental hospitals tend to perform more operations per bed, and hospitals with fewer than 100 beds perform relatively fewer operations (Figure 1-4).

Effect of Government Regulation

Development of evidence-based guidelines for surgical operations is necessary before reliable estimates of appropriate surgical rates can be based on population statistics. Despite this caveat, some health care planners believe that it is possible to establish the correct number of hospital beds, ORs, and complex diagnostic equipment—such as computed tomographic (CT) scanners and magnetic resonance imaging (MRI) units—that a given community requires, based on size of the community and its demograph-

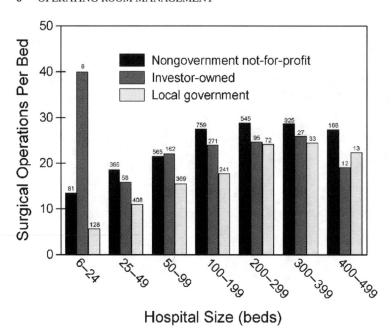

Figure 1-4. Number of operations per hospital bed for hospitals of various sizes in 1993. The number at the top of each bar represents the number of hospitals in that category. (Data from American Hospital Association Hospital Statistics, 1994–95 Edition. Chicago: American Hospital Association, 1995;8.)

ics, including age, ethnicity, and educational profiles. This idea is the basis for governmental regulation of capital expenditures via certificate-of-need (CON) programs, which force health care facilities to secure government approval for capital expenditures greater than a certain amount.

Both New York and Massachusetts used these methods heavily in the 1980s. However, neither state was able to demonstrate anticipated major reductions in health care costs when compared to less highly regulated states. California has attempted aggressive utilization management. Although this effort resulted in a reduction in the total number of inpatient beds, attempts to reduce the number of expensive programs such as cardiac surgery failed. In 1995, more California hospitals offered cardiac surgery, with smaller numbers of cases per program, than ever before.

Effect of Managed Care

Managed care (discussed in more detail in Chapter 2, Influence of Managed Care) offers the potential for improving efficiency and productivity by bringing the forces of a competitive free-market economy to bear on the medical marketplace. One of the most dramatic effects of managed care so far has been to reduce inpatient days (Figure 1-5). The decreased need for hospital beds has led to hospital mergers, consolidations, downsizing, and closures. Whether

managed care will produce a comparable long-term reduction in the number of operations performed is not clear (see Figures 1-1 and 1-5). Managed care may initially decrease surgical rates, but if significant patient queues develop, the demand for prompt surgery may push the rate back up to pre–managed care values. Although managed care is likely to reduce rates in high-utilization areas, the introduction of managed care to a wider population may actually increase the volume of surgery in geographic areas that currently have low rates of utilization.

Managed care organizations (MCOs) scrutinize expensive therapies such as surgery and may place pressure on physicians to substitute less expensive non-surgical forms of therapy when they exist. Most current surgical therapy has never been subjected to rigorous scientific scrutiny to prove efficacy. Although no effective alternative to surgery is available for certain medical conditions (e.g., appendectomy), some types of surgery might be replaced by less costly, equally effective alternatives. MCOs are powerfully motivated to identify and mandate the use of less expensive therapies.

MISSION OF THE OPERATING ROOMS

Everyone in an organization must clearly understand its mission and what the organization hopes to be like in the future (its vision). Crafting mission and vision

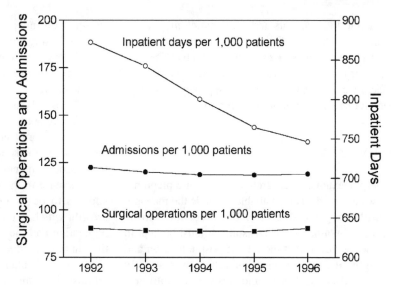

Figure 1-5. Remarkable reduction of inpatient days per 1,000 patients despite relatively stable numbers of hospital admissions and surgical operations. (Data from American Hospital Association Hospital Statistics, 1998 Edition. Chicago: Healthcare InfoSource Inc., a subsidiary of the American Hospital Association, 1998;9.)

statements that are neither trite nor platitudinal is not an easy task. One of the primary roles of leadership is to define the mission and vision of an organization in ways that are more productive and more effective than the organization's current, often unstated, ways of doing things. The leadership must then make certain that the mission and vision become ingrained in the daily culture of the organization.

Mission statements are not an instant cure for organizational problems. However, the process of developing a focused mission statement can be useful for bringing all the staff of a facility together. The mission statement for an OR suite should be consistent with the mission of the institution. A mission statement for the ORs of a community hospital may be inappropriate for an academic medical center, and vice versa. When OR managers begin to develop a mission statement, they must keep in mind who the customers are (both internal and external) and how customer satisfaction can be assured (Case Study 1-1).

The mission statement for the OR suite of an academic medical center might be "The mission of the ORs is to provide facilities in which state-of-the-art surgical care can be provided to the patient population and high-quality medical education can be pro-

CASE STUDY 1-1. Mission Statement for Community Medical Center's Operating Rooms

Surgeons have recently been complaining about the lack of available OR time at CMC and about difficulty in scheduling cases at desirable times. Approximately 3,500 cases are performed annually in CMC's three functioning ORs. The nursing staff has recently voiced concerns that the surgeons are scheduling cases at times that are convenient for the surgeons but often require overtime for nursing staff.

The hospital's CEO has asked each area of the hospital to develop a mission statement. The OR nurse manager is trying to decide what approach she should use. Her initial thought was to quickly write a mission statement herself, because she thought she really did not have time for protracted discussion. On second thought, she decided to use the writing of the mission statement as an opportunity to address some of the problems in the OR suite.

Who should she get together to write a mission statement for the ORs? Who should lead the group? What result should the nurse manager hope for? How can the mission statement meld together the community orientation of CMC with the desires of its for-profit owners?

vided to the residents and students learning at the University Medical Center." The mission statement for a freestanding surgical center might be "The mission of this center is to be the ambulatory surgical facility of choice for the surgeons, patients, and payers for health care in our community."

SUMMARY

Despite extensive research in health care planning, few empiric data are available to guide the manager in planning the size of or the procedures to be offered by a particular OR suite. It must be kept in mind, however, that the rate of hospitalization and length of stay of inpatients has dramatically declined in the 1990s, and this trend continues. Wide variations in rate of hospitalization exist under different forms of managed care. As outpatient surgery continues to grow, the need for "patient friendly," "surgeon friendly," and "payer friendly" ambulatory surgical facilities will increase. All three of these characteristics require a high degree of efficiency.

Other trends are more difficult to discern. The rates for some types of surgery may decrease (e.g., gastrectomy for ulcer disease), while rates for many types of minimally invasive surgery increase (e.g., laparoscopic cholecystectomy). Overall, the continuing increase in the number of surgical operations appears to be exceeding the rate of population growth, which is probably caused by aging of the population and the increased availability of effective surgical treatment. No matter what the national trends are, OR managers must consider local conditions—both the demographics of the population and the potential for market share—when deciding on appropriate sizing of the OR suite.

Chapter 2
Influence of Managed Care

If it be now, 'tis not to come,
if it be not to come, it will be now;
if it be not now, yet it will come: the readiness is all.

—*William Shakespeare (1564–1616):*
Hamlet, *Act V, Scene 2*

Health care delivery is going through profound evolution, if not revolution, as health care administrators, physicians, nurses, and others caught up in the changes are well aware. The shift to managed care has been likened to the industrial revolution, in which workshops of individual craftsmen were eliminated by the introduction of mechanized production. However, just as the industrial revolution brought an unprecedented increase in wealth and improved standard of living to some segments of society while exploiting others, the current health care revolution has profound implications, both good and bad. Whether this analogy is accurate will have to be decided by future historians. In any case, today's OR managers must be able to design strategies that will help their institutions thrive in newly competitive markets.

Managed care (or managed competition) attempts to impose control on the cost of health care by providing incentives for cost-effective care. Problems occur because measuring costs is much easier than measuring the effectiveness of less costly treatments. Changes in the market for health care provision that accompany the growth of managed care are profound and are proceeding at varying rates across the country. Table 2-1 lists some of the changes that can be expected as managed care penetrates a particular geographic region.

A wide diversity of MCOs are forming, usually referred to by a confusing array of initials. Whatever they are called, organizations involved in the delivery

of health care are becoming exceedingly complex and interrelated, with alliances that frequently shift. Substantial cultural differences often lie between the partners in these organizations: for-profit versus not-for-profit; fee-for-service payment versus capitated payment (defined in Reimbursement Methods); budget-managing hospital administrators versus entrepreneurial private practice physician groups; physicians in community-wide independent practice associations (IPAs) versus physicians employed by HMOs.

OR managers must function within this complex and rapidly changing environment and must learn how managed care affects the need for and the use of surgical services in their particular markets. Because groups within a single health care organization may have different outlooks and financial incentives, successful OR managers must have a clear understanding of the incentives that underlie behavior.

REIMBURSEMENT METHODS

Traditional fee-for-service payment systems offer incentives that usually increase the volume of medical care. Newer systems attempt to reduce these incentives. For example, capitation provides a fixed payment to a provider (or group of providers) for supplying specified medical services to a population of patients. The payment is not adjusted for

Table 2-1. Stages of Managed Care

Stage*	Providers	Use	Buyer Expectations	Insurers
Stage 1: Unstructured	Independent hospitals and physicians	High use of specialty and inpatient services	Low hospital and physician prices	Minimal penetration of health maintenance organizations (HMOs)
Stage 2: Loose Framework	Physicians organized in small groups	Use down 10–15%; increased use of ambulatory health care services as a substitute for inpatient care	Greater price predictability	Up to 30% HMO penetration
Stage 3: Consolidation	Hospital systems and large multi-specialty physician groups	Use down 25–30%; inpatient days per 1,000 patients fewer than 200 (non-Medicare)	Evidence of cost-effectiveness	Consolidation of HMOs and preferred provider organizations; up to 50% HMO penetration
Stage 4: Managed Competition	Integrated hospital/physician systems	Use down as much as 40%; inpatient days per 1,000 patients as low as 100 (non-Medicare)	Capitated price per enrollee for all services	Fewer major systems owing to mergers into integrated hospital/physician systems; more than 50% HMO penetration

*Although a market may fit into one of these stages, it need not have progressed through the sequence to get there. Some markets may be relatively stable in one stage for a long period.
Source: Adapted from LR Burns, GJ Bazzoli, L Dynan, DR Wholey. Managed care, market stages, and integrated delivery systems: is there a relationship? Health Affairs 1997;16:214.

volume or type of service but is based on a negotiated or fixed rate per member per month. Capitation clearly provides strong incentives for the efficient provision of health care and, in some instances, for a reduction in volume of health care.

Staff-model HMOs like the Kaiser Permanente system (in which physicians are employed) also provide cost-reducing incentives. What is generally needed is a method of paying for health care that provides an incentive to render the best affordable care, although all financial payment systems may have unintended consequences. Remnants of all types of reimbursement methods exist in every health care market (see Table 2-1), and all markets will likely continue to have multiple payment systems.

Traditional Insurance Plans

Indemnity insurance attempts to protect consumers from catastrophically large, unexpected medical bills. By spreading risk across a large population, the "average" cost of health care (with an administrative fee and a little profit added) is charged as a premium

to each subscriber. Use is higher when consumers do not directly pay for health care services. Furthermore, indemnity insurance is usually combined with fee-for-service payments to physicians, which further increases use because fee-for-service providers assume no risk through providing additional care. They may, in fact, gain financial benefits from increasing the volume of health care. Finally, the inclination in medicine to "do something" has traditionally been strong. All of these factors undoubtedly contributed to the unrestrained increase in health care expenditures in the United States during the 1980s.

The payment system illustrated in Figure 2-1 shows a lack of connection between the fixed revenues of insurance companies, based on fixed numbers of subscribers, and the variable expenses associated with paying for their health care. (However, the illustration does not account for the substantial income derived by insurance companies from investing reserves.) In this system, the insurance company bears all financial risk associated with uncertain future costs of health care. Because consumers are insulated from most direct costs of additional health care purchases, the incentives to

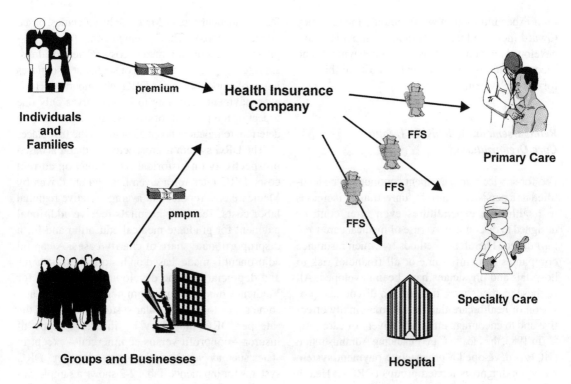

Figure 2-1. Payment under traditional health insurance is made to providers according to fee-for-service (FFS). The services provided by hospitals can be measured in a variety of ways (e.g., diagnosis, days, cost). (pmpm = per member per month.)

Table 2-2. Typical Medicare Case Payment Calculation for a Medicare Diagnosis-Related Group (DRG) with a Weight of 1.0000*

Inpatient case rate payment—non-capital		
Labor component		$ 2,782.84
Wage equalization factor (multiplier)		× 0.9649
Adjusted labor component of rate		$ 2,685.16
Non-labor component		+ $ 1,125.64
Hospital DRG Medicare rate		$ 3,810.80
Disproportionate share payment:	$3,810.80 × 0.1005 =	$ 382.99
Indirect medical education payment:	$3,810.80 × 0.4599 =	+ $ 1,752.59
		$ 5,946.38
DRG weight (multiplier)		× 1.0000
Total DRG non-capital payment		**$ 5,946.38**
Inpatient case rate payment—capital		
Hospital component		$ 168.77
Federal component		+ $ 264.68
Hospital DRG capital rate		$ 433.45
Capital disproportionate share payment:	$264.68 × 0.2037 =	$ 53.92
Capital indirect medical education payment:	$264.68 × 0.0525 =	+ $ 13.90
		$ 501.27
DRG weight (multiplier)		× 1.0000
Total DRG capital payment		**$ 501.27**
Inpatient total case rate payment		**$ 6,447.65**

*This calculation does not include other federal payments to hospitals, such as direct medical education payments and bad debt allowances.

limit expenditures are few. To counter the tendency toward increased use, insurance companies have developed methods, such as patient copayments and second opinions, to try to control costs in this fee-for-service system.

Reimbursement Methods for Health Care Organizations

Fee-for-service reimbursement continued to be identified as a persistent cause for unrestrained increases in health care expenditures even after controls designed to discourage overuse of medical care were introduced. Therefore, methods by which insurance companies can shift some or all financial risk to hospitals and physicians have been developed. All of these methods were designed to discourage provision of health care that is only marginally effective and to encourage efficient delivery of care.

In 1983, the Health Care Financing Administration (HCFA) developed a prospective payment system based on diagnosis-related groups (DRGs). Health care organizations subsequently have been paid a flat fee for inpatient care of Medicare beneficiaries, based on their diagnoses. This system not only focuses hospital managers on minimizing costs related to admissions (e.g., by reducing length of stay), but also makes issues of market share and DRG mix important. However, payment according to DRGs solves only one aspect of the problem of overuse. It fails to act as a deterrent to inpatient hospitalization in the first place.

The DRG system is prospective in that it is based prospectively on historical rather than on current costs. DRG rates for a given hospital are driven by Medicare cost reports and average relative regional labor costs. Teaching hospitals receive additional payment for graduate medical education and for a disproportionate share of charity cases. A capital adjustment is made, based on historical investments and depreciation. The development of DRGs for Medicare has led some commercial insurers and some states to adopt similar systems. However, the rate per DRG may vary by insurer or type of insurer—nonprofit versus commercial—except in states such as New York that have "all payer" DRG systems for inpatients. Table 2-2 shows a sample calculation for a Medicare DRG with a multiplier of

Table 2-3. Common Surgical Diagnosis-Related Groups (DRGs), Their Relative Weights
for Calculating Medicare Case Payments, and Typical Case Payments*

DRG	Description	DRG Weight	Total Case Payment
5	Extracranial vascular procedures	1.5143	$ 9,763.68
75	Major chest procedures	3.1951	$20,600.89
106	Coronary bypass with cardiac catheterization	5.5564	$35,825.72
107	Coronary bypass without cardiac catheterization	4.0685	$26,232.26
110	Major cardiovascular procedures with cc	4.1589	$26,815.13
148	Major small- and large-bowel procedures with cc	3.3710	$21,735.03
209	Major joint and limb reattachment procedures of lower extremity	2.2606	$14,575.56
210	Hip and femur procedures, except major joint age >17 yrs, with cc	1.8460	$11,902.36
214	Back and neck procedures with cc	1.9255	$12,414.95
478	Other vascular procedures with cc	2.2883	$14,754.16

cc = complications or comorbidities.
*See Table 2-2.

1.0000. Table 2-3 lists some common surgical DRGs and their relative weights. However, absolute weights vary for each health care organization.

Another common system for paying health care organizations for inpatient care is per diem payment. The per diem rate for a given condition may be constant, or it may decrease over the course of a hospital stay. Like DRG payments, this system provides an incentive to minimize expensive treatment provided during a hospitalization.

Medicare payment for ambulatory surgery is based on a different system than that used for inpatient surgery. HCFA has developed nine outpatient surgery groups based on the *International Classification of Diseases, Ninth Revision (ICD-9)* classification of procedures (Table 2-4). Each group has a different reimbursement rate. Total reimbursement is made up of this base rate plus a component based on the institution's historical Medicare costs.

Reimbursement Methods for Physicians and Other Providers

Physician payments have generally remained fee-for-service, although restrictions on services for which insurance plans will pay have been increasing. Specialty services must often be preapproved, and they may require a second opinion or may be available only through referral from primary care providers who have financial incentives to minimize specialty referrals. In response to patient pressures, some HMOs have begun allowing patients direct access to highly selected panels of efficient specialty providers. The fee-for-service system is commonly modified by contractual discounts for specific groups of patients. Providers who accept these discounts are often grouped into preferred provider organizations that are run by insurance plans. This arrangement permits groups of physicians in independent private practice to accept common fee schedules legally, without running afoul of federal antitrust regulations. Patients are usually charged a lower copayment or none at all when services are provided by physicians on the plan's preferred-provider list.

Discounted fee schedules create incentives for physicians to increase volume of services to preserve income. Consequently, insurance companies have developed mechanisms that attempt to prevent increased use. One method is to restrict physician panels to physicians who have utilization profiles that are financially favorable to the health plan. This tactic is called economic credentialing.

HMO plans are often highly restrictive for both patients and providers of health care. Restrictions are often generically referred to as *managed care*. In staff-model HMOs, physicians are full-time employees of the health plan, and the facilities used in providing ambulatory care are frequently owned by the HMO. (Some staff-model HMOs also own hospitals.) Salary

Table 2-4. Medicare Ambulatory Surgery Facility Payment Rates (Fiscal Year 1998)

Ambulatory Surgery Group	Sample Procedure	Medicare Payment Rate
1	Excision of benign lesion, diameter 3.1–4.0 cm	$ 314
2	Excision of benign lesion, diameter more than 4.0 cm	$ 422
3	Removal of leg veins	$ 482
4	Repair inguinal hernia	$ 595
5	Breast reconstruction, immediate or delayed, with tissue expander, including subsequent expansion	$ 678
6	Insertion of intraocular lens prosthesis (secondary implant), not associated with concurrent cataract removal	$ 789
7	Repair of recurrent inguinal hernia	$ 941
8	Intracapsular cataract extraction with insertion of intraocular lens prosthesis (one-stage procedure)	$ 928
9	Extracorporeal shock-wave lithotripsy	$1,150

and productivity bonuses can be structured to provide whatever financial incentives the HMO decides are needed. More common is the open-model HMO, in which panels of physicians contract for their services with the HMO. Physicians on HMO panels often join together in IPAs, which contract with the HMO on a capitated basis (fixed payment per HMO member). The IPA then pays member physicians by the fee-for-service method, often involving a "withhold" through which the IPA shares risk with the physicians. The withheld funds are paid to the physicians only to the extent that the IPA meets its financial goals.

Many variations of the HMO model exist. Different plans variably restrict the providers chosen for their panels and the types of care for which the insurer will pay. Physicians can assume substantial financial risk by agreeing to receive payment through capitation or by participating in "risk pools." Most HMOs try to have a strong network of primary care providers who tightly control access to specialty services.

Point-of-service (POS) plans are hybrids, resting between HMOs and unrestricted indemnity insurance plans. They allow patients more freedom to select providers and facilities but impose substantial financial penalties when such service is given by out-of-network providers. POS plans have enjoyed rapid growth because they help to control use but still allow subscribers the option of using out-of-plan providers—particularly specialists—without referral or preapproval (Figure 2-2).

Managed care is rapidly evolving, and OR managers must be fully informed about the variety of payment methods used in the local community. Because OR managers often have a broad interface with the community—with local health care organizations, employed physicians, private practice groups, and individual private practitioners—they must be well informed about the ways in which different payment methods affect each player. It is particularly important for them to ensure that excellent patient care is the dominant driving force and that potentially adverse effects of various financial incentives are recognized and minimized.

ORGANIZATIONAL STRUCTURES

Because providers control most health care expenditures, a fundamental premise of managed care is that financial risk should be shifted away from insurance companies toward providers, who then have an incentive to control costs. This shifting is often accomplished by some form of capitation (discussed earlier under Reimbursement Methods). Clearly, a single provider or small group practice cannot withstand such risk. (A single patient requiring liver transplantation would bankrupt a primary care provider who accepted responsibility for the total cost of that patient's care.) Consequently, providers affiliate with organizations that distribute capitated risk among many parties.

Figure 2-3 illustrates a relatively mature model of managed care. MCOs are vehicles for financing, whereas integrated delivery systems are vehicles for

Figure 2-2. Decline in the percentage of insured workers having conventional insurance and growth in the percentage of insured workers enrolled in managed care plans, 1993–1995. (HMO = health maintenance organization, PPO = preferred provider organization.) (Redrawn with permission from GA Jensen, MM Morrisey, S Gaffney, DK Liston. The new dominance of managed care: insurance trends in the 1990s. Health Affairs 1997;16:126. Copyright © 1997, The People-to-People Health Foundation Inc., all rights reserved.)

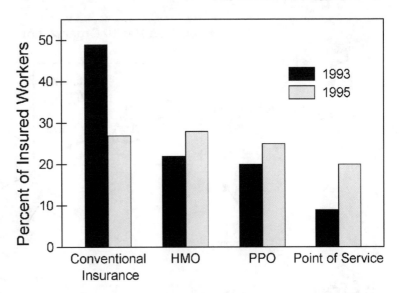

health care delivery. Both financing and delivery functions can be assumed by a single entity—an integrated health organization.

An integrated delivery system is formed when a health care organization and its providers develop a collaborative relationship in patient care. Such a collaborative grouping of a hospital with its medical staff is called a *physician hospital organization.* Many physicians have been wary of these organizations because of the financial clout wielded by hospitals and because of the hospitals' access to professional managers. However, the medical staff needs the hospital to forge an alliance attractive to payers and to generate the substantial amounts of capital needed to form a network. Because hospital medical staffs are often dominated by specialists, physician hospital organizations may have trouble attracting sufficient numbers of primary care providers.

INTEGRATION: VERTICAL AND HORIZONTAL

The development of Medicare's prospective payment system (i.e., DRG-based payments) in 1983 led hospitals to explore both vertical and horizontal integration. *Horizontal integration* refers to links between like elements (e.g., hospital mergers), and *vertical integration* refers to links between elements in the continuum of care (e.g., hospital acquisition of primary care clinics and nursing homes).

Horizontal integration is usually implemented to create economies of both scope and scale by forming comprehensive health care systems. Some mergers are made between unequal partners, as when a large medical center buys smaller community hospitals. Such acquisitions are often distant hospitals (suburban or rural) that are purchased to "feed" an urban medical center.

Mergers may have important implications for OR managers. Sometimes, to capitalize on economies of scale, a single manager is appointed to assume responsibility for all the ORs in a system. An opportunity may exist to reorganize clinical services so that certain facilities specialize in specific procedures. For example, cardiac surgery is sometimes consolidated in one facility when two or more hospitals, each offering cardiac surgery, merge. Because different physician groups, particularly hospital-based physicians, may have worked in the component facilities, the OR manager may have to work with these groups to help ensure financial equity through distribution of cases. Surgeons are likely to have strong preferences about where their surgery is performed. Convenience regarding office practices and other professional duties is usually an important consideration for surgeons. Referring physicians may prefer that certain patients have surgery at one facility or another to simplify postoperative visits. When cases are moved from one facility to another to improve efficiency for the health care organization, the OR manager must understand how the pro-

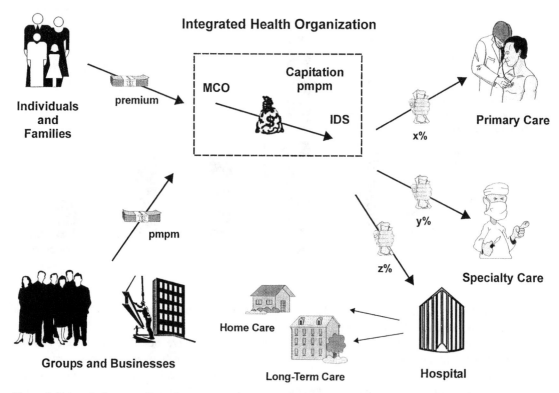

Figure 2-3. A typical revenue flow when a managed care organization (MCO) pays for medical care through capitation. Distribution of the capitated payment within the integrated delivery system (IDS) is shown as a percentage, although many other types of compensation arrangements exist. Capitation is intended to put providers at financial risk and thus to provide incentives for efficient practice. (pmpm = per member per month.)

posed changes will affect physicians and patients alike. Institutional risks can be substantial, because many surgeons and referring physicians may have a choice as to whether to use the merged facility.

Many for-profit hospital chains have followed an aggressive strategy of horizontal integration. The largest, Columbia/HCA, has facilities in 36 states and employs more than 285,000 people. By 1997, only 8 years after its founding, Columbia/HCA was the nation's ninth largest private employer. In early 1998, however, owing to regulatory and financial problems, Columbia/HCA began to permit more regional autonomy and to divest itself of some hospitals. Business practices common in other industries, such as frequent splitting and recombining of corporate divisions, have reached health care.

Vertical integration involves connecting elements of a production system that precede and follow an organization's core technology. For a predominantly inpatient health care organization, vertical integration might include primary and preventive ambulatory care, urgent care, emergency care, ambulatory surgery, skilled nursing facility, and home health care. Although less common, vertical integration can include vendors of health care products such as drugs, supplies, and equipment. Some pharmaceutical companies have become involved in health care delivery.

As vertical integration proceeds, the health care organization should continue to understand what its core competencies are and who its primary customers are. Internal customers become critically important in vertically integrated systems. Vertical linkages in health care do not perform the same function as in industrial production lines, where one process regularly follows another. Rather, necessary services for individual patients occur nearly randomly. Breakdowns in efficient patient care often occur at points of transfer (e.g., at the interface between primary care physicians and the emergency department [ED], and between the hospital and the skilled nursing facility). Vertical integration succeeds only to the extent that such points of transfer are made efficient and reliable.

Horizontal or vertical integration often requires re-engineering for the new, larger organization to realize cost savings. Re-engineering for the sake of cost containment often affects the OR suites of newly associated organizations. The OR manager may be in a special position to help the organization make decisions about which operative services to offer and at which locations. OR managers must always be aware of the trade-offs between institutional efficiency and possible inconveniences to the customers, both patients and physicians. In most environments, surgeons are able to perform surgery at a number of institutions. Therefore, the OR suite should be user friendly. The OR manager and the senior hospital leadership should agree on a set of business objectives for the OR suite that are consistent with the strategic plan of the parent organization (see Chapter 3 for a discussion of developing a business plan for an OR suite).

COMPETITION FOR PATIENTS

Providers have always competed for patients to some degree. In fee-for-service environments, additional revenues could be generated by physicians and health care organizations by increasing the number of patients cared for or by increasing the volume of services provided. In some geographic locations, the patient-to-physician ratio was high enough that many well-established physicians closed their practices to new patients. Because patients were, with few exceptions, unrestricted in the choice of a physician, primary care physicians built their practices not only on their medical skills, but also on their ability to provide a high level of patient satisfaction. Referral practices were built by providing prompt, highly accessible services to referring physicians. Surgeons chose to work in facilities that made their operations safe and convenient and that provided them with desired technology.

That idealized description is tempered by some not-so-ideal realities: patients' recollections of long waits in doctors offices, of fragmented care with referrals to multiple specialists, and of long lead times for appointments. Insurers and payers were faced with continually rising premiums, because

health care costs annually exceeded by several percentage points the rate of general inflation. At the same time, politicians and public policy analysts saw a continued rise in the number of patients with inadequate insurance and, thus, inadequate access to health care. Because of failure at the national level to develop a consensus on forming a government-sponsored health care system, solving problems in the cost of and access to health care has been relegated to the private sector.

Managed care (managed competition) was the private sector's solution to problems in cost and access. This new paradigm transformed the informal collegial competition among providers for patients into fierce competition for "covered lives." More covered lives means more revenues for the health delivery system. Provision of medical care has become an expense for the health care system, rather than a primary mission, as it was when physicians and local hospitals defined priorities. For-profit companies often refer to the ratio of medical expenses to revenues as the *medical loss ratio*. As competition for patients shifted to the system level, relationships have changed. Whereas patients previously had a primary relationship with their personally chosen physicians, they increasingly have a primary relationship with their health plans, and physicians are chosen from among those associated with the plan. Patient choice is further restricted by the fact that employers usually choose the health plan.

Only a few years ago, advertising for patients was thought to be unethical. Now, however, because for-profit systems expend large sums on advertising and marketing (Columbia-HCA reportedly spent $100 million on these activities in 1996), nonprofit hospitals, academic health centers, and networks must also expend considerable resources on marketing to remain competitive.

OR suites, whether freestanding or within traditional hospital structures, are important elements in the marketing of health care systems. Such marketing involves not only traditionally important health outcomes such as mortality and morbidity, but also patient satisfaction scores that depend on everything from convenience and cost of parking to courtesy and friendliness of support staff. Dramatic headlines in local newspapers about successes and failures of medical care, sometimes involving events occurring in ORs, serve to heighten public awareness of health systems. Although messages from the senior management of health care organizations to the OR manager may sound like a continual drone for cost reduction, the OR manager should take a positive view, seeking opportunities to compete for patients through publicity about new procedures and successes in patient care arising in the OR suite. (See Developing a Competitive Strategy on page 25.)

However, competition for patients is not based exclusively or even largely on outcomes measures. Commercial marketing and advertising methods virtually ensure that biased information is presented to the public. An important part of marketing is to target desirable consumers. In a capitated health care market, the most desirable consumers are those expected to require the least health care. Although managed care should accomplish this in the long term by its focus on preventive measures, a quest for short-term profits motivates plans to market their health care products to already healthy subscribers. This tendency is bolstered by frequent movement of people to different jobs, locations, and health care plans. Managers in not-for-profit environments may be left with patients who are sicker and who need more services. In this situation, OR managers may be under intense pressure to reduce costs without being able to emphasize services that are attractive for marketing.

EFFECTS ON THE OPERATING ROOM SUITE

The trappings of managed care—changes in institutional management, building of integrated health care networks, requirements that costs be reduced, and competition for patients—all hold the potential for having a profound impact on the OR suite. Although ORs may have been perceived in the past by hospital administrators to be substantial revenue generators that easily covered costs, the OR suite now may be seen as a place where large portions of capitated fees are spent. Pressure to collect OR statistics regarding not only quality outcomes but also the costs of providing quality care is likely to follow. (See Costing Methods for Patient Care Services on page 61.)

The greatest potential impact of managed care on the OR suite could be through the OR manager's involvement in the health care organization's "economic credentialing" of physicians (Case Study 2-1).

Credentialing physicians for certain procedures is deeply rooted in the traditional medical staff structure, but the use of cost data to determine who has permission to perform certain operations may become common. As might be expected, economic credentialing is a highly controversial and contentious issue. Such credentialing may be explicit, as when a health care organization (an IPA for example) chooses its surgeons by analyzing both the cost of individual operations (e.g., cost of supplies, duration of surgery, length of inpatient stays) and the volume of surgery performed on the health plan's patient population. Implicit economic credentialing may occur when health plans provide primary care physicians with information about the relative costs (to the plan) of referrals to certain surgeons, because such costs are shared through common risk pools. The old days of basing referrals on personal knowledge of another physician's skills appear to be gone forever.

OR managers may have to work closely with physicians (surgeons and anesthesiologists) to help them understand the economic impact of their medical decisions. Sound OR management may mean limiting the choices that these physicians have (e.g., in the types of drugs available to anesthesiologists and the types of sutures available to surgeons). The affected physicians should be involved in such standardization. (See Standardization of Supplies on page 124.) OR managers must ensure that these decisions do not adversely affect the quality of patient care or the attractiveness of the facility to efficient providers.

The ability to become more efficient may allow some OR suites, particularly freestanding surgical centers, to provide highly specialized services at costs well below market average and thus carve part of the market away from full-service providers. This trend has been seen in the automobile repair business. Although new automobile dealers clearly have the expertise and factory support for minor as well as major repairs (although many people think of the dealer only for warranty repairs—a market segment unavailable in the health care industry), most routine service is conducted by a multitude of efficient specialty providers (e.g., for oil and lube service, mufflers, and tires). Similar market fragmentation into specialty providers is also seen in health care, although to a much smaller extent. For example, cataract surgery may be more efficiently performed in ASCs that specialize in ophthalmic surgery.

CASE STUDY 2-1. Global Fee Schedules and Economic Credentialing at Freestanding Surgical Center

FSC has been facing a declining volume of surgery, even though its margin has increased. As competing hospitals in town have seen their inpatient volumes drop, they have aggressively moved into ambulatory surgery. Some surgeons prefer to perform ambulatory surgery in hospitals, because there they can conveniently mix outpatient and inpatient surgery (including operations on patients admitted on the day of surgery). As managed care has become more common in the community, many surgeons who use FSC have experienced a reduction in referrals. HMOs, through their IPAs, have been selecting only surgeons who provide services at lowest cost. Additionally, the IPAs place primary care physicians who make specialty referrals at financial risk.

The administrator and the president of the three-member physician anesthesia group that provides all the anesthesia services at FSC have been discussing ways to increase the volume of referrals to FSC. The anesthesiologist is an interested party, because most of the anesthesia group's income is based on discounted fee-for-service, and recent decreases in volume have hurt the group. The administrator has proposed bundled package pricing—bundling facility fees and anesthesiology professional fees—for some procedures.

The administrator and the anesthesiologist are brainstorming on how to structure their proposal. The administrator has explained to the anesthesiologist that most of FSC's facility fees are based on a system similar to Medicare's DRG payment system. Within each grouping, the administrator has calculated the facility's fixed and variable costs by *CPT* and *ICD-9* codes. Knee arthroscopy is a common procedure, but volume has recently dropped. Average variable cost for arthroscopy is $288, based on an average operating time of 48 minutes at $6 per minute, and the indirect cost is estimated to be $200. Currently, $623 is paid per procedure, giving a $135 profit margin. The administrator is worried that his fixed costs are actually being spread over fewer cases, and thus his indirect cost for arthroscopies may be higher than $200.

The anesthesiologist stated that the anesthesia group's average charge for arthroscopies is $360. The anesthesiologists are concerned that some of the orthopedic surgeons are substantially slower than others. How is FSC going to ensure that it attracts the faster surgeons with the best outcomes? The administrator suggested that they approach several faster surgeons about developing a global, inclusive price for both facility and professional fees—for surgery and anesthesia—to market to the local insurance companies and to the largest employer in the city, which is self-insured.

Who has the most to gain from a global pricing arrangement? Why would surgeons want to participate? Who should be most interested in discounting cost? Who has the least to gain? How can the administrator avoid offending slower surgeons if they are not included in the package?

The drive toward regional centers for high-cost items, such as cardiac surgery and organ transplantation, has in the past carried a quality label ("centers of excellence"), but future markets may push such specialization because of economic more than quality considerations. Many OR suites may have the right combination of facilities and efficient providers to be able to carve out a substantial share of a local or regional market. Recognizing these combinations and helping to organize them on a system-wide level can be an important role of the OR manager. Specialty areas to consider are cardiovascular services, total joint replacement, back surgery, and women's services. Although *centers of excellence* has historically described these carved-out services, a more germane contemporary term might be *centers of efficiency*.

ETHICS OF MANAGED CARE

Although traditional fee-for-service medicine has engendered many ethical concerns, managed care—particularly as implemented by for-profit health plans—has presented physicians, patients, and public policy makers with new challenges. Concerns have been expressed that managed care is eroding the physician-patient relationship and may be reducing the quality of patient care. Ethical issues arise from decisions in which the perceived best interests of all parties (including the patient) cannot simultaneously be accommodated. Balancing expenditures for the care of individual patients against the resources available to the entire population of patients enrolled in a health plan leads to conflicts of interest. Additional conflicts arise when financial incentives are held out to institutions and physicians to reduce the volume and cost of health care services. The foundation of the physician-patient relationship is the patient's trust that the physician is committed to serving the patient's best interests. "Doing something" is often thought to be indicated even when no firm scientific evidence indicates that available treatment is likely to be effective. When reimbursement to physicians was volume-driven (more payment for more visits and more procedures), the financial incentives of physicians were aligned with cultural expectations. However, managed care—particularly when it involves capitation—is altering these incentives considerably.

Managed care should embrace evidence-based medicine (i.e., the idea that medical therapy should be offered only when strong evidence shows that the potential benefits exceed the potential harms of treatment), which requires the development of treatment guidelines and protocols. Furthermore, money should not be needlessly spent when no health care benefit accrues to the patient. Although in the abstract, this approach seems appropriate and uncontroversial, in reality great passions can be aroused. For example, good evidence may be available that hospital discharge within 24 hours of a normal, uncomplicated delivery saves money and does not increase morbidity in either mother or newborn. However, adoption of this practice by many managed care companies caused such a political outcry that several states have legislated that managed care companies must pay for

at least 48 hours of in-hospital maternity care. Other piecemeal legislative solutions to perceived abuses by HMOs include mandated inpatient hospital stays for patients undergoing mastectomy.

Although few concerns are raised when physician income is independent of the services provided (as in staff-model HMOs), ethical concerns arise when physicians have a financial stake in for-profit systems that generate more profits when fewer patient services are provided. This type of conflict also occurs when primary care physicians receive larger payments when making fewer referrals to specialists.

Another ethical problem occurs when managed care contracts restrict physicians from discussing and recommending therapies that are not covered by the patient's managed care contract. This limitation is often coupled with restrictions on what physicians can tell patients about the quality of a particular HMO. Although HMOs frequently deny the existence of such policies, enough well-documented examples have been brought to light that several states have passed laws forbidding such practices (instituting, for example, a "managed care bill of patient rights" that forbids gag rules).

Laws cannot substitute for a strong code of professional ethics. The medical profession, which has always prided itself on having higher standards than are legally required, is now being put to the test by managed care. The ethical practice of medicine must always put the interests of patients ahead of personal gain.

FURTHER READING

Council on Ethical and Judicial Affairs, American Medical Association. Code of Medical Ethics. Chicago: American Medical Association, 1997.

Council on Ethical and Judicial Affairs, American Medical Association. Ethical issues in managed care. JAMA 1995;273:330–335.

Eddy DM. Clinical Decision Making: From Theory to Practice. A Series of Essays from the Journal of the American Medical Association. Sudbury, MA: Jones and Bartlett Publishers, 1996.

Jolt H, Leiovici MM. Managed Care: Principles and Practice. Philadelphia: Hanley and Belfus, 1996.

Kongstvedt PR. Essentials of Managed Health Care (2nd ed). Gaithersburg, MD: Aspen Publishers, 1997.

Chapter 3
Strategic Management in a Competitive Environment

The concept is interesting and well-formed, but in order to earn better than a "C," the idea must be feasible.

—A Yale University management professor commenting on student Fred Smith's paper proposing reliable overnight delivery service. (Smith went on to found Federal Express Corporation.)

OR suites, as competitive business enterprises, must be able to deliver products and services at a competitive advantage (e.g., price, quality, or ease of access) compared to other OR suites in the same market. Without a competitive advantage, the OR suite and its parent health care organization risk being outcompeted by rivals and relegated to mediocre performance, both financial and operational, or even to extinction. Only with a sustainable competitive advantage can a health care organization continue to generate sufficient income to prosper and, ultimately, to survive.

Business analysts often group ideas and techniques used to develop a competitive advantage under the heading *strategic analysis*. Originally developed for commercial business enterprises, the methods and concepts of strategic analysis discussed in this chapter may be applied by OR managers and senior management of health care organizations to generate a competitive advantage for the OR suite. Because application of such formal business methods to OR management is not yet commonplace, much of this discussion describes what should be done rather than what usually is done.

STRATEGIC MANAGEMENT

Strategic management, which is concerned with the future performance of an organization, generally addresses problems expected to be important to the organization in 1–10 years. This long time frame is meant to allow managers sufficient time to identify and respond to opportunities and threats resulting from changing market conditions. The length of the time frame also directs attention to trade-offs between short-term and long-term performance. Strategic management stands in contrast to operations management, which is directed toward improving the efficiency and effectiveness of current operations. The goal of strategic management is for the health care organization, as a business, to outperform the competition in terms of growth in earnings and assets. This growth is necessary because not-for-profit health care organizations would be unable to achieve their missions without these funds (see Mission of the Operating Rooms on page 6), and for-profit health care organizations must fulfill an obligation to their shareholders.

The OR manager and senior managers of the health care organization should collaboratively develop the institution's surgical services strategy. Some large health care organizations have formal strategic planning mechanisms that address problems at the level of the parent organization. Corporate-level strategic planners attempt to allocate corporate resources among the different business units (e.g., the OR suite, the ED, and the cancer center) to maximize the performance of the total enterprise and to ensure that the business strategies of the parts are compatible with each other and with the strategic plan of the overall organization.

STRUCTURAL ANALYSIS

The first step in developing a strategic plan is to examine the nature of the competitive environment in which the OR suite is situated. The formal system called *structural analysis* developed by business professor Michael Porter identifies five economic and competitive forces acting on a business that should be considered in the development of a business strategy:

1. Threat of entry by new competitors
2. Rivalry among existing competitors
3. Pressure from substitute services
4. Bargaining power of buyers
5. Bargaining power of suppliers

The collective strength of these forces sets limits on the potential financial performance of a business in its market.

Threat of Entry by New Competitors

Existing OR suites should do what they can to minimize the threat of new competitors entering their market. The most important barriers to entry of new competitors are the superior reputation and established customer base of an existing OR facility, which result from such factors as tradition, a long record of excellent customer service, and political or religious affiliations. Because there are few national "brands" in the surgical market, newcomers are forced to build their local reputations from ground zero, and competing with a well-established local reputation is difficult.

Beyond reputation, existing facilities may have substantial cost advantages from such factors as proprietary knowledge, favorable access to supplies and labor skills, favorable locations, government subsidies, and knowledge of and experience with community values. Of these, proprietary knowledge may be the most important, because costs tend to decrease significantly as experience grows, and experience is difficult to replicate. New entrants may attempt to overcome this disadvantage by copying an existing competitor's processes, hiring the competitor's employees, or purchasing know-how from consultants.

Despite the apparent advantage of experience, a health care organization should not rely too heavily on experience to deter new entrants. New technology, equally novel to all competitors, can quickly erase an advantage based on old technology. An institution that has successfully mastered a particular technology may be reluctant to abandon it when better technology becomes available. The strong tendency to stay with familiar and historically successful methods may cause managers to be negatively biased when they assess new devices or techniques or even to miss the arrival of innovations that are essential to remaining competitive.

A substantial competitive advantage is enjoyed by existing health care systems that have enrolled large numbers of patients in long-term contracts with large employers. Newcomers are at a considerable disadvantage if they must attract patients one by one. The need to invest in advertising and marketing, service discounts, and extra services to gain contracts with employers and attract new enrollees or patients may strongly discourage entry to the market.

On the other hand, some market circumstances favor entry of new competitors. First, a market in which existing facilities are unable to meet demand, as sometimes develops when a population is rapidly growing, attracts expansion-minded health care organizations. Second, a market in which existing health care organizations have poor community support is fertile ground for new entrants who wish to attract business. Third, a new entrant with a unique product or procedure may exploit a niche market that existing organizations have neglected or been unable to enter because of limitations in available personnel or technology. Fourth, a new entrant with the ability to get access to important marketing channels (e.g., a new HMO sponsored by the region's largest employer) has a substantial advantage in entering the market.

The best strategy to deter entry of competition is prevention. If case backlogs are large and growing, an existing facility must immediately add capacity. If community support and approval are weak, the institution should find out why and correct the problem. OR managers should continuously be aware of new technological and scientific developments that offer opportunities to establish new lines of business. Finally, existing health care organizations should always seek to meet or exceed the needs of large employers to prevent that business from shifting to new competitors.

Rivalry among Existing Competitors

Competitors invariably seek to improve their relative market positions through tactics such as reducing prices, improving customer service, introducing new services, and advertising. These competitive moves frequently incite retaliation, which, when effective, negates the efforts of the instigating competitor and consumes valuable resources without a net change in market share. For example, price cuts can be quickly and easily matched by rivals. Except for an unusual circumstance in which price cuts release a large, pent-up demand, they are likely to leave the entire market worse off. On the other hand, advertising battles may increase demand for certain services throughout the market, benefiting all health care organizations. Intense rivalry for market share often exists in slowly growing markets, because in this situation, taking market share from competitors is the only way to grow.

In markets where the services of many health care organizations are similar, or where competition among health care providers is intense, purchasers may be able to treat health care as a commodity— interchangeably provided by many health care organizations—and simply seek the lowest-priced service. This tactic may create rapid fluctuations in the relative positions of various health care organizations as they seek to match each other's prices. Only organizations with substantial financial resources are able to survive protracted price competition.

In contrast, in markets where health care services are highly differentiated, purchasers' preferences and loyalties to services or organizations may create

a layer of insulation against competition. Competitors may be remarkably diverse (e.g., an academic medical center may identify itself with the newest and most advanced technology or may claim superior expertise in the management of rare or complex diseases, and the community hospital may focus on highly efficient and empathetic patient care).

Competitors may be tempted to abandon unprofitable lines of business to improve their financial positions. However, exit barriers, whether economic, strategic, or emotional, may rule out this approach. Fixed economic costs of exit, such as labor agreements, resettlement costs, and facility costs, may keep marginally profitable activities alive. Additionally, strategic inter-relationships with other business units in the health care system may exist that protect unprofitable activities. Exit barriers may be based on image, marketing strategies, continuity of patient care, or government regulations.

Pressure from Substitute Services

Rapid advances in medical science continually provide new therapeutic alternatives. One characteristic that clearly distinguishes medicine as a business is the speed with which improved treatments can displace existing ones. Of particular interest to OR managers is how medical therapies are increasingly replacing certain surgical therapies. For example, chemotherapy regimens are beginning to offer reasonable alternatives to surgery for certain types of cancers. Similarly, radiologic or endoscopic interventions are displacing surgical treatment of some types of coronary artery stenoses and bile duct obstructions. Countering this trend, new surgical therapies can treat conditions formerly amenable only to medical therapy (e.g., total joint replacements for arthritis, implantable cardiac defibrillators for dysrhythmias, and epilepsy surgery for seizures) or not previously treatable at all (e.g., reimplantation for traumatic amputations of limbs).

Patients and health care purchasers increasingly favor alternatives to inpatient hospital care. For instance, freestanding ASCs are good substitutes for hospital-based OR suites for relatively minor surgical procedures. They often offer superior convenience and access for patients as well as substantial cost savings for health care payers. Carrying this trend even further, payers in many markets are putting pressure on physicians to deliver surgical services in the lowest-cost facility, which increasingly is the physician's office.

OR managers should always be on the lookout for opportunities to increase services that are not subject to competition from substitute types of therapies or sites of service. Such opportunities often lie in high-technology surgical care that requires state-of-the-art equipment (e.g., robot-controlled invasive techniques) or in treating the elderly, a progressively increasing proportion of patients in most health care markets.

Bargaining Power of Buyers

High-volume purchasers of health care, such as large corporations, are likely to shop for the most cost-efficient and cost-effective health care. When health care services in a community are not strongly differentiated, purchasers routinely select the lowest-cost alternative. Because health care purchasers seldom incur large switching costs when transferring care between health care organizations, long-term relationships may offer few incentives.

Purchasers of health care often attempt to play competitors against one another to force down prices while demanding higher quality or more services. This manipulation may happen through contract negotiations between purchasers (employers, insurance companies, state and federal agencies) and health care organizations. The relative negotiating power of purchasers is even greater when provider organizations, particularly those with large facilities, have high fixed costs that can only be covered by a large volume of services.

Health care organizations can attempt to improve their positions by engaging in "buyer selection"—directing marketing efforts toward relatively price-insensitive purchasers or smaller purchasers with less bargaining power. However, health care organizations can rarely influence the bargaining power of most buyers.

Bargaining Power of Suppliers

A relatively small number of powerful companies provide most medical supplies, equipment, and services to OR suites, leaving little opportunity to substitute for their products. Powerful suppliers often have a large, diverse national and international customer base, limiting the bargaining power of single health care organizations in price negotiations. Several large health care suppliers offer to contract with health care organizations for complete ordering, purchasing, warehousing, and distribution systems. This highly differentiated service places the health care organization at the mercy of high switching costs should it desire to change suppliers. Most suppliers have pricing structures that directly impose costs on health care organizations for switching sources.

To counter the strength of suppliers, many hospitals have joined purchasing cooperatives, which negotiate with suppliers on behalf of the cooperative's members. Because cooperatives purchase in large volumes, they often acquire more favorable pricing from vendors than individual health care organizations can. Suppliers whose products have not been selected by one or more of the national cooperatives are forced to compete on the basis of either significant product differentiation or considerably lower prices.

Having analyzed the position of the OR suite in its market in the light of Porter's five competitive forces, the OR manager can proceed to evaluate ways to develop one or more sustainable competitive advantages, or to modify and improve the existing ones.

SUSTAINABLE COMPETITIVE ADVANTAGE

Four general characteristics of an organization usually confer sustainable competitive advantage: (1) large size, (2) easy access, (3) long experience, and (4) core competencies. Other characteristics, such as excellent products, outstanding service, superior production methodology, and exceptional marketing, though important to the success of the organization, may be mimicked by competitors and thus do not confer unique competitive advantage.

Large size endows an organization with considerable sustainable advantage. A large organization can restrict competitors' strategic options to market segments in which the large organization has no interest. For example, a large trauma center is likely to receive almost all regional trauma patients, and would-be competitors are unlikely to attempt to enter the business. Size is even more valuable when economies of scale and efficiencies of experience are considered. A trauma center can realize economies of scale by treating enough trauma patients to cover the costs of 24-hour staffing of services such as MRI, intensive care units (ICUs), and the OR suite. These services may also be used by other highly technical clinical programs (e.g., heart surgery and organ transplant services) to realize both economy of scope and economy of scale.

Because patients and physicians generally prefer facilities with convenient access, an advantage may be established by locating health care facilities close to the homes, schools, or workplaces of target patient populations. Proximity of a health care facility to physicians' offices is a strong incentive for physicians to care for patients there. Similarly, proximity of a health care organization to resources such as laboratories, sources of equipment and supplies, and rehabilitation units can produce advantages of convenience and rapid response. Being close to the homes of hospital personnel is also advantageous in recruiting skilled help. A large organization may establish a network of points of service that a competitor will have difficulty matching.

Successful experience in developing methods for cost-effective care may confer substantial cost advantage. Standardized processes and services, backed by capital investment in equipment and in data acquisition and analysis, are most likely to show experience-based cost savings. An example from surgical support services is the unit cost of cleaning and sterilizing surgical instruments, which decreases with experience. The cost of preoperative evaluation of ambulatory patients provides a clinical example; an experienced group of clinicians contributes materially to the efficiency and effectiveness of the preoperative evaluation process. Many steps in the evaluation (e.g., history, physical examination, and laboratory studies) can be automated through clinical practice guidelines. Patient education can also be automated with videotapes and printed materials.

Core competencies, defined as areas of broadly based special abilities, can contribute to a sustainable competitive advantage. For example, the existence of a core competency in cardiac care involving experienced diagnostic and invasive cardiologists, cardiac surgeons, anesthesiologists, OR nurses, and critical care physicians, as well as other frontline ancillary staff, confers a powerful competitive advantage. Not only are the respective clinical abilities of the participants well established, but their collective management and operational functions are integrated into a strong unit. To develop a core competency requires superior communication, mutual respect, and a deep commitment to working across traditional organizational boundaries. It involves

many levels of people and functions and is facilitated by a flat organizational structure. The skills that collectively constitute a core competency usually come from individuals who view their personal roles broadly and who are able to recognize opportunities for blending their personal expertise with that of others in new and interesting ways.

Competitive advantage of core competencies is derived in the short run from efficient and effective patient care. For this type of competitive advantage to be sustainable in the long run, it must be readily expandable to new clinical services at lower cost and with more alacrity than competitors. Existing core competencies enable an organization's leadership to consolidate organization-wide knowledge, technology, and production skills into new core competencies that empower individual units to adapt quickly to changing opportunities. Many such core competencies involving the OR suite can be developed (e.g., cardiac care, organ transplantation, and women's and children's health services).

DEVELOPING A COMPETITIVE STRATEGY

After determining the position of the OR suite in its market in terms of Porter's five structural forces and assessing the extent to which the OR possesses (or lacks) the four characteristics that are primarily responsible for sustainable competitive advantage, the OR manager can begin to develop a strategic plan. Although the OR manager should shoulder most of the responsibility for developing the OR suite's competitive strategy, this activity must take place in collaboration with senior managers of the organization and the chairs of the surgical departments to ensure that the OR suite's strategic plan is consistent with overall organizational goals.

There are three major approaches to developing an advantage over competitors:

1. Strive to be a low-cost provider, aiming for a cost-based advantage.
2. Establish differentiation from competitors based on advantages such as quality of care, customer service, and technological superiority.
3. Focus on a market niche, catering to purchasers' and patients' needs and preferences.

These three approaches are not mutually exclusive; they can be combined in various ways.

Formulation of a strategy involves identifying tactics that match the strengths and distinctive competencies of the organization to opportunities in the marketplace. Tactics should be identified to reduce exposure of the organization to market risk in areas of relative weakness. This process is repeated for each of Porter's five competitive forces.

Table 3-1 lists potential strategies that could be part of an OR's strategic plan.

COMPETITIVE MOVES

When the OR suite's general strategic plan has been developed, it must be put into action. The strategy is implemented through a series of competitive moves made by the OR manager. Brute-force competition involves using superior resources and capabilities to force an outcome favorable to the organization by overcoming and outlasting any retaliation. An OR suite wishing to attract surgeons might guarantee a 7:30 AM start time to all surgeons, even though such a move might lead to reduced overall OR utilization (usually undesirable). This approach is sustainable only if the organization possesses clearly superior competitive attributes (e.g., a sufficient number of ORs and staff) and can tolerate the cost disadvantage that results from the lowered efficiency. Such a strategic move is stable only as long as the organization maintains these superior attributes. Superior attributes may not be enough to

ensure the desired outcome if the competitors are tough, desperate, or irrational in their responses.

A threatening move is intended not only to improve the organization's position, but also to threaten the financial performance of competitors. An example of a threatening move—the development of a new outpatient arthroscopy service—is described in Case Study 3-1. If a competitor effectively retaliates, the move and the retaliation may damage everyone's performance. In trying to forecast the effects of retaliation, managers should assess its likelihood and, if it is highly likely, the expected speed, effectiveness, and strength of the retaliation. The organization provoking retaliation must be prepared to counter it. For example, an organization may respond to a threat from a competitor with a full-scale advertising campaign, which the competitor must be ready to match.

Some moves increase the chances of heightened competition or even outbreaks of competitive warfare. A high degree of market instability (e.g., heightened competition caused by the entry of a national chain through acquisition or rapid market penetration of a new HMO) increases the likelihood of an outbreak of warfare in response to a competitive move. Trust between competitors, based on a history of controlled competition and continuity of interaction among the competitors, decreases the likelihood of outright war. Additionally, organizations that have joint ventures or nonbusiness associations, such as shared postgraduate medical education programs (residencies and fellowships) tend to avoid outbreaks

Table 3-1. Potential Competitive Strategies

Cost position: The operating room (OR) suite seeks to be the low-cost provider of OR services. Large size and long experience with cost-control measures favor this approach.

Price policy: The OR suite distinguishes itself from others by the (lower) price it charges patients and payers. This strategy may easily be matched by competitors.

Marketing: The OR suite attempts superior marketing, whether by preferred access to certain channels, as with long-term contracts with managed care plans or large employers, or by careful selection of advertising campaigns. Marketing also may easily be matched by competitors.

Relationships: The OR suite develops and sustains relationships with physicians, payers, and other health care units and organizations to gain referrals for surgical services. This is another form of marketing.

Name identification: The OR suite seeks name identity instead of competition based on price or other variables.

Service breadth: The OR suite offers ancillary customer services to patients or payers in addition to providing surgical services.

Service quality: The OR suite attempts to offer the highest level of service quality, measured both in terms of patient satisfaction and clinical outcomes.

Specialization: The OR suite chooses to focus its efforts on a limited number of specific surgical services (preferably highly profitable ones).

Technology leadership: The OR suite seeks to develop and maintain technological leadership.

CASE STUDY 3-1. Freestanding Surgical Center Strategic Plan for Ambulatory Orthopedic Surgery

The administrator of FSC has decided to enhance service levels and service differentiation for certain services. Ambulatory arthroscopies represent an attractive service for development within the orthopedic segment. This service benefits from FSC's 10 years of experience in ambulatory gynecologic surgery, which includes endoscopic procedures (laparoscopies and pelviscopies) that involve equipment similar to that used in arthroscopies.

FSC plans to promote its new ambulatory orthopedic service to payers, employers, patients, and orthopedic surgeons. The administrator plans to work closely with orthopedic surgeons and the facility's nurses to develop a low-cost, high-efficiency, rapid-recovery ambulatory orthopedic service. He also plans to propose a global pricing arrangement to the anesthesiologists and some of the faster orthopedists currently using the surgical center (see Case Study 2-1 on page 19) and to discuss negotiated contracts with large payers for global orthopedic case rates. Estimates show that investments in the OR plant and equipment and OR personnel education and training should be paid back within 3 years by gaining 20% of the current ambulatory orthopedic surgery market.

How can the FSC administrator determine whether this move will be threatening to either the nearby academic medical center or to a cross-town community hospital currently providing orthopedic service in its ambulatory ORs? Both hospitals have recently recognized the potential for augmenting income through increasing their volume of ambulatory orthopedic surgery. Both have response capability to launch sustained price wars and other retaliatory moves. What can the administrator do to try to avoid competitive retaliation?

---

of war. Risks of unrestrained competitive attack are emphasized here because managers of health care organizations, who often have little experience in organizational competition, may believe that attack is the norm in the business world, when just the opposite is true.

Nonthreatening moves are preferred in the execution of a strategic plan. Moves that, when matched by a significant number of competitors, improve the position of all competitors are fairly common. For example, if all health care facilities initiate POS patient copayments, then most facilities would realize increased revenues. However, not all organizations should necessarily endorse such a move. A tertiary-care hospital would realize fewer benefits, because it has a lower proportion of ambulatory patients. In contrast, a competitive ambulatory center would realize considerable benefit from copayments collected at the point of service. In selecting this type of move, the manager should try to forecast the impact of the move on each competitor, including pressures on competitors to forego the benefits of cooperating in favor of the possible benefits of breaking with the ranks.

OR managers must be prepared to defend against competitors' moves. A credible defense inhibits competitors from even considering threatening moves. For example, a history of immediate and effective retaliation to previous threatening moves is a highly credible defense. This defense is enhanced by clearly possessing the resources to retaliate and the will to use them. A strategic battle may thus be prevented from developing in the first place, because competitors are likely to conclude that initiating an offensive would not ultimately be in their best interests—a business equivalent of the military doctrine of mutually assured destruction.

BUSINESS PLAN

Developing and implementing a theoretically beneficial competitive strategy is not sufficient. After the strategy has been put into action, its effects must be measured, which requires the development of specific goals and objectives as part of the strategic plan that are based on expected improvements over the status quo. The analyses displayed in Table 3-2

Table 3-2. Steps in Formulating a Business Plan for the Operating Room Suite

1. Assess current performance of the operating room suite.
2. Assess potential performance in important market segments.
3. Evaluate moves to increase profit and market share in existing segments.
4. Consider eliminating poorly performing services.
5. Develop short-term performance objectives.
6. Identify areas in which current performance could be improved.
7. Identify new patient-care services and market segments in which excess resources might be invested.
8. Assess methods for lowering unit costs.
9. Assess methods for lowering the cost of capital.
10. Determine cash requirements of strategic moves and potential sources of funds.
11. Forecast financial or operational performance for the strategic moves under consideration.
12. Generate a concrete and specific statement of strategy and measurable objectives for presentation to the health care organization's senior management.

can be helpful. They are used to assess the current status and future potential performance of a business unit and to help determine whether strategic moves will be or have been beneficial.

Step 1: Assess Current Performance of the Operating Room Suite

Relevant financial and operational measurements for the assessment of current performance are discussed in Financial Performance on page 39 and Operational Performance on page 42. Market measures include market share for specific surgical procedures, ambulatory surgical procedures, and surgical specialty procedures; customer service measures include overall patient satisfaction, perceived quality of care, perceived access to care, perceived cost of care, and waiting times. These measurements should be evaluated in terms of absolute values and trends as well as against benchmarks. For many OR managers, information about the performance of competitors may be impossible to get, and few benchmarks with which to compare the OR suite's performance may be available. Despite such limitations, an honest attempt should be made to assess current performance as a foundation for developing a sound business plan.

Step 2: Assess Potential Performance in Important Market Segments

For each market segment of interest, the OR manager should assess the strengths and current market share of the OR suite and compare it to competitors' performance in the same segments. Competitors' strategies should be identified to whatever extent is possible. To determine the financial attractiveness of each segment, a prediction of profit margin and overall market demand for surgical services should be made, even if it is only crudely accurate.

For example, cardiac surgical services might be highly valued in the strategic plan of the health care organization, owing to existing strengths in cardiology services. With an aging population, demand for cardiology and cardiac surgical services would be expected to increase substantially over time. The strategic plan of the OR suite should then include development of methods for capturing a higher market share of cardiac surgery by enhancing its clinical performance and volume capacity to attract more referrals and to accommodate increasing demand.

In contrast, organ transplantation services might not be highly valued by the hospital, owing to proximity of a well-established, high-volume (and probably lower-cost) regional competitor that has excellent clinical outcomes. Hence, the hospital would logically choose to concentrate on the cardiology/cardiac surgery strategic group, while the regional competitor focuses on the organ transplantation strategic group.

Step 3: Evaluate Moves to Increase Profit and Market Share in Existing Segments

Tactics that may increase profit and market share in already existing segments include price reductions to increase volume, price increases to raise profit margins, and service enhancements and service differentiation to better serve specific customer needs. Other tactics include advertising and promotion to payers, patients, and other key decision makers to increase awareness of services. Negotiated contracts can also be used to capture market share. Decisions are based on analysis of the relationships among volume, margin, and investment.

Step 4: Consider Eliminating Poorly Performing Services

Discontinuing a poorly performing service is a reasonable option when resources used by the discontinued service can be profitably redistributed to other services and when the shift can be expected to improve the overall performance of the OR suite. For example, the pediatric surgery service of a hospital or ASC might be experiencing declining volume and poor financial performance because of aggressive marketing by the region's children's hospital. The high cost of maintaining pediatric equipment, facilities, and training for a small and declining volume of patients might be seen as a reason to eliminate pediatric surgery and reallocate resources to ambulatory surgical services having better financial performance. The decision to abandon a particular line of business must be consistent with the health care organization's strategic plan. Some money-losing services (*loss leaders*) may be necessary to support the organization's strategic plan.

Step 5: Develop Short-Term Performance Objectives

Short-term performance objectives allow OR managers an opportunity to achieve reasonable objectives within an acceptable time frame. Under most circumstances, an "acceptable time frame" is considered to be 1–2 years, but in volatile markets, it may be as brief as a few months. As always, the OR suite's performance objectives must be consistent with the corporate strategic plan.

The strategic plan of a community hospital might emphasize growth in ambulatory patient care. As part of the hospital's plan, the OR suite would focus on ambulatory surgical procedures. The OR plan for year 1 might include development of a preoperative evaluation clinic to prepare patients for ambulatory surgery. The short-term performance

objective might be to have 33%, 67%, and 100% of all ambulatory surgery patients evaluated in the clinic at 6, 12, and 18 months, respectively. The business plan would include a system for measuring operational factors, such as cost per clinic visit and staff hours per clinic visit, as well as provisions for measuring customer service, such as clinic waiting times and overall patient satisfaction.

Step 6: Identify Areas in Which Current Performance Could Be Improved

Specific areas in which improvement is desirable should be identified and targeted. For example, the OR manager might believe that performance of a new preoperative evaluation clinic should be based on that of one or more best-performing clinics, but estimates obtained from internal and external information sources show a gap between the performance of the hospital's preoperative evaluation clinic and that of the best-performing clinics. The OR manager should initiate efforts to analyze reasons for the gap as a preliminary step to improving operational performance of the local clinic. This analysis depends on benchmark information that may be difficult to obtain or may be based on data from systems that are so dissimilar that comparisons are not meaningful. Nonetheless, pressure should be exerted to upgrade performance to achieve realistically high standards.

Step 7: Identify New Patient-Care Services and Market Segments in Which Excess Resources Might Be Invested

New patient-care services and market segments in which an organization might invest excess resources should be sought out. The primary distinction between investing in new services and enhancing existing services is that new services are subject to potential barriers to entry, whereas existing services are not (Case Study 3-2).

Step 8: Assess Methods for Lowering Unit Costs

Simple cost reduction (e.g., through reduction in staff) may have a negative impact on quality of patient care and could lead to loss of business

CASE STUDY 3-2. Community Medical Center's Strategic Plan for Women's and Children's Health Care

CMC's strategic plan includes developing a new center for women's and children's health care, a new clinical specialization for the organization. The OR manager expects to include in the OR suite's strategic business plan the need to build, equip, and staff ORs to enlarge and enhance obstetric, gynecologic, and pediatric surgical services. A special budget must be prepared that details investments and anticipated expenses for the new services.

Resources liberated from improved OR efficiency could be applied to this new patient-care service. However, allocation of additional resources through CMC's organizational strategic plan is likely to be necessary.

Responses from competitors that already have women's and children's services in their strategic groups could range from no response at all to competitive warfare against CMC's entrance into this sector of the local health care market. Responses might include aggressive advertising campaigns and efforts to convince obstetrician-gynecologists and pediatricians to use the facilities that already have substantial, specialized experience in women's and children's health care. What can the OR manager do to try to counter this potential retaliation?

rather than to growth. However, unit costs can be effectively reduced through creating economies of scope and of scale.

Economies of scope and scale can be achieved in areas of core competencies. For example, if the strategic plan of a hospital is focused on cardiac services, the OR suite would be expected to support a strong cardiac surgical service. The organization would invest heavily in educating clinicians, developing clinical protocols, and establishing case management methods to develop or improve core competency in cardiac surgery. By attracting surgical referrals and increasing surgical volume, clinicians would gain greater experience, helping to achieve decreased case costs and increased clinical quality. These improvements, along with increasing case volume, could be expected to lead to a favorable overall cost position compared to existing competitors and potential new entrants in cardiac surgery.

Step 9: Assess Methods for Lowering the Cost of Capital

The potential for reducing the amount of capital used for present and projected volumes of services must be evaluated. Alternatives to capital expenditures include leasing or renting equipment and facilities or stocking high-cost supplies on consignment. Addi-

tional alternatives include partnerships, collaborations, and affiliations with other health care providers (sometimes competitors) to share capital costs.

For example, hospitals performing cardiac surgery must maintain a large inventory of expensive cardiac valves of various types and sizes. An OR manager might contract with a supplier for a consigned valve inventory, thus avoiding the cost of maintaining a purchased inventory, or the OR managers of two or more competing hospitals might agree to share a consigned inventory to increase the supplier's volume and consequent profit. Based on this arrangement, the supplier might agree to a price discount linked to the combined volume of valves purchased each month. The savings could then be shared among the health care organizations in proportion to their respective uses of the valves.

Step 10: Determine Cash Requirements of Strategic Moves and Potential Sources of Funds

Cash requirements for strategic moves include initial cash investments for new equipment and new staff as well as ongoing cash requirements for supplies and staff training. Funds may originate from external sources or from ongoing services provided in the OR suite, if the hospital's accounting system is able to attribute revenues and expenses directly to OR services.

For example, through concerted efforts by the OR manager, OR efficiency might be increased 10% by decreasing OR turnover times, improving the scheduling of cases, decreasing cancellations, and modifying support staff work hours. Analysis of cost accounting variances would show that the labor cost variance has decreased by 10%, liberating a substantial amount of cash for investment in another facet of the OR suite's strategic plan, such as developing a preoperative assessment clinic.

Step 11: Forecast Financial or Operational Performance for the Strategic Moves under Consideration

The performance of a proposed new unit is difficult to predict, but forecasting is necessary for rational evaluation of strategic alternatives. For example, an OR manager may set performance objectives for the proportion of patients to be seen in a new ambulatory preoperative evaluation clinic, and these goals might be considered attainable by the anesthesiologists, surgeons, and nurses who will staff the unit. Using the best available external data (perhaps by analyzing other ambulatory clinics in the same health care organization), an attempt should be made to forecast operational and customer service measures such as cost per clinic visit, staff hours per clinic visit, overall patient satisfaction, and clinic waiting times.

Step 12: Generate a Concrete and Specific Statement of Strategy and Measurable Objectives for Presentation to the Health Care Organization's Senior Management

The presentation should

1. Identify, for each relevant segment and service, (1) current performance, (2) performance objectives, and (3) time frames.
2. Propose changes in the mix of market segments and surgical services.
3. Eliminate poorly performing services and redirect resources to stronger ones.
4. Develop new services that have a high probability of becoming profitable.
5. Invest capital in new services, forecasting short-term and long-term profitability.

6. Ensure consistency between the OR suite's strategic plan and the corporate strategy and demonstrate how the OR suite's plan supports corporate goals.

SUMMARY

The OR suite is an essential business unit that should be highly profitable in most health care organizations. Traditional views of the OR suite have focused on physical areas, operational functions, and clinical practices (i.e., operations management). The OR suite's business plan must reflect a broader perspective that is consistent with the goals of the parent health care organization. This perspective must recognize the needs and expectations of purchasers, as well as the activities of competing health care entities. Although strategic management does not discount the importance of operations management, it deals with the bigger picture, seeking to identify and respond to opportunities and threats in the evolving health care market.

Porter's structural analysis of the marketplace is a powerful tool for assessing competitive forces: threat of entry, rivalry of competitors, pressure from substitute services, bargaining power of buyers, and bargaining power of suppliers. The business strategy of the OR suite must be flexible enough to respond to market changes. It should include competitive moves capable of producing sustainable advantages for the OR suite and for the parent health care organization.

To produce sustainable competitive advantage, the OR manager and organizational leaders must decide where the OR suite and the parent organization have the best chance to win a competitive edge. Such an advantage is achieved by the development of health care services and attributes that appeal to purchasers and patients, that set the organization apart from its rivals, and that counter competitive moves from rival organizations.

FURTHER READING

Porter ME. Competitive Strategy: Techniques for Analyzing Industries and Competitors. New York: The Free Press, 1998.

Shortell SM, Morrison EM, Friedman B. Strategic Choices for America's Hospitals. San Francisco: Jossey-Bass Publishers, 1992.

Chapter 4

Analyzing Financial and Operational Performance

It has been said that figures rule the world. Maybe. But I am sure that figures show us whether it is being ruled well or badly.

—*Johann Wolfgang von Goethe (1749–1832)*

ORs are usually profitable, in the sense that the revenues generated by providing OR services exceed the cost of providing them. In some health care facilities, the ORs may be the most profitable part of the organization. Hospital leaders have traditionally expected OR managers to improve financial performance by optimizing charges for OR services while attracting as many surgeons as possible to generate an essential revenue stream for the hospital. In managed care environments, ORs, although necessary for patient care, have come to be regarded as major consumers of resources that must be managed as efficiently as possible. Under these circumstances, hospital leaders expect OR managers to improve financial performance by optimizing operational performance.

Except when OR managers run freestanding ASCs, they are not responsible for the overall financial and operational performance of the entire organization. However, OR managers must be aware of the critically important relationship between the financial and operational performance of the OR suite and the performance of the larger institution. In most instances, this relationship is understood only in a qualitative sense—organizational financial performance is improved by reducing OR costs, by increasing OR operational efficiency, or by increasing OR patient volume. Organizations rarely have a financial model that is sophisticated enough to quantitatively predict the impact of operational changes in the OR suite on the financial performance of the organization (e.g., organizational financial performance will be improved by 2% if OR utilization is increased by 10%).

Nevertheless, OR managers must be active decision makers—they must be the driving force behind efforts to improve the financial and operational performance of the OR suite. OR managers should use organizational financial and operational data in conjunction with other information to make sound decisions that focus on operational improvements leading to improved financial and operational performance.

The major function of information in general, and of financial information in particular, is to improve the quality of decisions. Decision making in business is fraught with uncertainty, error, and unexpected consequences. Accurate, timely, and relevant information can help OR managers reduce uncertainty by analyzing past and present performance to forecast the future. Managers can then rationally select courses of action based on their analyses and forecasts. Actions can range from allowing existing policies to continue (changing nothing) to making major policy changes, even completely reversing existing policies.

USES OF FINANCIAL INFORMATION

OR managers should understand the five basic uses of financial information that provide a foundation for evaluating financial and operational performance of an organization: to assess financial condition, stewardship, efficiency, effectiveness, and compliance.

Financial Condition

Financial information about a health care organization is most commonly used to evaluate the organization's viability—its financial capacity to continue pursuing operational goals at a consistent level of activity. Financial information is used by persons inside and outside the organization to make short- and long-term decisions regarding the organization. For example, suppliers may be interested in an organization's short-term ability to pay for shipments, and civic leaders may be interested in the organization's long-term ability to provide health care for the community. In both cases, the financial condition can be evaluated by reviewing financial and operational performance ratios (discussed in detail in the sections Financial Performance Ratios, page 39, and Operational Performance Ratios, page 42).

Stewardship

Financial information was originally generated in large measure for purposes of stewardship, to prevent and detect loss of assets and resources through employee malfeasance. Although employee fraud and embezzlement are now uncommon, understanding the values of various categories of assets can help in managing inventory and supplies and can guide further investments.

Efficiency

Financial information is used to compute and evaluate the efficiency of operations. *Efficiency*, defined

as the ratio of output to input, measures quantity but not quality of output. Efficiency in health care focuses on producing the greatest quantity of patient care (output) with the least quantity of labor and materials (input). This focus is a major concern for health care organizations in managed care environments. Measured efficiency or cost should be compared or contrasted to a standard or expectation. Such standards or expectations are formalized in the budgetary process. Many financial and operational indicators are measures of efficiency, which OR managers can influence through making decisions and implementing changes.

Effectiveness

Financial information is used to evaluate the effectiveness of operations management. *Effectiveness* is defined as the extent to which established objectives are attained through production of outputs; it is not concerned with the relationship of outputs to inputs (efficiency). Measuring operational effectiveness is more difficult than measuring efficiency, because objectives may not be quantitative. Institutions may therefore focus on efficiency rather than on effectiveness. Effectiveness is often measured in terms of the goals of the organization's mission statement and is closely related to quality of health care. Because conflicts can arise between efficiency and effectiveness, part of the OR manager's job is to balance perceived trade-offs for the OR suite.

Compliance

Financial information can be used to determine whether budgets have been maintained and whether internal contracts between management areas have been honored. Financial information can also be used by outside parties that have an interest in the organization (e.g., bond holders) to ensure that their investments remain sound.

USERS OF FINANCIAL INFORMATION

Many people need financial information to assess the financial and operational status of the health

Table 4-1. Groups Requiring Financial Information about Health Care Organizations

Boards of trustees or directors: to evaluate solvency and viability of their organization and to guide decisions on pricing, financing, and investing.

Creditors: to determine amounts and terms of credit to be granted to the organization and to evaluate the security of outstanding debt obligations.

Employee unions: to assess the financial status of the organization for meeting demands for higher salaries and wages, as well as for fulfilling contractual obligations to unionized employees.

Regulators: to evaluate existing and proposed payment rates and (in some cases) to approve capital expenditures.

Public and private granting agencies: to determine the organization's ability to continue providing services supported by grants and to assess the need for additional funds.

Managers (in general): to understand financial implications of the health care operations and activities in their respective domains.

OR managers (in particular): to understand implications and contributions of the OR suite to the financial and operational performance of the parent health care organization.

OR = operating room.

care organization (Table 4-1). With so many demands for financial information, producing tailored information for each decision maker would be costly and time consuming. Hence, specific information is taken from general-purpose financial statements by the individuals who require it. Decision makers use the numerous values and notations on the financial statements, as well as analytical tools such as ratios, to evaluate the financial and operational performance of single units or of the organization as a whole.

FINANCIAL ACCOUNTING VERSUS MANAGERIAL (COST) ACCOUNTING

Financial accounting provides general-purpose financial statements to aid in a wide variety of decisions. Financial accounting follows "generally accepted accounting principles" that shape and define the four financial statements that are the primary products of financial accounting (see following section). Use of these principles creates a uniformity that enables readers to compare financial information among organizations.

In contrast to financial accounting, managerial or cost accounting is primarily concerned with preparing financial information for specific purposes, usually for internal users (see Chapter 5). Because this information is used within the organization, formal and uniform principles of preparation are not necessary. If questions regarding interpretation arise, those preparing the information are read-

ily available to the decision makers. Uniformity and comparability of information, which are desired goals of financial accounting, are less important in managerial accounting.

FINANCIAL STATEMENTS

Financial statements consist of four distinct but interrelated parts: the balance sheet, the income statement, the cash flow statement, and notes to the financial statements. The notes indicate the accounting principles used in preparing the statements and may also provide valuable information about the financial and operational status of the organization, such as refinancing agreements, asset acquisitions or divestitures, and unique or extraordinary charges.

Balance Sheet

The *balance sheet*, also known as the *statement of financial position*, is the first part of the financial statement. The balance sheet consists of a categorized list of the organization's assets and financial obligations at the end of an accounting period. It is, in effect, a picture of the organization's financial status at one point in time. Assets include money on hand; money owed to the organization; and the value of property, equipment, and other tangible objects owned, reduced by the effects of depreciation. Liabilities of the organization are debts owed to other entities, whether long-term or short-term, regardless of the type of creditor. Thus, accounts payable to suppliers and loans from a bank are treated equally as liabilities. The categories of assets and liabilities that make up a balance sheet are listed in Tables 4-2 and 4-3.

The balance sheet is regarded by some as the best single indicator of the financial condition of the organization. It indicates whether the organization is strong enough to support future growth or withstand periods of financial adversity.

Tables A4-1A and A4-1B on page 48 contain the two segments of a balance sheet (assets and liabilities, respectively) for the hypothetical CHCS.

Table 4-2. Typical Balance Sheet Definitions: Assets

Current assets: cash or items of value that can be converted into cash within 1 year.

Cash and cash equivalents: assets that are readily used for daily payments. Cash and cash equivalents include currency, deposited funds, savings accounts, certificates of deposit, other readily marketable securities, and negotiable instruments (i.e., checks, money orders, and bank orders).

Accounts receivable: amounts due from customers (patients and payers) for services that have been provided (or products that have been delivered). Revenues from these services (or products) have been earned, but cash has not yet been received. In reality, some portion of the accounts receivable eventually turns out to be uncollectable for one reason or another. Therefore, allowances must be made. An allowance is defined as a predicted reduction from an established charge. Several types of allowances are

    Uncollectable allowance: the difference between established charges and lower settlements

    Charity allowance: the difference between established charges and special charges extended to indigent patients

    Courtesy allowance: the difference between established charges and special charges extended to patients such as employees, physicians, and clergy

    Doubtful allowance: the difference between established charges and unrecoverable payments

    Contractual allowance: the difference between established charges and contracted payer payments

Inventory and supplies: materials used in the delivery of health care services, such as supplies used for various activities (e.g., direct patient care, laboratory testing, office support, and housekeeping).

Prepaid expenses: expenditures for future services, such as prepaid insurance premiums and prepayment on rented facilities and leased equipment.

Non-current assets: assets held for longer than 1 year that are not expected to be converted to cash in the immediate future, if ever.

Property, plant, and equipment: tangible, permanently held assets used in operations. These assets are often termed fixed assets, capital assets, or property, plant, and equipment. These assets are valued on the balance sheet at their historical cost of acquisition, reduced by an allowance for depreciation. Property and equipment that are not used in operations are categorized as investments.

    Land and improvements: permanently held real estate assets used for health care operations. These assets include not only land, but also roads, parking lots, sidewalks, fences, and water and sewer systems. Land is, by convention, not depreciated.

    Buildings and equipment: permanently held real estate structures and permanently held tangible assets used for health care operations. Equipment is divided into three categories: (1) equipment that is affixed to the building, such as elevators, furnaces, and generators; (2) major movable equipment that is usually stationary but can be moved, such as radiology or laboratory equipment; and (3) minor equipment that is usually relatively inexpensive and has a relatively short useful life, such as office equipment (e.g., desks, typewriters, and computers) and some patient-care items (e.g., beds, linens, and wheelchairs).

    Construction in progress: money expended on construction projects that are not complete. When a construction project is completed, value of the improvement is transferred from the construction in progress account to the building and equipment account.

    Allowance for depreciation: accumulated depreciation of an asset over the useful life of the asset. At acquisition, allowance for depreciation of an asset is zero; at the end of the useful life of the asset, allowance for depreciation should equal the acquisition cost.

Restricted assets: assets with limitations imposed on their use by the health care organization. The board of directors sometimes restricts certain assets to specific uses, such as replacing plant or equipment. Third parties may restrict use of certain funds to selected activities, such as research and education.

Other assets: investments (including real estate and marketable securities) or intangible assets (which may include balance sheet goodwill and organization costs).

Table 4-3. Typical Balance Sheet Definitions: Liabilities and Equity

Liabilities are either obligations for goods and services already received or amounts owed in the form of debt.

Current liabilities: obligations that are expected to be paid within 1 year or before the end of the current operating cycle, whichever is longer.

    Accounts payable: obligations to pay cash for goods or services already received.

    Accrued liabilities: obligations that result from previous operations that will be paid within 1 year.

    Accrued payroll expense

    Accrued vacation pay

    Accrued tax deductions

    Accrued rent

    Accrued insurance costs

    Accrued workers' compensation claims

    Current portion of long-term debt: the portion of a long-term debt that will be repaid within the next year.

Non-current liabilities or long-term debt: obligations that will not be paid for at least 1 year. They generally consist of long-term debt owed to banks and other lenders, including whatever bonds or other obligations the organization has issued. The portion of debt that is due within 1 year appears under current liabilities in the current portion of long-term debt.

Equity: the difference between assets and liabilities. Equity increases by adding income. It represents potential for future investments on behalf of the organization. In for-profit organizations, equity is owned by the shareholders. In not-for-profit organizations, equity is used to pay for future investments to be made for community benefit.

Income Statement

The income statement shows how much money the organization has made (or lost) during a defined time span, usually 1 year (in contrast to the balance sheet, which shows the financial resources and obligations of the organization at a given point in time). *Income*, also called *profit* (or *loss*), is defined as the difference between total revenues and total expenses—the "bottom line." The income statement lists revenues generated by providing clinical services and goods (e.g., drugs from the pharmacy) and revenues from nonclinical enterprises (e.g., parking, the cafeteria, and television rentals). It also lists the expenses of providing goods and services and running the organization. Income shown on the income statement directly affects the retained earnings shown on the balance sheet. Profits are added to and losses subtracted from retained earnings.

Revenues reported in the income statement are realized in the accounting period when the service is provided (or the goods are delivered), not when payment for the service (or goods) is received. Similarly, expenses are realized when they are incurred, not when payment is made. The reason for this "accrual" method is that inconsistent and variable delays may arise between the time at which revenues or expenses are realized and the time at which payment is received or made. The goal of accrual accounting is to temporally match expenses with the revenues they generate, regardless of actual cash flows. Many existing hospital accounting systems (particularly in academic hospitals) cannot easily generate accrual reports.

Table 4-4 summarizes the components of revenues and expenses found in an income statement. Table A4-1C on page 49 contains an income statement for the hypothetical CHCS.

Cash Flow Statement

The cash flow statement, the third major part of the financial statement, provides an evaluation of cash-producing and cash-consuming transactions for the accounting period. It explains changes in amounts of cash that appear between the beginning and end of the accounting period. The cash flow statement reports cash flows related to operating, financing, and investing activities of the organization. It shows the financial status of the organization in terms of cash flow, rather than according to revenues and expenses in the income statement or accounting entries in the balance sheet. Table 4-5 defines the components of a cash flow statement.

Table A4-1D on page 50 contains a cash flow statement for the hypothetical CHCS; Table A4-1E on page 51 contains notes that offer general information about the principles and context from which the CHCS financial statements were drawn.

Analyzing Financial Statements

Financial statements include an abundance of information about the state of the organization at a particular point in time. For decision making, however,

Table 4-4. Typical Income Statement Definitions

Revenues: money received from patient-care operations and non–patient-care activities.

Patient-care revenues: money generated from provision of health care services to patients. These revenues are usually shown as a net value, after allowances, which often appear in the notes section of the statement. For example, charity care represents services provided for which payment is neither expected nor sought. However, values attributed to the charity care allowance enable the organization to assess charitable contributions. Patient-care revenues are shown as a net value, after the charity care allowance. On the other hand, bad debt represents payment expected and sought for patient services but not forthcoming. Bad debts are reported as an expense rather than as an allowance to be subtracted from revenues. When reporting patient-care revenues, factual information and estimations are used. Charges that have been billed and payments that have been received are factual information, whereas charges that have not been billed or payments not yet received are estimated. Estimated values are dependent on contracts with payers, volume of patient-care services, and duration of the accounting period.

Other revenues: money generated from non–patient-care operations. They include
   Educational programs
   Research and grants
   Rentals of space or equipment
   Sales of medical and pharmacy items to non-patients
   Cafeteria sales
   Auxiliary fund raising and gift shop sales
   Parking
   Investment income on malpractice trust funds

Expenses: value of resources consumed in operations. They include
   Salaries and wages
   Employee benefits
   Professional fees
   Supplies
   Interest
   Bad debt expenses
   Depreciation and amortization
   Restructuring costs

Nonoperating gains (losses): money generated from incidental or peripheral transactions. They include
   Contributions or donations unrelated to income from endowments
   Revenues from rentals or facilities unrelated to patient-care operations
   Gains (losses) from investment of unrestricted funds
   Gains (losses) from sale of property

Income: difference between revenues and expenses. Positive income represents a gain (profit), negative income a loss.

Table 4-5. Typical Cash Flow Statement Definitions

Income: income is equal to revenues in excess of expenses, a value that comes from the income statement. Positive income is profit, and negative income is loss (i.e., expenses in excess of revenues).

Adjustments to reconcile income to net cash provided by operating activities: these adjustments offset the influence of non-cash expenses on income. Certain expenses are realized at the time they are incurred but are not paid until later, sometimes after the end of the accounting period. Therefore, to account for such expenses, certain adjustments are made to the cash flow statement. They include
   Provision for bad debt
   Depreciation and amortization

Change in assets and liabilities: these adjustments offset the influence of changes in balance sheet accounts that consume or generate cash. They are additions to and subtractions from cash flow, depending on changes in the balance sheet account from the previous to the current accounting period. These adjustments include changes in
   Patient accounts receivable, with provision for bad debt
   Inventory and supplies
   Prepaid expenses
   Restricted assets
   Other assets
   Accounts payable
   Accrued payroll and employee benefits
   Accrued insurance
   Other liabilities

Cash flows from investing activities: these adjustments offset the influence of investments that consume cash. The adjustments are additions for sales of assets and subtractions for purchase of assets. They include
   Purchase of property, plant, and equipment

Cash flows from financing activities: these adjustments offset the influence of financing activities that consume or generate cash. The adjustments are additions for cash received in financing activities and subtractions for cash paid in financing activities. They include
   Repayments of long-term debt

Net increase (decrease) in cash and cash equivalents: the change in cash and cash equivalents produced by activities during the accounting period. The value may be positive or negative, depending on whether more cash was received or paid out during the period. Positive values are generally better than negative ones. In interpreting either positive or negative values, however, activities that consume or generate large amounts of cash, such as purchase or sale of property, plant, and equipment, must be considered.

much of the benefit derived from financial statements results from tracking trends in values from one accounting period to the next. For example, sequential balance sheets provide information on changes in the organization's assets and liabilities, which might prompt further financial investigation. Similarly, sequential income statements show trends in revenues, expenses, and income. A decline in revenues should prompt investigation into which market segments have not met expectations according to historical data. An increase in expenses should prompt investigation into what operating activities experienced costs in excess to those forecast from historical data. Sequential cash flow statements can demonstrate trends in the organization's sources and uses of cash for operations, which may be useful for making decisions about financing and investing activities.

FINANCIAL PERFORMANCE

Beyond general observations about trends reflected in financial statements, many standardized indicators of an organization's financial performance are available. They measure the organization's ability to generate resources to fulfill the organization's mission. Although no single indicator summarizes the organization's complete financial or operational performance, selected indicators may yield a reasonably complete assessment.

Health care organizations must be able to generate either debt or equity funds to finance resources. (Equity funds are funds generated from ongoing business activity.) In the short-term, debt financing can be used to obtain necessary resources. However, for long-term growth, health care organizations must be able to generate equity funds to finance resources. Slow growth in equity may compromise the ability of health care organizations to replace aging physical assets. With slow equity growth, an organization may eventually be unable to provide necessary health care services and to fulfill its mission. Therefore, rate of equity growth is one of the most important indicators of financial performance.

Indicators of financial performance are usually expressed as ratios, making the information easier to interpret and facilitating benchmarking between similar institutions. Numerators and denominators are taken from the standardized financial statements. Ratios can be tracked over time, yielding trends that can be used to evaluate management decisions. Indicators describing a particular institution can be compared to industry standards. Many health care consultants maintain financial and operational performance records for a large number of health care organizations to facilitate comparisons. These records can give decision makers, both internal and external to the organization, lead time for taking appropriate corrective actions. Many indicators have been tested to determine their validity in predicting business failure, and some have been shown to be capable of predicting financial problems as early as 5 years in advance.

Performance ratios are divided into four types, each of which measures different aspects of an organization's financial status. *Liquidity ratios* measure ability to meet short-term obligations. *Capital structure ratios* measure ability to meet long-term obligations. *Profitability ratios* measure ability to generate retained earnings and thus to increase assets. *Activity ratios* measure the efficiency with which assets are used to generate revenues.

Financial Performance Ratios

Liquidity Ratios

Liquidity ratios measure an organization's ability to pay its current bills with its current assets. The amount by which current assets exceed current liabilities is called working capital. The amount of working capital is a measure of an organization's ability to meet its short-term obligations. The more liquid an organization, the better able it is to meet short-term obligations or current liabilities. Liquidity is central to the financial health of an organization. Organizations often experience financial problems because of a liquidity crisis that causes them to be unable to meet financial obligations when due.

Current Ratio. The current ratio is arrived at by dividing current assets by current liabilities. Although the current ratio is a widely used measure, it does not take into account the relative liquidity of various components of current assets. Cash and marketable securities are very liquid, but accounts receivable and inventory are much less so. Relative liquidities may reflect the organization's ability to pay short-term obligations.

Acid Test. Acid test is the ratio of cash and cash equivalents to current liabilities. Because this ratio includes only the most liquid of current assets, acid test avoids the problem of neglecting relative liquidities that is intrinsic to the current ratio.

Days in Patient Accounts Receivable. Days in patient accounts receivable is the ratio of net patient accounts receivable (accounts receivable less allowances) to mean patient revenues per day (annual patient revenues divided by 365). It is a measure of the delay between the time at which services are performed and the time at which payment for those services is received. A lower value indicates increased liquidity. A higher value may indicate problems in collection owing to faulty billing or collection.

Days of Cash on Hand. Days of cash on hand is the ratio of cash and cash equivalents to daily operating expenses, excluding depreciation. It measures the number of days an organization could meet its average daily expenditures with existing cash and marketable securities. This ratio is an indicator of the maximum period an organization could safely withstand an acute shortfall in cash income.

Capital Structure Ratios

Capital structure ratios measure the long-term solvency or liquidity of an organization. These ratios are used by long-term creditors and bond-rating agencies to determine an organization's ability to repay long-term debt. Since the 1980s, health care organizations (and the health care industry in general) have substantially increased their levels of debt, which makes capital structure ratios extremely important. These ratios measure not only an organization's ability to finance asset growth through debt, but also the organization's ability to grow.

Long-Term Debt-to-Equity Ratio. The long-term debt-to-equity ratio is the ratio between total long-term debt and total equity. It measures an organization's ability to carry additional long-term debt. Low values indicate that the organization may be able to carry additional long-term debt.

Times Interest Earned Ratio. In contrast to the long-term debt-to-equity ratio, which focuses on the amount of debt, the times interest earned ratio measures an organization's ability to make interest payments on the debt. It is defined as the sum of income (the difference between revenues and expenses) and interest expense divided by interest expense. A high value is desirable. Ability to pay interest is important, because bond covenants may severely restrict management actions if interest is not paid. A bond covenant may require repayment of the entire remaining principal balance if interest is not paid according to the bond terms.

Cash Flow-to-Debt Ratio. The cash flow-to-debt ratio is calculated by dividing the sum of income and depreciation by the sum of current liabilities and long-term debt. This ratio measures an organization's ability to meet future debt payments by gauging the total funds available to the organization without additional financing and the attendant need for future funds to retire debt. A low value indicates a potential problem in meeting future debt obligations. The cash flow-to-debt ratio has been shown to be an excellent predictor of financial failure.

Debt Service Coverage Ratio. Debt service coverage ratio is the number of times the debt service requirement can be met from existing funds. It measures an organization's ability to make both interest and principal payments. Higher values indicate greater ability to meet financing obligations.

Profitability Ratios

Profitability ratios measure an organization's ability to generate profit or income. Both for-profit and not-for-profit health care organizations require income to invest in new assets such as buildings and equipment. Profitability is a function of the organization's revenues and expenses. Constraints on the production of revenues are produced by the fierce price competition in which many health care organizations are currently engaged. Such constraints on revenue production commonly lead organizations to intensely scrutinize expenses and to initiate cost reduction efforts to improve (or at least preserve) financial performance. Because crash efforts to reduce costs are usually disruptive to normal functions and may lead to reduced quality, continually and gradually improving the efficiency of revenue production is generally preferable. (Recall that efficiency is the ratio of output to input.)

Total Margin Ratio. The total margin ratio is the percentage of total revenues produced by operating activities (related to patient care) and by nonoperating activities (not related to patient care) that is profit. Total margin does not delineate which activities are more profitable.

Operating Margin Ratio. Operating margin ratio is the percentage of operating revenues (related to patient care) that is profit. Operating margins can be increased either by increasing revenues or by reducing costs. In managed care markets, health care organizations have limited opportunity to increase revenues by raising prices. Therefore, reducing costs is the predominant method for increasing operating margin.

Return on Equity Ratio. The return on equity ratio is the income expressed as a percentage of equity. Many financial analysts consider return on equity to be the primary test of profitability. For organizations without access to donor funds, government funds, or other sources of equity, long-term sustainable growth is funded only by return on equity.

Activity Ratios

Activity ratios measure the relationship between revenues and assets. They can be regarded as measures of efficiency, with revenues as the outputs and assets the inputs. Investments in assets should lead to generation of revenues. Generation of revenues in excess of expenses requires efficient use of assets.

Asset Turnover Ratio. The asset turnover ratio is calculated by dividing total operating revenues by total assets. A high value indicates that an organization's investment in assets is being used efficiently to generate revenues or to provide patient services. Like profitability ratios, the asset turnover ratio is susceptible to distortion, because older assets may be less efficient than newer assets in producing revenues.

Fixed Asset Turnover Ratio. The fixed asset turnover ratio is similar to the asset turnover ratio, but fixed assets, a subset of total assets, are used as the denominator. Therefore, this ratio measures efficiency in using fixed assets. Because fixed assets usually represent the largest category of investments made by health care organizations, measuring efficiency of their use is particularly important. Low values may be caused by excessive investment in fixed assets, inadequate volume for existing capacity, or low prices for services. A weakness of this ratio is that it does not distinguish between older, less efficient assets and newer, more efficient assets.

Current Asset Turnover Ratio. The current asset turnover ratio measures efficiency in use of current assets (i.e., cash, marketable securities, accounts receivable, and inventory) to generate revenues. In contrast to the asset turnover and fixed asset turnover ratios, the current asset turnover ratio does not consider older assets.

Limitations of Financial Performance Ratios

Analysis of financial ratios can help assess the financial condition of health care organizations. However, comparisons using financial ratios are not necessarily straightforward. First, financial ratios can vary according to many factors, such as region of the country. The uneven spread of managed care throughout the country has lead to variations by city, state, and region. Various health care markets present different circumstances on which managers must act, and these differences are reflected in standard financial ratios. Second, inflation can have an adverse effect on financial ratios. For example, unadjusted historical costs reported in balance sheets can confound the comparison of organizations to each other or to national norms. This problem is most pronounced in ratios dealing with fixed or total assets. Third, different accounting methods used by various health care organizations can confound comparisons using financial ratios. Even when underlying financial events are identical, significant differences in financial ratios can result when different accounting methods are used. Therefore, financial ratios can be more dependable for judging the financial condition or analyzing trends in the financial condition of one health care organization than for comparing the financial conditions of several health care organizations.

Table 4-6 summarizes financial performance ratios, stating the formulas used to calculate them and giving some representative values for each.

Although OR managers in most health care organizations may not have ready access to the financial statements of the organization, unit managers should be familiar with the language, the terms, and the reasoning behind their use. OR managers should frequently interact with central administrators who use these terms and who make decisions based on them.

Table A4-1F on page 52 contains an analysis of the financial performance of the hypothetical CHCS.

OPERATIONAL PERFORMANCE

Just as financial indicators are used to judge a health care organization's financial performance, operational indicators are used to judge the organization's operational performance—how well the organization manages the deployment of equipment, supplies, and personnel (i.e., how efficiently the organization is converting resources to services). Many resources, including supplies, equipment, buildings, and other assets, are needed to fulfill an organization's mission. A well-managed health care organization accumulates and consumes neither too few nor too many resources in fulfilling its mission.

To improve operating income, operating revenues must be increased or operating expenses decreased. Health care revenues are derived from either traditional fee-for-service reimbursement or fixed-price capitation contracts. (See Reimbursement Methods on page 9.) Total fee-for-service revenues are determined by the number of services provided and the fee collected per service. Revenues from capitation are determined by the number of patients enrolled and the capitation premium per enrollee.

A health care organization that has both fee-for-service and capitated patients can improve operating revenues by reducing the number of capitated services or by increasing the capitated premium, the number of capitated enrollees, the number of fee-for-service services, or the fee collected per service. Because capitated premiums and fees collected per patient-care service are primarily determined by either market rates or rate-setting agencies, managers and clinicians usually focus on increasing the number of capitated enrollees and the number of fee-for-service patient-care services to improve operating income. Reducing the number of capitated services can be problematic, even when it can be done without decreasing the overall quality of care.

Most health care organizations attempt to increase or preserve operating income by decreasing operating expenses. Aggressive management of resources can reduce operating expenses for both fee-for-service and capitated patients.

Operational Performance Ratios

Operational indicators, like financial indicators, are usually expressed as ratios. Health care organizations function in different environments and may deliver different mixes of services to their patient populations. To make operational indicators between such diverse organizations more nearly comparable, many operational indicators are adjusted for case mix and prevailing local wages. Case mix adjustment is a mathematical correction made to account for differences in severity of illness between patient populations. Wage index adjustment is a mathematical correction made to account for differences in employee wages between geographic areas. Each geographic area has a specific wage index that may change annually. The national wage index is 1. Although case mix and wage index adjustments improve comparisons between organizations, benchmarking experts advise restricting comparisons to organizations that have similar characteristics (i.e., patient populations, patient-care operations, facilities, medical equipment, equity financing, debt financing, and lease contracts).

A basic set of operational performance ratios is discussed in the sections immediately below. Formulas and typical values for each ratio are found in Table 4-7. Although these formulas were developed for use in evaluating inpatient facilities, some can be adapted for freestanding and hospital-based ASCs.

Occupancy

Occupancy measures the use of inpatient hospital beds. The financial implications of a particular value for occupancy depends on the method of reimbursement. In fee-for-service reimbursement, high occu-

Table 4-6. Financial Performance Ratios: Formulas and Typical Values

Ratio	Formula	Typical Values		
		Low	Middle	High
Liquidity				
Current	$\dfrac{\text{Current assets}}{\text{Current liabilities}}$	1.5	2.0	2.5
Acid test	$\dfrac{\text{Cash + Cash equivalents}}{\text{Current liabilities}}$	0.2	0.25	0.3
Days in patient accounts receivable	$\dfrac{\text{Patient accounts receivable}}{\text{Total patient revenues/365 days}}$	40	55	70
Days of cash on hand	$\dfrac{\text{Cash + Cash equivalents}}{\left(\text{Total operating expenses} - \text{Depreciation}\right)/365 \text{ days}}$	20	26	32
Capital structure				
Long-term debt-to-equity	$\dfrac{\text{Long-term debt}}{\text{Equity}}$	0.6	0.7	0.8
Times interest earned	$\dfrac{\text{Income + Interest expense}}{\text{Interest expense}}$	2.4	2.7	3.0
Cash flow-to-debt	$\dfrac{\text{Income + Depreciation}}{\text{Current Liabilities + Long-term debt}}$	0.1	0.2	0.3
Debt service coverage	$\dfrac{\text{Income + Depreciation + Interest expense}}{\text{Principal payment + Interest expense}}$	3.0	3.5	4.0
Profitability				
Total margin	$\dfrac{\text{Income} \times 100\%}{\text{Total revenues}}$	3%	4%	5%
Operating margin	$\dfrac{\left(\text{Operating revenues} - \text{Operating expenses}\right) \times 100\%}{\text{Total revenues}}$	2%	3%	4%
Return on equity	$\dfrac{\text{Income} \times 100\%}{\text{Equity}}$	5%	7.5%	10%
Activity				
Asset turnover	$\dfrac{\text{Total operating revenues}}{\text{Total assets}}$	0.8	0.9	1.0
Fixed asset turnover	$\dfrac{\text{Total operating revenues}}{\text{Total fixed assets}}$	1.5	2.0	2.5
Current asset turnover	$\dfrac{\text{Total operating revenues}}{\text{Total current assets}}$	3.0	3.5	4.0

pancy is good, indicating higher use of facilities and correspondingly higher revenues to cover overhead costs. In capitated reimbursement, low occupancy is more likely to be good, indicating fewer services provided and correspondingly lower expenses. On the other hand, low occupancy may also indicate over-capacity and, unless the number of capitated enrollees can be increased, income may be insufficient to cover fixed expenses. Having a combination of patients covered by fee-for-service, capitated, and other reimbursement methods in the same facility makes interpreting occupancy difficult.

Length of Stay, Case Mix Adjusted

Length of stay, case mix adjusted, measures the average duration of an inpatient stay. With any type of fixed-fee-per-case (DRGs) or per-patient reim-

Table 4-7. Operational Performance Ratios: Formulas and Typical Values

Ratio	Formula	Typical Value
Occupancy	$\dfrac{\text{Patient days} \times 100\%}{\text{Number of licensed beds} \times 365 \text{ days}}$	50%
Length of stay, case mix adjusted	$\dfrac{\text{Number of patient days}}{\text{Number of discharges} \times \text{Case mix index}}$	4.5 days per discharge
Revenue per discharge, case mix and wage index adjusted	$\dfrac{\text{Net inpatient revenues}}{\text{Number of discharges} \times \text{Case mix index} \times \text{Wage index}}$	$5,000
Revenue per visit, wage index adjusted	$\dfrac{\text{Net outpatient revenues}}{\text{Number of visits} \times \text{Wage index}}$	$225
Cost per discharge, case mix and wage index adjusted	$\dfrac{\text{Inpatient operating expenses}}{\text{Number of discharges} \times \text{Case mix index} \times \text{Wage index}}$	$5,000
Cost per visit, wage index adjusted	$\dfrac{\text{Total outpatient costs}}{\text{Number of visits} \times \text{Wage index}}$	$225
Inpatient staff hours per discharge, case mix and wage index adjusted	$\dfrac{\text{Inpatient FTEs} \times 2{,}080 \text{ hours*}}{\text{Number of discharges} \times \text{Case mix index} \times \text{Wage index}}$	135
Outpatient staff hours per visit	$\dfrac{\text{Number of outpatient FTEs} \times 2{,}080 \text{ hours}}{\text{Number of visits}}$	6
Salary per FTE, wage index adjusted	$\dfrac{\text{Salaries}}{\text{Number of FTEs} \times \text{Wage index}}$	$33,000
Capital costs per discharge, case mix and wage index adjusted	$\dfrac{\text{Inpatient capital costs}}{\text{Number of discharges} \times \text{Case mix index} \times \text{Wage index}}$	$400
Outpatient revenue percentage	$\dfrac{\text{Net outpatient revenues} \times 100\%}{\text{Total revenues}}$	33%

FTE = full-time-equivalent employee.
*2,080 is the number of hours worked in a year consisting of 260 working days.

bursement (capitation), higher values are associated with higher costs and decreased profitability. Consequently, length of stay has become a central concern of hospital administrators. OR managers can assist in reducing length of stay by taking steps to ensure timely availability of the OR for patients already in the hospital. (See Scheduling Considerations on page 101.)

Revenue Per Discharge, Case Mix and Wage Index Adjusted

Revenue per discharge, case mix and wage index adjusted, measures the average revenue realized per discharge. OR managers should understand this ratio so that they can ensure proper allocation of organizational resources to the OR suite to cover the expenses of the OR facility and its management, including the cost of supplies and equipment.

Revenue Per Visit, Wage Index Adjusted

Revenue per visit, wage index adjusted, measures the average revenue realized per outpatient visit. Although OR managers usually have no responsibility for traditional outpatient clinics, they may control preoperative assessment clinics. ASCs may be included in this measure or may be separated out.

Cost Per Discharge, Case Mix and Wage Index Adjusted

Cost per discharge, case mix and wage index adjusted, measures the average cost per discharge.

Although the OR contribution to cost per discharge may be large, many organizations do not have accounting systems sophisticated enough to separate the OR portion of cost per discharge from the other costs of hospitalization.

Cost Per Visit, Wage Index Adjusted

Cost per visit, wage index adjusted, measures the average cost per outpatient visit. Its usefulness to OR managers is similar to that of revenue per visit.

Inpatient Staff Hours Per Discharge, Case Mix and Wage Index Adjusted

Inpatient staff hours per discharge, case mix and wage index adjusted, measures overall inpatient labor productivity. Lower values indicate greater labor productivity, but not necessarily lower costs. In benchmarking between organizations, it is important to understand that an organization may have lower inpatient staff hours per discharge but a higher overall cost of labor if it uses fewer, higher-cost, more skilled, more productive workers than another organization that uses a larger number of lower-cost, less skilled, less productive workers. Additionally, inpatient staff hours per discharge does not take into account differences in length of stay independent of case mix severity, which can be important because longer stays require more staff hours. The OR suite, with its labor-intensive services, can account for a disproportionately large number of staff hours per discharge, particularly as length of stay is decreased.

Outpatient Staff Hours Per Visit

Outpatient staff hours per visit measures the average amount of labor required for an outpatient visit. Because this indicator is not adjusted for case mix differences, managers must use caution when using it to make comparisons to other organizations. Determining whether ambulatory surgery is included in this measure is particularly important, because outpatient surgery differs from the outpatient activity that occurs in typical clinics. Furthermore, outpatient staff hours per visit is subject to the same caveat as inpatient staff hours per discharge regarding the mix of higher-paid, more productive workers and lower-paid, less productive workers.

Salary Per Full-Time-Equivalent Employee, Wage Index Adjusted

Salary per full-time-equivalent employee (FTE), wage index adjusted, measures the average unit cost of labor, which is usually the largest component of an organization's expenses. Several caveats should be understood for this measure, especially when it is used for benchmarking between organizations. First, labor mix influences this measure; an organization using more highly skilled, higher-cost labor will have higher average salaries than an organization using less-skilled, lower-cost labor, even though the overall employee productivity and salary expenses of the two organizations may be comparable. Second, use of contracted labor services may affect reported salaries, because its costs do not appear as salary expenses. Organizations that contract lower-paid labor services, such as housekeeping, usually have a higher average salary. However, such organizations may have offsetting savings in human resource costs. OR managers should understand the influence of OR salary and wage structures on the salary per FTE measure. They may need to scrutinize high salaries (paid per pay period) and wages (paid per hour) and justify them. In addition, OR managers should understand the influence of altering labor skill mixes on overall labor costs. To reduce labor costs, some health care organizations have implemented programs to match employee skill mixes to the intensity and complexity of patient care. In the OR suite, this sometimes translates into the use of fewer RNs and more OR technologists.

Capital Costs Per Discharge, Case Mix and Wage Index Adjusted

Capital costs per discharge, case mix and wage index adjusted, measures the total amount of interest and depreciation expense per discharge. The age of the facility and its equipment influence the value of this indicator. Newer facilities and equipment usually have higher depreciation and interest costs, which translate to higher values for capital costs per discharge. Newer facilities may permit more efficient use of personnel, however, thus offsetting some or all of the higher capital costs. Additionally, the use of debt financing increases interest costs, which in turn increases capital costs. Finally, use of operating leases for facilities or equipment reduces capital costs. When benchmarking between organizations, managers should be careful to assure that organizations being compared have facilities and equipment of similar age as well as similar personnel costs per activity and similar capital financing structures.

Outpatient Revenue Percentage

Outpatient revenue percentage measures the relative contribution of outpatient care to the organization's total revenues. This indicator must be interpreted in conjunction with inpatient information. Increases in the percentage of revenues from outpatient services are not necessarily good, because the cause may be a decrease in inpatient revenues. On the other hand, an increase in the outpatient revenue percentage combined with stable or increased inpatient revenues is usually favorable.

Analyses of the Operational Performance of the Hypothetical CHCS

Tables A4-1G and A4-1H on page 53 contain analyses of the operational performance of the hypothetical CHCS. Table A4-1I on page 54 contains the financial ratios that would occur if CHCS's operating margin were 0% or 3% rather than 0.06%.

SUMMARY

The financial and operational performance of an organization can be assessed by analyzing financial statements and financial and operational performance indicators. Analyses may include examining organizational trends and benchmarking to similar organizations. The analyses can identify inpatient and outpatient areas that need perfor-

mance improvement. Such analyses also help the organization's leaders set financial and operational goals. These goals usually include improving operational efficiency to ensure that the organization survives financially and can continue to achieve its missions.

Although OR managers are not directly responsible for the financial and operational performance of the organization, their decisions and actions contribute substantially to the organization's financial and operational performance. Organizational leaders are likely to hold OR managers accountable for financial and operational performance within the OR suite. Hence, OR managers should understand how to analyze financial statements and financial and operational performance indicators as they apply to their responsibility centers.

FURTHER READING

Anthony RN, Young DW. Management Control in Nonprofit Organizations (5th ed). Burr Ridge, IL: Irwin Professional Publications, 1994.

Bandler J. How to Use Financial Statements: A Guide to Understanding the Numbers. Burr Ridge, IL: Irwin Professional Publications, 1994.

Berman HJ, Kukla SF, Weeks LE. The Financial Management of Hospitals (8th ed). Ann Arbor, MI: Health Administration Press, 1994.

Cleverley WO. Essentials of Health Care Finance (4th ed). Gaithersburg, MD: Aspen Publishers, 1997.

Gapenski LC. Understanding Health Care Financial Management: Text, Cases, and Models (2nd ed). Chicago: AUPHA Press/Health Administration Press, 1996.

Stickney CP, Weil RL. Financial Accounting: An Introduction to Concepts, Methods, and Uses (9th ed). New York: The Dryden Press/Harcourt Brace Jovanovich College Publishers, 1997.

Appendix 4-1

Community Health Care System: Analysis of Financial Statements and Performance Indicators

The financial statements and performance measures for CHCS are shown in Tables A4-1A through A4-1H. A comparison of the 1997 and 1998 data shows that the organization has experienced many changes, many of them not favorable.

ANALYSIS OF FINANCIAL STATEMENTS

CHCS's balance sheet (see Table A4-1A) suggests a very difficult year for financial and operational performance. Individual asset accounts show significant changes. In particular, the contractual allowances under accounts receivable, which reflect discounts from regular pricing for contracted customers, have increased dramatically. This implies that shifts have occurred in payer populations from traditional reimbursement mechanisms to managed care contracts. The decrease in inventory and supplies suggests improved inventory control methods, and the decrease in prepaid expenses may reflect improved temporal matching of purchases to consumption of services provided; both are favorable changes. The value of property, plant, and equipment has increased, primarily in the land and improvements and building and equipment accounts. Construction in progress has decreased, suggesting that new facilities may soon be operational and profitable.

Significant changes have also occurred in the liability accounts (see Table A4-1B). Decreases in most individual components of the accrued liabilities suggest improved management of purchased services, products, and personnel. The large increase in current portion of long-term debt, in conjunction with the decreased accrued liabilities, indicates larger debt payments.

The retained earnings account has increased only $898,000 (down 71% from the previous year) for the accounting period, suggesting financial and operational difficulties for CHCS in 1998.

The income statement (see Table A4-1C) further indicates financial and operational difficulties. The good news is that total expenses decreased dramatically by approximately $4.5 million, from $149.5 million to $145 million, indicating aggressive cost reduction efforts. The bad news is that revenues decreased even more, by approximately $6.5 million, again suggesting large discounts from managed care contracts and perhaps other shortfalls in billing and collections. The combination of an increase in contractual allowance of $3.5 million and a decrease in revenues of $6.5 million strongly suggests that CHCS is entering an aggressive managed care environment.

The cash flow statement (see Table A4-1D) shows a decrease in cash and cash equivalents of $910,000, which is consistent with contraction of retained earnings and generally poor financial and operational performance.

Table A4-1A. Community Health Care System Balance Sheet: Assets

Assets (in thousands)	1998	1997
Current assets		
Cash	$ 3,364	$ 5,990
Cash equivalents	6,032	4,316
Accounts receivable	21,655	22,622
Uncollectable allowances	766	1,046
Charity allowances	921	1,257
Courtesy allowances	98	136
Doubtful allowances	144	201
Contractual allowances	4,665	1,086
Inventory and supplies	1,745	2,147
Prepaid expenses	1,309	1,544
Non-current assets		
Property, plant, and equipment	62,730	62,452
Land and improvements	4,545	3,967
Buildings and equipment	116,997	109,648
Construction in progress	336	1,087
Allowance for depreciation	59,148	52,250
Restricted assets	12,344	12,121
Other assets		
Miscellaneous assets	1,392	830
Total assets	**$110,571**	**$112,022**

ANALYSIS OF FINANCIAL PERFORMANCE RATIOS

Financial performance ratios for CHCS, which were calculated from its financial statements (see Tables A4-1A through A4-1D), are listed in Table A4-1F.

The ratios indicate financial and operational difficulties in 1998 that are consistent with information in the financial statements. First, the liquidity ratios show a mixed picture compared to typical values. The current ratio and acid test show favorable trends between 1997 and 1998, indicating that CHCS is improving its ability to pay for current liabilities.

Table A4-1B. Community Health Care System Balance Sheet: Liabilities and Equity

Liabilities and Equity (in thousands)	1998	1997
Current liabilities		
Accounts payable	$ 7,406	$ 7,895
Accrued liabilities		
Payroll expenses	2,393	3,684
Employee benefits	2,253	2,936
Other liabilities	2,583	2,823
Insurance costs	1,768	1,941
Current portion of long-term debt	1,453	670
Non-current liabilities		
Long-term debt	37,577	37,833
Equity		
Retained earnings	55,138	54,240
Total liabilities and equity	**$110,571**	**$112,022**

Table A4-1C. Community Health Care System Income Statement

Revenues and Expenses (in thousands)	1998	1997
Revenues		
Patient-care revenues	$134,101	$140,684
Other revenues		
Educational programs	887	886
Research and grants	973	2,417
Rentals of space or equipment	2,421	971
Sales of medical and pharmacy items to non-patients	2,592	2,587
Cafeteria sales	802	801
Auxiliary fund raising and gift shop sales	1,143	1,141
Parking	1,058	1,056
Investment income on malpractice trust funds	973	971
Total revenues	**$144,950**	**$151,514**
Expenses		
Salaries and wages	67,165	67,893
Employee benefits	13,961	16,217
Professional fees	8,803	12,048
Supplies	33,269	33,316
Interest	4,004	3,857
Bad debt expenses	5,406	6,583
Depreciation and amortization	6,898	8,022
Restructuring costs	5,275	628
Taxes	252	913
Total expenses	**$145,033**	**$149,477**
Nonoperating gains (losses)		
Revenues from activities unrelated to patient care	812	833
Gains (losses) from investment of unrestricted funds	703	621
Gains (losses) from sale of property	(534)	(360)
Total nonoperating gains (losses)	**$ 981**	**$ 1,094**
Excess of revenues and nonoperating gains (losses) over expenses	**$ 898**	**$ 3,131**

However, days in accounts receivable and days of cash on hand show slightly unfavorable trends, suggesting problems with billing and collections.

The capital structure ratios show mostly unfavorable trends and some unfavorable comparisons to typical ratios. Most ominously, the trends of the cash flow-to-debt ratio, which can predict bankruptcy as early as 5 years before the fact, and times interest earned and debt service coverage are unfavorable. CHCS has an average amount of debt similar to comparable organizations but has a declining ability to make debt payments. This dangerous combination can place CHCS in financial peril.

CHCS has significantly lower profitability ratios than comparable organizations. Lower profitability was evident in 1997 and was much worse in 1998, when the operating margin was actually negative.

The declining profitability is consistent with decreased operating revenues that probably resulted from lower net income derived from managed care contracts. This trend is particularly dangerous in combination with its reliance on debt in the capital structure.

The turnover ratios indicate reasonable efficiency in generating revenues relative to investments in assets. However, the trends are unfavorable.

During recent accounting periods, CHCS has experienced a reduction in the value of assets and equity, decreasing income, and significantly decreasing profitability, combined with a highly leveraged capital structure, increasing debt payments, and declining asset turnover. This combination is alarming. CHCS managers and clinicians must immediately and drastically reduce costs.

Table A4-1D. Community Health Care System Cash Flow Statement

Cash Flow (in thousands)	1998
Cash flows from operating activities and gains and losses	
Revenues and gains greater than (less than) expenses and losses	$ 898
Adjustments to reconcile revenues and gains in excess of expenses and losses with net cash provided by operating activities and gains and losses	
Provision for bad debts	5,406
Depreciation and amortization	6,898
Change in assets and liabilities	
Patient accounts receivable with provision for bad debt	4,439
Inventory and supplies	402
Prepaid expenses	235
Restricted assets	(223)
Other assets	(562)
Accounts payable	(489)
Accrued payroll and employee benefits	(1,974)
Accrued insurance	(173)
Other liabilities	(240)
Net cash provided by operating activities	14,617
Cash flows from investing activities	
Purchase of property, plant, and equipment	(14,074)
Net cash used by investing activities	(14,074)
Cash flows from financing activities	
Repayments of long-term debt	(1,453)
Net cash provided by (used by) financing activities	(1,453)
Net increase (decrease) in cash and cash equivalents	(910)
Cash and cash equivalents at beginning of year	10,306
Cash and cash equivalents at end of year	9,396

ANALYSIS OF OPERATIONAL PERFORMANCE RATIOS

Operational data for CHCS are shown in Table A4-1G, and operational performance ratios are shown in Table A4-1H. Examination of the ratios reveals operational difficulties that are consistent with the conclusions drawn from analysis of the financial statements in Tables A4-1A through A4-1D and the financial performance ratios in Table A4-1F. First, length of stay at CHCS is much greater than typical values. Because CHCS is entering an era of aggressive managed care, it must find a way to reduce length of stay and to begin using lower-cost alternatives to inpatient care (e.g., ambulatory or home care).

CHCS's cost per discharge, inpatient staff hours, salary per FTE, and capital costs per discharge are higher than typical values. The magnitude and consistent direction of the differences indicate severe operational inefficiencies.

Although CHCS has initiated cost reduction efforts, as evidenced by lower expenses in 1998, the efforts have not been adequate to offset lower revenues.

The CHCS cost per visit and staff hours per visit are higher than typical values for outpatient care. The high values reveal operational inefficiencies in the CMC Ambulatory Clinic and Community Ambulatory Health Centers.

In summary, CHCS has severe operational problems in both inpatient and outpatient areas. CHCS managers and clinicians must improve efficiency, in terms of unit costs and intensity of use, if CHCS is to remain financially viable.

INFLUENCE OF OPERATIONAL PERFORMANCE ON FINANCIAL PERFORMANCE

CHCS has severe operational inefficiencies in both inpatient and outpatient areas that have adversely

Table A4-1E. Community Health Care System (CHCS): Notes to Financial Statements

Basis of presentation

The combined financial statements for CHCS cover accounts for the controlled entities that include

Community Medical Center (CMC) (175 licensed acute care beds)

Community Skilled Nursing Facility (75 licensed skilled nursing facility beds)

Community Home Health Care

Community Medical Transport and Emergency Response

CHCS Property and Investment Management (CMC Ambulatory Clinic, Community Ambulatory Health Centers, and Community Professional Arts Building)

Summary of significant accounting policies

The accounting policies that CHCS follows in the accompanying combined financial statements are as follows:

Principles of combination: The combined financial statements include the accounts of CHCS. All significant inter-entity accounts and transactions have been eliminated in the combination.

Net patient revenues: Net patient service is reported at the estimated net realizable amounts from accountable payers for services rendered. Retroactive adjustments for prepaid services are accrued on an estimated basis during the period that related services are rendered and will be adjusted in future periods for tentative and final settlements.

Charity care: CHCS provides care to patients who meet certain criteria under its charity care policy without charge or at amounts less than its established rates. Payments for charity care are not pursued and are not reported as revenues.

Statement of revenues and expenses: For purposes of display, transactions deemed by management to be ongoing, major, or central to the provision of health care services are reported as revenues and expenses. Transactions that management has deemed incidental to operations are reported as nonoperating gains and losses.

Cash and cash equivalents: Cash and cash equivalents include depository accounts and cash management funds at local banks and short-term investments, including investment trust funds. Realized gains and losses are based on cost.

Investments: Investments in real estate, U.S. government obligations, and other interest-bearing accounts are carried at cost, and investments in mutual funds, bonds, and stocks are carried at cost or market value, whichever is lower. Realized gains and losses on sales are based on cost.

Inventories: Inventories of pharmaceutical and medical supplies are stated at cost or market value, whichever is lower, based on the first-in, first-out method. Durable medical equipment, owned for lease to others, is valued at cost, net of depreciation, or net realizable sale value, whichever is lowest.

Property, plant, equipment: Property, plant, and equipment are stated at cost. Depreciation is computed using the straight line method over the estimated useful lives of the assets. Gains and losses resulting from the sale are included in nonoperating gains (losses).

Fair value of financial instruments: CHCS discloses estimated fair value for cash, cash equivalents, accounts receivable, accounts payable, and long-term debt according to Statement of Financial Accounting Standards.

Accrued insurance costs, professional liability, and workers' compensation: These costs consist of reserves for claims that are incurred but not reported.

Taxes: CHCS is a for-profit health care organization.

Long-term debt

Long-term debt (in thousands) as of June 30 consisted of

	1998	1997
CHCS refunding bonds, series 1994	$26,351	$27,738
CHCS variable rate bonds	6,712	5,235
Term loan	2,561	2,804
Mortgages and capitalized leases	1,953	2,056
Total long-term debt	**$37,577**	**$37,833**

influenced financial performance of the organization. The effects of operational performance on financial performance can be estimated by assuming different operational scenarios. Conversely, operational changes necessary to achieve various financial targets can be estimated.

In the example shown in Table A4-1I, the CFO of CHCS estimates the operational changes required to achieve two different financial targets: operating margins of 0% and 3%. The CFO decides to seek the financial goals through reducing the number of employees. To calculate the number of

Table A4-1F. Community Health Care System Financial Performance Ratios and Interpretation

Ratio	Typical Values			Community Health Care System		Standard	Trend
	Low	Middle	High	1998	1997		
Liquidity							
Current	1.5	2.0	2.5	1.91	1.84	Favorable	Favorable
Acid test	0.2	0.25	0.3	0.53	0.52	Favorable	Favorable
Days in patient accounts receivable	40	55	70	58.9	58.7	Favorable	Unfavorable
Days of cash on hand	20	26	32	24.8	26.6	Favorable	Unfavorable
Capital structure							
Long-term debt-to-equity	0.6	0.7	0.8	0.68	0.70	Favorable	Unfavorable
Times interest earned	2.4	2.7	3.0	1.22	1.81	Unfavorable	Unfavorable
Cash flow-to-debt	0.1	0.2	0.3	0.14	0.19	Favorable	Unfavorable
Debt service coverage	3.0	3.5	4.0	2.16	3.32	Unfavorable	Unfavorable
Profitability							
Total margin	3%	4%	5%	0.62%	2.07%	Unfavorable	Unfavorable
Operating margin	2%	3%	4%	(0.06%)	1.34%	Unfavorable	Unfavorable
Return on equity	5%	7.5%	10%	1.63%	5.77%	Unfavorable	Unfavorable
Activity							
Asset turnover	0.8	0.9	1.0	1.31	1.35	Favorable	Unfavorable
Fixed asset turnover	1.5	2.0	2.5	2.31	2.43	Favorable	Unfavorable
Current asset turnover	3.0	3.5	4.0	4.25	4.14	Favorable	Favorable

Table A4-1G. Community Health Care System Operational Data

Operational Data	Inpatient[a]	Outpatient[b]	Other[c]	Total
Revenues (in thousands)				
Patient-care revenues	$73,755	$20,519	$39,827	$134,101
Other revenues	5,966	1,660	3,223	10,849
Total revenues	**$79,721**	**$22,179**	**$43,050**	**$144,950**
Operating expenses (in thousands)				
Salaries and wages	$36,941	$10,075	$20,149	$ 67,165
Fringe benefits	7,679	2,094	4,188	13,961
Professional fees	3,961	1,320	3,522	8,803
Supplies	18,298	4,990	9,981	33,269
Interest	2,202	600	1,202	4,004
Bad debt	2,974	810	1,622	5,406
Depreciation and amortization	3,794	1,034	2,070	6,898
Total expenses	**$75,849**	**$20,923**	**$42,734**	**$139,506**
Other data				
Total discharges	8,277	—	—	8,277
Licensed beds	175	—	75	250
Inpatient hospital days or skilled nursing facility days	52,707	—	13,001	65,708
Outpatient visits or paraprofessional encounters	—	43,799	12,776	56,575
Full-time employee equivalents	916	145	604	1,665
Case mix index	1.09	—	—	—
Wage index	1.14	1.14	1.14	—

[a]Community Medical Center.
[b]Community Medical Center Ambulatory Clinic and Community Ambulatory Health Centers.
[c]Community Skilled Nursing Facility, Community Home Health Care, Community Medical Transport and Emergency Response, and Community Professional Arts Building.

Table A4-1H. Community Health Care System Operational Performance Ratios and Interpretation

Ratio	Typical Value	1998	Interpretation
Occupancy	50%	83%	*
Length of stay, case mix adjusted	4.5 days	5.84 days	Unfavorable
Revenue per discharge, case mix and wage index adjusted	$5,000	$7,751	*
Revenue per visit, wage index adjusted	$225	$444	*
Cost per discharge, case mix and wage index adjusted	$5,000	$7,375	Unfavorable
Cost per visit, wage index adjusted	$225	$419	Unfavorable
Inpatient staff hours per discharge, case mix and wage index adjusted	135	185	Unfavorable
Outpatient staff hours per visit	6.0	6.9	Unfavorable
Salary per full-time-equivalent employee, wage index adjusted	$33,000	$35,385	Unfavorable
Capital costs per discharge, case mix and wage index adjusted	$400	$583	Unfavorable
Outpatient revenue percentage	33%	15%	*

*Some operational performance indicators must be judged in terms of the local health care environment and cannot be assigned favorable or unfavorable interpretation out of context.

Table A4-1I. Community Health Care System: Influence of Operational Performance on Financial Performance (Financial Reporting Period 1998)

Financial Ratios	Operating Margin			Typical Range	
	No Change	0%	3%	Low	High
Current	1.91	1.91	2.16	1.5	2.5
Acid test	0.53	0.53	0.77	0.2	0.3
Days in patient accounts receivable	58.9	58.9	58.9	40	70
Days of cash on hand	24.8	25.1	37.8	20	32
Long-term debt-to-equity	0.68	0.68	0.63	0.6	0.8
Times interest earned	1.22	1.25	2.33	2.4	3.0
Cash flow-to-debt	0.14	0.14	0.22	0.1	0.3
Debt service coverage	2.16	2.18	2.97	3.0	4.0
Total margin	0.62%	0.68%	3.68%	3%	5%
Operating margin	(0.06%)	0%	3%	2%	4%
Return on equity	1.63%	1.78%	8.95%	5%	10%
Asset turnover	1.31	1.31	1.26	0.8	1.0
Fixed asset turnover	2.31	2.31	2.31	1.5	2.5
Current asset turnover	4.25	4.24	3.76	3.0	4.0
Cost reduction (in thousands)	—	($83)	($4,432)	—	—
Change in number of employees	—	(2.3)	(125)	—	—
Percent change in number of employees	—	(0.1%)	(7.5%)	—	—
Cost reduction per discharge	—	($10.03)	($535.46)	—	—

employees that must be eliminated, he uses the reduction in wages required to achieve each of the financial targets.

To produce an operating margin of 0%, the CFO finds that a cost reduction of $85,000 is necessary. This can be achieved by eliminating two to three employees, which results in a cost reduction of only $10.27 per patient discharge. To produce an operating margin of 3%, the CFO determines that a cost reduction of $4.4 million is required. This number is equivalent to the combined salaries of approximately 134 employees—15% of the employee pool—and represents a cost reduction of $536.43 per patient discharge.

The CFO also calculates other financial performance ratios for each financial target. Achieving an operating margin of 3% corrects many of the serious problems with financial performance previously discussed. Many of the liquidity, capital structure, profitability, and activity ratios are dramatically improved in this scenario. Values for some of the more seriously deranged financial indicators move into ranges that are typical for similar health care systems.

Chapter 5

Managerial (Cost) Accounting

Asked by a waitress whether he would like his pizza cut into four or eight slices:
"Better make it four. I don't think I can eat eight."

—*Yogi Berra (1925–)*

Managerial (cost) accounting is an essential tool for managing a complex organization such as an OR suite. The information provided by a well-designed accounting system can assist in making fundamental and necessary decisions. The accounting system should be able to distinguish domains in which the OR suite is performing well from domains in which it is not. Information from the accounting system can offer early warning of adverse trends and can be used to predict the probability of success of new initiatives.

Despite the critical role routinely played by the cost accounting system in most business enterprises, many hospitals are poorly equipped in this area. Hospitals are notorious for their sparse investment in information-processing equipment and personnel. In addition, medically trained personnel frequently are poorly informed about the techniques of managerial accounting and tend to underestimate its usefulness.

Difficulties facing hospitals that have primitive cost accounting systems can be traced and explained historically. During the mid-1960s, most hospitals were nonprofit businesses, charging patients or their insurers for the cost of each health care service delivered plus a small margin. For most patients, the cost of hospital care was covered by indemnity insurance, which reimbursed the patient all or a portion (typically 80%) of out-of-pocket expenditures. When the first major federal programs

that directly paid for medical care—Medicare for the elderly and Medicaid for the poor—were introduced in the 1960s, it seemed reasonable for the government, like private insurers, to cover cost of care plus a small margin.

Under this cost-plus system, the price charged by hospitals was determined by the volume of care provided. Each day of hospitalization, each laboratory test ordered, and each medication dispensed created a charge that increased the eventual reimbursement. Hospital managers had to establish a charge for each reimbursable service provided (e.g., by laboratories, the pharmacy, the blood bank, or the OR suite). Some charges were time based, such as the number of days in the hospital or in the ICU. In the OR suite, higher payments were made for longer cases, and little or no attention was paid to the nature of the actual surgical operations performed or the supplies and equipment required. Whether the charges bore a close relationship to the actual cost of providing the services did not seem to matter. As long as the total reimbursements met the total cost of running the hospital and the individual charges met the insurer's and the government's accounting standards, hospital managers, insurance companies, and government auditors seemed satisfied. Consequently, over the years the relationship between costs and charges has become vague and inconsistent, with large overestimates and underestimates for individual services.

Cost-plus payment encouraged hospital managers to capture every detail of supplies used and services rendered to maximize charges and subsequent reimbursements. It also encouraged managers to concentrate on efficient billing and collection systems to maximize revenues. This system provided little incentive to reduce costs or to provide services in an efficient manner. Furthermore, it neither encouraged accurate determination of the true cost of individual services nor placed any pressure on hospital managers to develop sophisticated systems for managerial accounting or cost control.

Problems with government-funded indemnity reimbursement appeared almost immediately after the advent of Medicare. The most substantial difficulty was that the unmet demand for medical care was far higher than Congress and the government planners anticipated. Consequently, from the outset expenditures routinely exceeded the amounts budgeted. In addition, because the ultimate consumers of medical care—patients—were largely insulated from cost, no cost-control pressure arose from consumers. Even today, patients do little or no cost-comparison shopping, and neither patients nor physicians pay much attention to assessing whether the benefit of a particular treatment is worth the cost.*

In an attempt to control rapidly increasing expenditures, the Medicare program replaced its cost-plus system with the DRG reimbursement method in 1983. Under this system, after each patient's discharge from the hospital, the billing department assigns the patient to one of approximately 200 DRGs, based on the discharge diagnosis. Payment to the hospital for each patient discharged with a given DRG is a fixed amount, regardless of the amount of resources expended.

Payers other than the federal government have also moved toward reimbursement mechanisms under which hospitals are at financial risk when expenses exceed revenues. Examples of these mechanisms are capitation (fixed payment to care for a group of patients for a fixed time interval), per diem rates, and case rates. (See Reimbursement Methods on page 9.) Hospital managers must adopt an entirely new strategy to deal with these new forms of payment. Whereas under a cost-based system additional patient-care services increased the hospital's revenues, under capitation or DRG reimbursement extra services reduce the hospital's margin. Health care managers—including OR managers—must focus attention on controlling costs to maximize financial gains or minimize losses.

To optimize financial performance, hospitals must know which DRGs make money (the "winners") and which DRGs lose money (the "losers"). The hospital's interest shifts from developing and maintaining systems designed to maximize charges to developing and maintaining systems designed to identify the true cost of providing health care services associated with each DRG. A hospital unable to distinguish the winners from the losers runs a serious risk of financial disaster. Therefore, hospital managers must develop accounting systems capable of determining and tracking the costs of all services provided each patient in each DRG. This process has two main elements. First, for each patient, the hospital must accurately track the relevant resources used throughout a hospital stay and be able to connect those resources with the patient's DRG. Many existing hospital charge systems can adequately perform this task. Second, the hospital must know the full cost of each service provided (e.g., meals, laboratory tests, physiotherapy sessions, surgical operations). This aspect of cost accounting is more difficult for most health care organizations to achieve.

COST BEHAVIOR

A fundamental principle of managerial accounting is the distinction between fixed and variable costs. *Fixed costs* are costs that do not change when the volume of service increases or decreases (Figure 5-1A). Fixed costs in a health care setting include the cost of such items as building-loan payments, property taxes, and depreciation, as well as the many other costs that continue to accrue no matter how many patient-care services are being provided. Fixed costs usually occur at fixed intervals (e.g., monthly loan payments). *Variable costs* change in proportion to changes in volume

---

*Highly insightful concepts regarding assessing the potential benefits and harms of alternative forms of patient care in the context of cost are found in Eddy DM. Clinical Decision Making: From Theory to Practice. A Collection of Essays from JAMA. Boston: Jones and Bartlett, 1996.

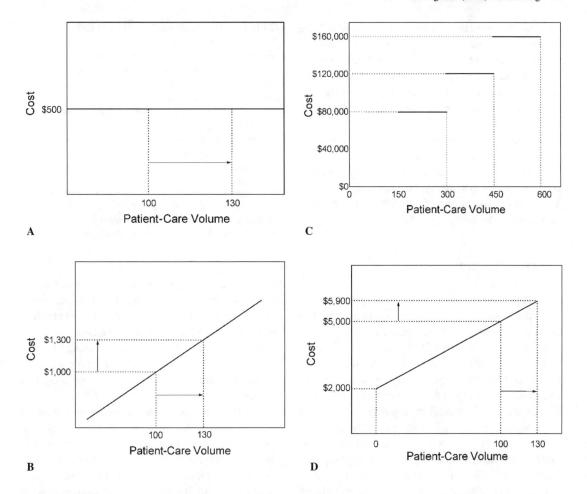

Figure 5-1. Cost behavior. **A.** Fixed costs do not change with changes in patient-care volume. **B.** Variable costs change in direct proportion to changes in volume. **C.** Semi-fixed costs (step costs) change in incremental steps. **D.** Semi-variable costs have elements of fixed and variable behavior.

of service (Figure 5-1B). If the number of surgical procedures increases by a given percentage, then the costs of such things as dressings, sutures, pharmaceuticals, and many other supplies will change roughly proportionally. Fixed and variable costs are at extreme ends of the continuum of cost behaviors.

Semi-fixed costs (step costs) vary with the volume of output, but they change in large incremental steps (Figure 5-1C). For example, two perfusion technicians may be able to manage the needs of the cardiac surgery program until a volume of 300 cases per year is reached, at which point a third perfusionist must be hired. The cost of perfusion technicians is semi-fixed, because changes occur in relatively large, discrete units.

Finally, semi-variable costs involve relatively small incremental costs or may be proportional in some ranges (Figure 5-1D). For example, utility costs are semi-variable. The costs of basic utilities, such as climate control and lighting, are fixed. Other utility costs, however, are proportional to the number of patients cared for in the OR suite, because additional patients require more monitoring by electronic devices, more sterilizing of surgical instruments, and more cleaning of ORs.

In contrast to the relative ease of allocating fixed costs to hospital functions, special techniques must be used to estimate variable costs. Linear regression is the most accurate method and the easiest to understand. Assume a semi-variable cost behavior such as that depicted in Figure 5-1D, in which the departmental cost of a service or product is plotted against volume of output. When the line of best fit is mathematically calculated, the y-axis intercept represents the fixed cost, and the slope of the line represents the variable cost of each additional unit of service or product. In this example, the slope shows that increasing patient-care volume by 100 units increases cost by $3,000 (from $2,000 to $5,000) and that increasing volume by 30 units more increases cost by $900. Therefore, the variable cost is $30 per unit of service or product. The fixed cost is the y-intercept: $2,000.

CONTROLLABLE COSTS

In a typical management control process, the responsibility for controlling costs is assigned to managers of responsibility centers, who usually control some but not all of the costs incurred by the centers. *Controllable costs* are costs that can be influenced by a manager's decision making. For example, OR managers usually control staffing levels for nurses. If hospital policy requires that one nurse be on duty in the OR suite at all times, however, the cost of the required nurse is an uncontrollable fixed cost from the OR manager's standpoint. In contrast, if the OR manager has the option of adding nurses to the OR staff when volume increases, the semi-fixed cost of additional nurses would be controllable. Similarly, the OR manager has some control over the cost of supplies (a direct variable cost). Although the manager could decide to reduce costs by purchasing cheaper supplies, the choice of supplies often depends on surgeon preference or on group purchasing contracts negotiated by the hospital. In neither of these cases does the OR manager have complete control of supply costs.

In medical facilities, six major factors determine controllable costs (Table 5-1). First is the mix of diagnoses, which determine the types of treatment received by patients. The various diagnoses in the facility's patient population are governed largely by the decisions of admitting physicians and the preferences of patients. These factors are influenced by the hospital's marketing department and by the provision of special facilities for particular types of cases.

Table 5-1. Principal Factors Determining Controllable Costs in a Medical Facility*

1. Mix of diagnoses, which determine the types of treatments received by patients
2. Numbers of patients having each diagnosis
3. Quantity and types of resources used to treat each patient having a given diagnosis
4. Fixed medical facility costs
5. Cost of resources needed to treat each patient having a given diagnosis
6. Efficiency with which resources are used in treatments

*The first four factors are controlled primarily by physicians and their leaders; the last two are controlled primarily by those who manage the health care organization's resources.

Decisions to develop special competence in particular types of cases (e.g., cardiac surgery or liver transplantation) are usually made by the clinical chiefs in conjunction with the hospital's managers.

The second major factor determining controllable costs is the number of each type of case, which is influenced by the same factors as the mix of diagnoses.

The third factor is the quantity and type of resources used to treat patients with given diagnoses. These choices are largely controlled by treating physicians, who may be influenced to some extent by cost-control measures initiated by the health care organization. Such initiatives may include clinical pathways that guide the treatment of patients having a particular diagnosis and that raise flags if the course deviates significantly from the norm. Although the health care organization may have some influence, the resource cost per case is primarily controlled by members of the medical staff—the clinical chiefs who make clinical pathways available and the physicians who either do or do not use the pathways.

The fourth factor determining controllable costs is fixed medical facility costs, which encompass a range of properties (often equipment) that are largely controlled by the judgments of attending physicians and their clinical chiefs. Whether the OR suite needs a new and improved operating microscope is an example of such a decision. Similarly, physicians control such variables as the need for intensive care for certain patient groups, for expanded laboratory capabilities, or for new radiology equipment. Although fixed medical facility costs are usually determined by individual physicians or by physician leaders, the costs are often subject to budget constraints set by facility managers.

These first four factors are all primarily under the control of the treating physicians and their leaders. Managers of hospital departments are only partially able to affect costs generated by these drivers. Methods for control include efforts to influence case mix through marketing (directed toward both patients and physicians), efforts to influence physicians' medical decision making, and budgetary constraints.

The fifth factor determining controllable costs is the cost of resources needed to treat patients who have given diagnoses. Whereas fixed medical facility costs and the quantity and types of resources may be largely controlled by members of the medical staff, physicians less frequently specify the exact details of the equipment and supplies used. (For example, surgeons may require that blood salvage equipment be available, but they would probably not specify the brand or the vendor.) Hospital administrators play two roles in determining prices paid for necessary resources. First, an important part of a hospital manager's responsibility is to educate physicians about the costs of various treatment choices. Physicians are frequently unaware of the relative costs of various therapeutic alternatives, and they also may be unaware of the availability of alternative equipment or supplies. Second, purchasing agents have a duty, sometimes in consultation with physician leaders and unit managers, to negotiate the lowest possible prices with vendors of equipment and supplies. (See Purchasing on page 127.) Many medically trained people may be surprised to learn that the prices a facility pays for many patient-care resources are subject to negotiation over broad ranges.

The final factor determining controllable costs is the efficiency with which patient-care resources are used. Such issues as levels of stock, wastage, outdating of supplies, damage to stock, and inventory shrinkage are the responsibility of unit managers. Similarly, unit managers must match personnel to the workload as much as possible, arranging for the work to be performed without excessive idle time. In fact, one of the most important aspects of the day-to-day management of an OR suite is ensuring

efficient use of the aggregate of resources comprising the OR suite (see Chapter 8).

Knowledge of costs, combined with predicted DRG reimbursements, allows realistic budgets to be constructed. However, few hospitals have accounting systems that are comprehensive enough to carry out such detailed cost analysis. The essential activities—identifying direct costs, appropriately allocating indirect costs, analyzing cost behavior, and identifying those responsible for controllable costs—represent a large undertaking that requires a level of management commitment and sophistication found infrequently in medical facilities.

FUTURE COSTS

In management decision making, future costs must be anticipated. Managers may use historical costs to estimate future costs. However, using only historical data to develop budgets for responsibility centers is often insufficient. Projected changes in types and volumes of services and methods for providing the services must be taken into consideration. When estimating future costs, four types of costs should be considered: *avoidable costs*, *sunk costs*, *incremental costs*, and *opportunity costs*.

Avoidable costs can be circumvented by a manager's decision. They can be reduced by decreasing the volume of services or products produced. These costs often have fixed and variable components. For example, if the number of procedures in an OR suite is reduced by 30%, then the variable costs of supplies proportionally decrease and the labor hours of nurses proportionally decrease stepwise. However, the fixed costs of administrative personnel remain fixed. Hence, the avoidable costs are the variable costs of supplies and semi-fixed labor hours of nurses and other clinical personnel.

Incremental costs are incurred owing to a manager's decision. They are the converse of avoidable costs. Incremental costs may also have fixed and variable components, which depend on how intensively existing resources are being used. For example, a manager may contemplate whether to accept a managed care contract that will substantially increase surgical volume. The manager can anticipate increases in variable costs for additional supplies and personnel and in fixed costs if additional equipment and instruments are required. Whether opening a new line of business or expanding an existing line will be profitable must be determined through careful analysis of incremental costs.

Sunk costs are unaffected by current managerial decisions. They are determined by past decisions that cannot be changed in the present or future. For example, costs incurred by the purchase of blood salvage equipment last year are unaffected by a decision to outsource blood salvage services this year. The costs of the equipment are sunk costs. If the blood salvage equipment were leased, however, the costs would not be sunk, because the decision to outsource could include terminating the equipment agreement.

Opportunity costs are incurred by allocating resources suboptimally from a financial standpoint. For example, if an ASC has an option to convert vacant building space into either additional ORs with an expected return of $5 million or additional procedure rooms with an expected return of $4 million, the opportunity cost of choosing the procedure rooms is $1 million. Of course, this decision will be influenced by other considerations, such as the degree of certainty that the estimated revenues generated by each type of facility will be realized.

DIRECT VERSUS INDIRECT COSTS

To control costs and to learn where opportunities for financial improvement exist, hospital managers must use accounting systems that recognize the full cost of services provided. A fundamental part of determining the full cost is to identify proportions of the cost called *direct* and *indirect costs* and to allocate these costs in a reasonable way.

Direct costs are costs that can be traced to a specific source. One source might be a given surgical operation, such as a thyroidectomy. (See a typical preference card for a thyroidectomy on page 118 to gain a sense of the supplies required for this operation.) The direct costs for most of the supplies and labor for which a hospital has established charges are relatively clear, although no system for capturing them may be available.

Indirect costs, on the other hand, cannot be easily traced to a specific source (cost object). For exam-

ple, such hospital costs as liability insurance premiums or hospital utility bills cannot be easily traced to a specific surgical operation. Other indirect costs include depreciation of the physical plant and the costs of housekeeping, security, and telecommunications. These types of costs are often referred to as *overhead*.

ALLOCATION OF INDIRECT COSTS TO THE OPERATING ROOM SUITE

The true cost of doing business can be determined only when indirect costs are included in each department's costs. To assign indirect costs, OR managers must perform two basic cost accounting maneuvers: accepting costs from responsibility centers that provide services to the OR suite and transferring costs to responsibility centers for which the OR suite provides services.

Costs are transferred according to a rational formula. A general accounting principle states that all indirect costs are allocated to direct departments (departments that can charge externally for their services). Suppose that the housekeeping department, an indirect department, devotes 20% of its housekeeping labor hours to the OR suite (a direct department). Consequently, 20% of the costs of running the housekeeping department should be allocated to the OR suite. Housekeeping costs are traceable, based on housekeeping labor hours and the cost of supplies and equipment used in the OR suite. When costs from indirect departments have been completely allocated to departments directly providing services to patients, full cost allocation has been achieved.

Three methods of cost allocation are generally accepted: step-down, double distribution, and simultaneous equations. The method used is usually chosen by the finance department of the health care organization.

Step-down is the simplest and most commonly used method for indirect cost allocation. It recognizes the costs rendered by indirect departments (e.g., housekeeping) to other indirect departments (e.g., the laundry), as well as to direct departments (e.g., the OR suite). The indirect department that incurs the smallest costs from serving other indirect departments and is responsible for generating the largest costs to direct departments allocates its costs first. Then the indirect department with the next smallest costs from other indirect departments and the next greatest costs to direct departments allocates its costs. This sequence is continued until all costs are allocated to the direct departments.

The double distribution method is a refinement of the step-down method. In the first step, each indirect department allocates its respective indirect costs to both direct and indirect departments. In the second step, the indirect costs allocated to the indirect departments from other indirect departments are reallocated to the direct departments.

In the simultaneous equations method, a series of equations is solved to allocate costs among the various departments, both indirect and direct. The equations are formulated to allocate all the services of indirect departments to direct departments, as in the other allocation methods.

Cost allocation should be equitable. For example, if the housekeeping department expends 40% of its budget but only 20% of its total labor hours on the OR suite, then allocating the housekeeping cost to different departments on the basis of labor hours is not equitable. Such allocation would force other hospital departments to assume too high a proportion of housekeeping costs, and apparent costs in those departments would be artificially high. To recover those apparent costs, some department managers might be forced to overprice their services. In contrast, the cost of running the OR suite would be artificially low, causing the OR manager to underprice OR services. Providing high volumes of underpriced services can lead to large financial losses, and providing high volumes of overpriced services can lead to loss of contracts with insurers and other payers.

For indirect costs like the laundry, which are relatively concrete, allocating indirect costs is usually straightforward. On the other hand, determining what proportion of the hospital's malpractice insurance payment should be assigned to the OR suite is difficult. Reasonable arguments can be made that liability insurance premiums should be divided evenly among all patients, or that patients undergoing high-risk procedures should bear a higher proportion of the costs. The method chosen for allocating indirect costs is usually determined by the finance or accounting department. Despite having little or no input into the

method used for allocation, however, OR managers have considerable responsibility for understanding indirect costs and for applying them to patient-care activities.

Appendix 5-1 on page 65 contains a simplified example illustrating the step-down and double distribution methods for allocating laundry and housekeeping costs to the OR suite and to other departments.

COSTING METHODS FOR PATIENT CARE SERVICES

OR managers may not be able to develop an accounting system more sophisticated than that of the parent institution. They must work with the hospital's finance department to develop accounting tools that allow rational management of the OR suite. The most significant element to be identified in an OR suite is the full cost of each case. When cost information is available at this level, cases can be aggregated in many ways to answer a variety of important questions: What are the relative costs of different types of cases, of different surgeons performing the same types of cases, or of different types of patients—older or younger, more or less healthy—undergoing the same procedures? Of course, knowing the answers to these questions is one thing, and putting the information to practical use is another.

Measuring direct costs of surgical cases is relatively straightforward in an OR suite with a computerized preference card system. (See Preference and Procedure Cards on page 115.) The cost of items contained on each preference card can be determined, and the time required to perform the surgery can be retrieved from the ORDB to determine labor costs for the case. (See Operating Room Cost Analysis on page 144.) Indirect costs in the OR suite can be assigned by a variety of methods, but the simplest is to assign them in proportion to the duration of each case. This method will probably underestimate the indirect costs of short cases, but it offers a reasonable approximation.

Appendix 5-2 on page 68 contains examples of the application of several methods for estimating the cost of an inguinal herniorrhaphy. Variations of this operation with different *CPT* codes are included to demonstrate how the different methods yield different results when conditions vary. (See the discussion of *CPT* codes under Procedure Codes on page 146.)

BUDGETING

The budget of an OR suite can be a useful tool if developed carefully and used appropriately. A well-constructed budget is an agreement between the OR manager and a senior facility administrator and should be developed through negotiation between the two parties. The budget should represent a pledge by the OR manager to run the OR suite for a specified time for a specified price. Many different types of budgets are used, but the most common for an OR suite are the discretionary budget and the standard or flexible budget.

The discretionary budget is fixed. This type of budget is appropriate when a manager directly controls most of the spending of a clinical unit. The discretionary budget is intended to place a limit on the facility resources that are allocated to the unit. The manager has a duty to ensure that the rate and spacing of expenditures are such that the unit can function throughout the budget period. Many OR suites use discretionary budgets, often developed by central hospital administrators with little or no input from the OR leadership. As resources available to hospitals shrink, a discretionary OR budget may decrease from the previous year's level, even when OR volume is increasing.

Preferable to the discretionary budget is the flexible budget, which attempts to predict the cost behavior of the OR suite. It contains fixed and variable elements that expand or contract with changes in OR volume, supplier prices, and other variables affecting OR costs. The flexible budget is most appropriate when the manager has little or no control over the cost drivers other than management efficiency. The OR suite is an almost textbook example of appropriate use of a flexible budget.

The budget should be used as a tool by the manager to determine whether costs and resource use are functioning as predicted. Variations from the budget (usually called *variances* in accounting terminology) should alert the manager that something unexpected has happened to invalidate predictions made when the budget was prepared. One of the duties of the OR manager is to determine causes of substantial variances from the budget and to report the findings to senior management when appropriate.

Well-developed techniques for analyzing budget variances are described in accounting textbooks. These methods can distinguish clearly among different causes of budget problems. Specifically, variance analysis can separate the effects of changes in case volume, changes in labor and nonlabor costs, and changes in intensity of labor and nonlabor use. Variance analysis is usually performed in consultation with personnel in the hospital's finance department.

SPECIAL CONSIDERATIONS FOR OPERATING ROOM MANAGERS

Knowing cost behavior is becoming increasingly critical for hospitals. When hospital managers are offered an opportunity to contract for a substantial number of new cases at a fixed price per case, they will not know whether the reimbursement is adequate without accurate knowledge of the full cost of the additional cases, which is determined by the cost behavior of the prospective cases. All fixed, variable, semi-fixed, and semi-variable costs should be estimated to determine the incremental cost, which is the cost of performing one case more than is currently done. The incremental cost (sometimes incorrectly referred to as *marginal cost*) determines whether the reimbursement for performing additional cases will be sufficient.

A highly simplified version of cost analysis involving fixed and semi-fixed costs appears in Case Study 5-1. (If an actual management decision were being made, the model would have to incorporate many more variables.)

One concept important to understanding fixed and variable costs is that as volume increases, the variable cost per case usually remains relatively constant, whereas the fixed cost per case decreases because fixed costs are spread over a larger number of cases (economy of scale). Although this rule is generally true, it fails in many situations. If a service is already operating at its full capacity, an increase in volume may force the construction of new capacity, thus substantially raising fixed costs (converting what was a fixed cost into a semi-fixed cost). The actual cost behavior of a complex system such as a hospital (or even an OR suite) is a composite of many interacting cost behaviors, which can be determined only by collecting data that show how the system operates over a considerable time interval (rarely less than 2 years).

CASE STUDY 5-1. Break-Even Analysis at Freestanding Surgical Center

The administrator of FSC is performing a break-even analysis of a new laparoscopic surgical procedure. He is evaluating various staffing and reimbursement scenarios to determine whether FSC should offer the procedure to surgeons and patients. He starts with the most basic scenarios and then adds additional complexity to understand various nuances.

Fee-for-Service

In the first scenario, the administrator assumes fee-for-service reimbursement. It costs $200,000 per year to lease the necessary laparoscopic equipment, and the assumption is made that this is the only direct cost. The fee-for-service reimbursement pays $500 per procedure. Therefore, a volume of 400 procedures per year is required to cover fixed costs, and this represents the break-even point. Volume greater than 400 procedures will lead to a profit of $500 per procedure. The management incentive is to meet the break-even point of 400 cases to cover fixed costs and to surpass the break-even point to make a profit of $500 per procedure.

In a second scenario, the administrator also assumes a fee-for-service reimbursement method but adds technical support to the costs of providing the service—a laparoscopic technician salaried at $20,000 per year to operate and maintain the equipment. The technician's salary is a semi-fixed cost. The administrator assumes that the technician can cover a maximum of 500 laparoscopic procedures per year. Therefore, for one to 500 procedures the technical labor cost is fixed at $20,000, and that cost must be added to the laparoscopy equipment fixed cost. Because the added labor cost increases costs to $220,000, the break-even point is raised to 440 procedures per year. An annual volume greater than 440 procedures leads to a profit of $500 per procedure, up to a maximum of 500 procedures, beyond which a second technician must be hired. In this scenario, the management incentive is to meet the break-even point of 440 cases per year to cover fixed costs of equipment and the technician, but not to exceed 500 cases, which would cap the potential profit at $30,000, or an average profit of $60 per procedure.

In the administrator's third scenario, he also assumes fee-for-service reimbursement and the need for technical support. He additionally assumes, however, that more than 500 procedures but fewer than 1,000 procedures will be performed each year, requiring that a second technician be hired at an annual salary of $20,000. With the additional semi-fixed labor cost, the cost becomes $240,000 and the break-even point increases to 480 procedures per year. An annual volume greater than 480 cases leads to a profit of $500 per procedure up to 1,000 procedures per year. The management incentive now is to meet the break-even point of 480 to cover fixed costs of equipment and technicians but not exceed 1,000 procedures per year. If the annual volume reaches 1,000 procedures, the annual profit would be $260,000, or an average of $260 per procedure. If the annual volume only reaches 500 cases, however, the annual profit would only be $10,000, or an average of $20 per procedure.

Capitation

In the last scenario, the administrator assumes capitated reimbursement, fixed costs of leasing equipment, and semi-fixed costs of required technical support. From an actuarial analysis, he predicts that the surgical center's capitated population base will require 525 laparoscopic procedures per year. He believes that the local insurance companies will pay annual capitated payments equivalent to the anticipated annual fee-for-service payments less a 10% discount. Hence, FSC will receive capitated

(continued)

CASE STUDY 5-1. (*continued*)

payments of $236,250 per year (525 procedures × $500 per procedure × 90%). From his previous scenarios, the administrator knows that the surgical center will need two technicians to cover the anticipated 525 procedures and that the fixed cost will be $240,000 per year. This analysis shows that the capitated payment will not cover the fixed costs and that FSC would experience a loss of $3,750 per year ($240,000 – $236,250) on the new laparoscopic procedure. The administrator thinks that the actuarial analysis overestimates use of the new procedure and that actual use will be less than 500 procedures per year, however, which would eliminate the need for a second technician. Under these circumstances, the surgical center would experience a profit of $16,250 per year ($236,250 – $220,000).

Predicting cost behaviors (trends in fixed and variable costs) is much more difficult than estimating costs of individual procedures. Data necessary for the analysis often are not available, and collecting the data is a major undertaking. Even if the data exist, they may be severely limited in their usefulness by referring to a constricted range of case loads. If the case load has always been relatively constant, as in many medical facilities, predicting the effect of a sudden increase in volume is not possible, because the necessary data do not exist. (Note that the analysis of the semi-variable cost behavior exhibited in Figure 5-1D on page 57 depended on a substantial number of cases of the type for which the cost analysis was performed.) Methods for estimating the incremental cost for a particular type of case are beyond the scope of this book.

SUMMARY

The primary purpose of managerial (cost) accounting is to provide managers with critical information

necessary for rational and efficient management of complex organizations. Sophisticated accounting can identify areas of strength that may be candidates for marketing. Accounting methods can also identify areas of weakness that require augmented resources or, in some cases, areas that should be abandoned. Finally, from the OR manager's standpoint, one of the most important uses of cost accounting is to provide information that can facilitate improvements in the efficiency with which resources are used in the OR suite and, ultimately, to increase profitability.

FURTHER READING

Berman HJ, Kukla SF, Weeks LE. The Financial Management of Hospitals (8th ed). Ann Arbor, MI: Health Administration Press, 1994.

Cleverley WO. Essentials of Health Care Finance (4th ed). Gaithersburg, MD: Aspen Publishers, 1997.

Horngren CT, Foster G, Datar SM. Cost Accounting: A Managerial Emphasis (9th ed). Englewood Hills, NJ: Prentice Hall, 1996.

Appendix 5-1

Comparison of Methods for Allocating Indirect Costs

Simplified hypothetical direct and indirect cost profiles are shown in Table A5-1A. In the step-down method, the order in which indirect costs are allocated to direct departments using the same drivers yields slightly different cost allocations (Tables A5-1B and A5-1C). The double distribution method first allocates among direct and indirect departments and then, as a second step, reallocates proportional shares of the indirect departments' indirect costs to direct departments (Table A5-1D). The methods yield different but comparable results (Table A5-1E). In this simplified example, the maximum difference of $365 between the highest and the lowest allocation to the OR suite represents only 0.22% of the total OR costs ($150,000 direct plus $13,000 indirect). This difference may become important if profit margins for OR service contracts or for capitated or case-rate contracts are extremely small, especially when the OR manager has direct responsibility for the profitability of the OR suite.

Table A5-1A. Simplified Hypothetical Direct and Indirect Cost Profiles

Department	Direct Costs	Laundry Pounds	Square Feet
Laundry	$ 20,000	—	25,000
Housekeeping	$ 30,000	7,500	—
Operating rooms	$150,000	20,000	50,000
Other departments	$300,000	72,500	125,000
Total	**$500,000**	**100,000**	**200,000**

Table A5-1B. Step-Down Method (Laundry Allocated First)

Laundry allocation (to direct and indirect departments)	
To housekeeping department	
(7,500 lb/100,000 lb) × $20,000	$ 1,500
To operating rooms	
(20,000 lb/100,000 lb) × $20,000	4,000
To other departments	
(72,500 lb/100,000 lb) × $20,000	14,500
Total laundry allocation	**$ 20,000**
Housekeeping allocation (to direct departments)	
To operating rooms	
(50,000 sq ft/175,000 sq ft) × ($30,000 + $1,500)	$ 9,000
To other departments	
(125,000 sq ft/175,000 sq ft) × ($30,000 + $1,500)	22,500
Total housekeeping allocation*	**$ 31,500**
Total direct costs after step-down allocation of indirect costs	
Operating rooms	
$150,000 [direct] + $4,000 [indirect laundry] + $9,000 [indirect housekeeping]	$163,000
Other departments	
$300,000 [direct] + $14,500 [indirect laundry] + $ 22,500 [indirect housekeeping]	337,000
Total direct costs	**$500,000**

*Includes $1,500 allocated from laundry.

Table A5-1C. Step-Down Method (Housekeeping Allocated First)

Housekeeping allocation (to direct and indirect departments)	
To laundry department	
(25,000 sq ft/200,000 sq ft) × $30,000	$ 3,750
To operating rooms	
(50,000 sq ft/200,000 sq ft) × $30,000	7,500
To other departments	
(125,000 sq ft/200,000 sq ft) × $30,000	18,750
Total housekeeping allocation	**$ 30,000**
Laundry allocation (to direct departments)	
To operating rooms	
(20,000 lb/92,500 lb) × ($20,000 + $3,750)	$ 5,135
To other departments	
(72,500 lb/92,500 lb) × ($20,000 + $3,750)	18,615
Total laundry allocation*	**$ 23,750**
Total direct costs after step-down allocation of indirect costs	
Operating rooms	
$150,000 [direct] + $7,500 [indirect housekeeping] + $5,135 [indirect laundry]	$162,635
Other departments	
$300,000 [direct] + $18,750 [indirect laundry] + $18,615 [indirect housekeeping]	337,365
Total direct costs	**$500,000**

*Includes $3,750 allocated from housekeeping.

Table A5-1D. Double Distribution Method

Laundry primary allocation (to direct and indirect departments)	
To housekeeping department	
(7,500 lb/100,000 lb) × $20,000	$ 1,500
To operating rooms	
(20,000 lb/100,000 lb) × $20,000	4,000
To other departments	
(72,500 lb/100,000 lb) × $20,000	14,500
Total laundry allocation	**$ 20,000**
Housekeeping allocation (to direct and indirect departments)	
To laundry	
(25,000 sq ft/200,000 sq ft) × ($30,000 + $1,500)	$ 3,938
To operating rooms	
(50,000 sq ft/200,000 sq ft) × ($30,000 + $1,500)	7,875
To other departments	
(125,000 sq ft/200,000 sq ft) × ($30,000 + $1,500)	19,687
Total housekeeping allocation[a]	**$ 31,500**
Laundry secondary allocation (to direct departments)	
To operating rooms	
(20,000 lb/92,500 lb) × $3,938	$ 851
To other departments	
(72,500 lb/92,500 lb) × $3,938	3,087
Total additional laundry allocation[b]	**$ 3,938**
Total direct costs after step-down allocation of indirect costs	
Operating rooms	
$150,000 [direct] + ($4,000 + $851) [indirect laundry] + $7,875 [indirect housekeeping]	$162,726
Other departments	
$300,000 [direct] + ($14,500 + $3,087) [indirect laundry] + $19,687 [indirect housekeeping]	337,274
Total direct costs	**$500,000**

[a]Includes $1,500 allocated from laundry.
[b]Accounting for allocation from housekeeping to laundry.

Table A5-1E. Results of Applying the Different Methods of Allocation

	Indirect Costs		
Method of Allocation	**Operating Rooms**	**Other Departments**	**Total**
Step-down method: laundry allocated first	$13,000	$37,000	$50,000
Step-down method: housekeeping allocated first	$12,635	$37,365	$50,000
Double distribution method	$12,726	$37,274	$50,000

Appendix 5-2

Comparison of Methods for Allocating Costs to Patient-Care Services

The following tables illustrate four methods for estimating cost of patient care in the OR: (1) actual costing (Table A5-2A), (2) normal costing (Table A5-2B), (3) standard costing (Table A5-2C), and (4) activity-based costing (Table A5-2D). The results of applying each method are compared in Table A5-2E.

Table A5-2A. Actual Costing*: Inguinal Hernia Repair

Procedure	Patient 1	Patient 2	Patient 3	Patient 4	Patient 5	Utilization/Unit Cost
	CPT 49505 Repair initial inguinal hernia; reducible	CPT 49505 Repair initial inguinal hernia; reducible	CPT 49507 Repair initial inguinal hernia; incarcerated or strangulated	CPT 49520 Repair recurrent inguinal hernia; reducible	CPT 49521 Repair recurrent inguinal hernia; incarcerated or strangulated	
Nurse hours at $25/hr	1.0 / $25.00	0.8 / $20.00	1.5 / $37.50	2.0 / $50.00	1.3 / $32.50	Actual / Actual
Technician hours at $12/hr	1.0 / $12.00	0.8 / $9.60	1.5 / $18.00	2.0 / $24.00	1.3 / $15.60	Actual / Actual
Sutures (pkg) at $5/pkg	1.0 / $5.00	1.0 / $5.00	2.0 / $10.00	3.0 / $15.00	2.0 / $10.00	Actual / Actual
Dressings (no.) at $5 each	2.0 / $10.00	2.0 / $10.00	3.0 / $15.00	1.0 / $5.00	3.0 / $15.00	Actual / Actual
Medications (no.) at $10 each	2.0 / $20.00	3.0 / $30.00	2.0 / $20.00	2.0 / $20.00	1.0 / $10.00	Actual / Actual
Housekeeping hours at $10/hr	0.5 / $5.00	0.5 / $5.00	0.4 / $4.00	0.6 / $6.00	0.5 / $5.00	Actual / Actual
Utilities hours at $1/hr	1.5 / $1.50	1.3 / $1.30	1.9 / $1.90	2.6 / $2.60	1.8 / $1.80	Actual / Actual
Administration hours at $30/hr	1.3 / $39.00	1.9 / $57.00	2.1 / $63.00	1.4 / $42.00	3.4 / $102.00	Actual / Actual
Total	**$117.50**	**$137.90**	**$169.40**	**$164.60**	**$191.90**	

CPT = Current Procedure Terminology.

*Actual utilization and actual unit cost rates are used for determining direct and indirect costs. At the time procedures are performed, indirect unit costs may not be available, which makes actual costing less feasible than other methods.

Table A5-2B. Normal Costing*: Inguinal Hernia Repair

	Patient 1	Patient 2	Patient 3	Patient 4	Patient 5	Utilization/Unit Cost
Procedure	CPT 49505 Repair initial inguinal hernia; reducible	CPT 49505 Repair initial inguinal hernia; reducible	CPT 49507 Repair initial inguinal hernia; incarcerated or strangulated	CPT 49520 Repair recurrent inguinal hernia; reducible	CPT 49521 Repair recurrent inguinal hernia; incarcerated or strangulated	
Nurse hours at $25/hr	1.0 $25.00	0.8 $20.00	1.5 $37.50	2.0 $50.00	1.3 $32.50	Actual Actual
Technician hours at $12/hr	1.0 $12.00	0.8 $9.60	1.5 $18.00	2.0 $24.00	1.3 $15.60	Actual Actual
Sutures (pkg) at $5/pkg	1.0 $5.00	1.0 $5.00	2.0 $10.00	3.0 $15.00	2.0 $10.00	Actual Actual
Dressings (no.) at $5 each	2.0 $10.00	2.0 $10.00	3.0 $15.00	1.0 $5.00	3.0 $15.00	Actual Actual
Medications (no.) at $10 each	2.0 $20.00	3.0 $30.00	2.0 $20.00	2.0 $20.00	1.0 $10.00	Actual Actual
Housekeeping hours at $10/hr	0.5 $5.00	0.5 $5.00	0.4 $4.00	0.6 $6.00	0.5 $5.00	Actual Budgeted
Utilities hours at $0.90/hr	1.5 $1.35	1.3 $1.17	1.9 $1.71	2.6 $2.34	1.8 $1.62	Actual Budgeted
Administration hours at $35/hr	1.3 $45.50	1.9 $66.50	2.1 $73.50	1.4 $49.00	3.4 $119.00	Actual Budgeted
Total	**$123.85**	**$147.27**	**$179.71**	**$171.34**	**$208.72**	

CPT = Current Procedure Terminology.
*Budgeted rather than actual unit costs are used for indirect cost determinations.

Table A5-2C. Standard Costing*: Inguinal Hernia Repair

Procedure	Patient 1	Patient 2	Patient 3	Patient 4	Patient 5	Utilization/Unit Cost	
	CPT 49505 Repair initial inguinal hernia; reducible	CPT 49505 Repair initial inguinal hernia; reducible	CPT 49507 Repair initial inguinal hernia; incarcerated or strangulated	CPT 49520 Repair recurrent inguinal hernia; reducible	CPT 49521 Repair recurrent inguinal hernia; incarcerated or strangulated		
Nurse hours at $25/hr	1.5 $37.50	1.5 $37.50	1.5 $37.50	1.5 $37.50	1.5 $37.50	Standard	Standard
Technician hours at $12/hr	1.5 $18.00	1.5 $18.00	1.5 $18.00	1.5 $18.00	1.5 $18.00	Standard	Standard
Sutures (pkg) at $5/pkg	2.0 $10.00	2.0 $10.00	2.0 $10.00	2.0 $10.00	2.0 $10.00	Standard	Standard
Dressings (no.) at $5 each	1.0 $5.00	1.0 $5.00	1.0 $5.00	1.0 $5.00	1.0 $5.00	Standard	Standard
Medications (no.) at $10 each	2.0 $20.00	2.0 $20.00	2.0 $20.00	2.0 $20.00	2.0 $20.00	Standard	Standard
Housekeeping hours at $10/hr	0.5 $5.00	0.5 $5.00	0.5 $5.00	0.5 $5.00	0.5 $5.00	Standard	Budgeted
Utilities hours at $0.90/hr	1.82 $1.64	1.82 $1.64	1.82 $1.64	1.82 $1.64	1.82 $1.64	Standard	Budgeted
Administration hours at $35/hr	2.02 $70.70	2.02 $70.70	2.02 $70.70	2.02 $70.70	2.02 $70.70	Standard	Budgeted
Total	**$167.84**	**$167.84**	**$167.84**	**$167.84**	**$167.84**		

CPT = Current Procedure Terminology.

*Standard (estimated) utilization and standard unit costs are used for direct cost determinations; standard (estimated) utilization and budgeted unit costs are used for indirect cost determinations.

Table A5-2D. Activity-Based Costing*: Inguinal Hernia Repair

	Patient 1	Patient 2	Patient 3	Patient 4	Patient 5	Utilization/Unit Cost
Procedure	CPT 49505 Repair initial inguinal hernia; reducible	CPT 49505 Repair initial inguinal hernia; reducible	CPT 49507 Repair initial inguinal hernia; incarcerated or strangulated	CPT 49520 Repair recurrent inguinal hernia; reducible	CPT 49521 Repair recurrent inguinal hernia; incarcerated or strangulated	
Nurse hours at $25/hr	1.0 / $25.00	0.8 / $20.00	1.5 / $37.50	2.0 / $50.00	1.3 / $32.50	Actual / Actual
Technician hours at $12/hr	1.0 / $12.00	0.8 / $9.60	1.5 / $18.00	2.0 / $24.00	1.3 / $15.60	Actual / Actual
Nurse hours for sutures at $7/nurse hr	1.0 / $7.00	0.8 / $5.60	1.5 / $10.50	2.0 / $14.00	1.3 / $9.10	Nurse hours / Budgeted
Nurse hours for dressings at $8/nurse hr	1.0 / $8.00	0.8 / $6.40	1.5 / $12.00	2.0 / $16.00	1.3 / $10.40	Nurse hours / Budgeted
Nurse hours for medications at $15/nurse hr	1.0 / $15.00	0.8 / $12.00	1.5 / $22.50	2.0 / $30.00	1.3 / $19.50	Nurse hours / Budgeted
Nurse hours for housekeeping at $3.50/nurse hr	1.0 / $3.50	0.8 / $2.80	1.5 / $5.25	2.0 / $7.00	1.3 / $4.55	Nurse hours / Budgeted
Nurse hours for utilities at $0.90/nurse hr	1.0 / $0.90	0.8 / $0.72	1.5 / $1.35	2.0 / $1.80	1.3 / $1.17	Nurse hours / Budgeted
Nurse hours for administration at $50/nurse hr	1.0 / $50.00	0.8 / $40.00	1.5 / $75.00	2.0 / $100.00	1.3 / $65.00	Nurse hours / Budgeted
Total	$121.40	$97.12	$182.10	$242.80	$157.82	

CPT = Current Procedure Terminology.
*Activity rates (nurse hours) are used for the utilization rates of both direct and indirect cost determinations. Actual and budgeted values are used for unit costs.

Table A5-2E. Comparison of Costing Methods*: Inguinal Hernia Repair

	Patient 1	Patient 2	Patient 3	Patient 4	Patient 5	Average
Procedure	*CPT* 49505 Repair initial inguinal hernia; reducible	*CPT* 49505 Repair initial inguinal hernia; reducible	*CPT* 49507 Repair initial inguinal hernia; incarcerated or strangulated	*CPT* 49520 Repair recurrent inguinal hernia; reducible	*CPT* 49521 Repair recurrent inguinal hernia; incarcerated or strangulated	
Actual costing	$117.50	$137.90	$169.40	$164.60	$191.90	$156.26
Normal costing	$123.85	$147.27	$179.71	$171.34	$208.72	$166.18
Standard costing	$167.84	$167.84	$167.84	$167.84	$167.84	$167.84
Activity-based costing	$121.40	$ 97.12	$182.10	$242.80	$157.82	$160.25

CPT = Current Procedure Terminology.

*Responsible managers choose a method for costing based on the trade-off between desired accuracy and the cost of achieving that degree of accuracy. Although actual costing is the most accurate, it is the most difficult and expensive to undertake. The other methods, though less accurate, are less costly to perform and are considered to be reasonable methods for allocating costs to patient-care services. In these simplified examples, the less-expensive costing methods generally overestimated total costs compared to actual costing. These differences reflect inherent errors in the less-accurate methods and would be reported as budget variances in the budget reconciliation process.

Chapter 6

Management Services

We can't solve problems by using the same kind of thinking we used when we created them.

—Albert Einstein (1879–1955)

An extremely complex organizational structure is required to provide surgical services. A multitude of skills from a mix of many types of personnel are needed. OR managers must organize and direct many types of skilled workers to produce highly efficient patient care.

A fundamental problem in management of the OR suite is that the goals of the people who inhabit it—surgeons, anesthesiologists, nurses, and others—are often not congruent with the goals of the hospital or of the OR suite itself. For example, surgeons may want to have the same nursing team assigned to every operation they perform. The nursing leadership, however, while supporting this concept in principle, may think that the quality of nursing care will be optimized if nursing teams are multiskilled and capable of assisting in many different types of surgery, thus facilitating cross-coverage when necessary during illness or vacations.

In an environment of conflicting goals, the OR manager may be forced into the role of a police officer whose duty is to enforce OR and hospital policy. Under these circumstances, the number of meetings grows, the process of problem resolution slows, and the OR and hospital strategic goals may not receive appropriate priority. The solution is to develop systems to align the interests of the OR users and personnel with those of the hospital and of the OR suite, thus motivating the users to act in ways that benefit the organization. With alignment of interests, polic-

ing functions are minimized, and management can focus on supporting the common interests of the users, the OR suite and its personnel, and the hospital.

MANAGEMENT AND LEADERSHIP

Total Quality Management

A set of management principles advocated by W. Edwards Deming, often referred to as *total quality management* (TQM), has become widely accepted. Quality is broadly defined as "meeting or exceeding the needs and expectations of the customer." This deceptively simple definition creates an essential focus on the customer—in an OR, the customers are patients, surgeons, and staff—and requires that quantifiable measurement of the customer's needs and expectations be used to measure quality. For example, patients and surgeons may expect that the start of surgery will never be delayed by more than 30 minutes. TQM emphasizes decision making based on data and advocates aligning all members of the organization to achieve common goals.

Another principle of TQM is that decision making should be driven down into the lower echelons of the organization. Only the personnel who are trying to make a process work can really understand what improvements are needed. The OR manager should assemble work groups that include all interested parties to arrive at proper conclusions. A work group trying to find a cure for late-starting ORs might conclude that poor performance by transportation workers is the problem if no representative of the transportation workers is in the group to identify systems problems that prohibit transportation workers from effectively performing their jobs. (See the example in Appendix 11-2 on page 165.)

TQM emphasizes that most problems are caused by inadequacies in systems rather than by deficiencies of workers performing their jobs within the constraints imposed by those systems. The manager's focus should generally be on improving processes and systems (composites of processes) rather than on correcting performance of individual workers.

Deming championed a set of "points for management" to help create a quality-focused organization (Table 6-1). Although these principles were developed for industrial organizations, the focus on systems and the emphasis on involving everyone at all levels of the hierarchy in redesigning systems are highly applicable to OR suites.

Table 6-1. Deming's 14 Points for Management

1. Create constancy of purpose toward improvement of product and service.
2. Adopt the new philosophy.
3. Cease dependence on inspection to achieve quality.
4. End the practice of awarding business on the basis of price tag.
5. Improve constantly and forever the system of production and service.
6. Institute training on the job.
7. Institute leadership.
8. Drive out fear, so that everyone may work effectively for the company.
9. Break down barriers between departments.
10. Eliminate slogans, exhortations, and targets.
11. Eliminate work standards (quotas) on the factory floor.
12. Remove barriers that rob the hourly worker of his right to pride of workmanship.
13. Institute a vigorous program of education and self-improvement.
14. Put everyone in the company to work to accomplish the transformation.

Source: Reprinted from Out of the Crisis by W. Edwards Deming by permission of MIT and the W. Edwards Deming Institute. Published by MIT, Center for Advanced Educational Services, Cambridge, MA 02139. Copyright © 1986 by The W. Edwards Deming Institute.

Because of broad acceptance of the principles of TQM, many consulting organizations will, for a price, assist in "re-engineering" or in developing a TQM program. However, adopting the language and jargon of TQM is not sufficient for success. An organization cannot simply buy a packaged TQM program and expect that a crash implementation will work. Although education and training are fundamental to improving the performance of an organization, simply requiring employees to go to TQM training is futile. Consultants can be helpful, but they cannot substitute for commitment throughout the organization to systems-oriented methods of improvement. That commitment must originate and be championed at the highest levels of management.

Although TQM appropriately focuses on process, it does not eliminate the need for performance evaluation. Managers must continue to set standards for performance not only of the system, but also of the individuals working within it. Appropriate feedback is required for individuals to achieve optimal performance.

Many of the concepts of TQM are derived from lessons learned in assembly-line environments. Although many assembly-line concepts can be translated to service industries, OR managers must guard against the unthinking application of general industrial models to the highly specialized and complex OR environment. (See When Things Do Not Go As Planned on page 111.)

Outcomes Assessment and Customer Satisfaction

Whereas TQM emphasizes process improvement, a more recent trend has been to focus on outcomes of health care. Outcomes are broadly defined to include not only changes in the health status of patients after medical interventions but also things such as the cost of health care and the satisfaction of patients with the process of health care.

Heightened concern about patient satisfaction is a manifestation of applying the definition of high quality previously mentioned—meeting or exceeding the needs and expectations of the customer. Items appearing near the top of prioritized lists that are generated when patients are asked about their concerns regarding upcoming surgery are surprising to some health care providers (e.g., fear of postoperative nausea and vomiting often appears higher on the list than fear of pain or fear of dying). Similarly, when patients are asked to evaluate their hospital stay, inconvenient parking and unpalatable food sometimes result in low patient satisfaction despite high-quality medical and nursing care. Consequently, health care organizations are making stronger efforts to identify issues that matter to patients and to intensify efforts to improve performance in these areas.

Surgeons are also customers of the OR suite, and their needs and expectations should be identified and efforts made to meet or exceed them. So long as health care organizations make more money when surgical volume is increased, the surgeon is a customer whose satisfaction is important to the organization. On the other hand, if capitation becomes a dominant method of paying for health care services, both surgeons and health care organizations are likely to seek to minimize surgical volume, which is an expense under capitation rather than an income generator, as it is in fee-for-service. In a highly capitated system, surgeons may no longer be highly valued customers of the OR suite.

Differences between Management and Leadership

Management and leadership are both needed in an organization. This applies to organizational components (the OR suite) and to the parent organization (the hospital). Management and leadership, although quite different, involve complementary and learnable skills. Managers must ensure that proper policies and procedures are in place to facilitate smooth organizational functioning and that the policies and procedures, once established, are followed. Another function of managers is to provide direction and feedback to the workers so that the goals of the organization can be achieved (Table 6-2).

In contrast, the role of an organization's leadership is to develop and communicate the strategic plan of the organization. Leaders must motivate members of the organization to "do the right thing" by enabling them to understand the long-range goals of the institution and to apply that understanding to their own tasks. Motivation comes from a leader's expressing the organization's vision in ways that stress the importance of each individual in achieving the organization's goals. Developing and communicating a vision in ways that are not so pedestrian as to evoke cynicism or so vague as to be useless is difficult. Clear communication of the organization's vision requires considerable time and effort. Table 6-3 describes some important responsibilities of leaders.

Industrial organizations typically spend considerable time and money in training their managers and leaders. In contrast, most health care organizations expect effective leaders and managers to rise spontaneously from the ranks of clinicians and administrators. Consequently, health care organizations may have difficulty finding new solutions to old problems ("this is how we've always done it"). Investing resources in training managers and hiring people who have fresh ideas from outside the organization are likely to be cost effective in the long run.

Neither leadership nor management is the process of making all the decisions—just the opposite. The people most impacted by decisions must be involved in the decision making to arrive at the best solutions for improving an organization's performance and to give the workers a sense of control. This principle is extremely important in managing the OR suite.

Use of Information in Management

Decisions that both managers and leaders must make require information about the organization. This information includes clinical, financial, and

Table 6-2. Managerial Duties

Focus on order
Develop policies and ensure compliance
Get things done cost effectively
Effect compromises to solve problems
Provide feedback to the workers

Table 6-3. Leadership Duties

Focus on results
Think strategically
Develop and communicate a shared vision
Create an agile and improving organization
Create a sense of urgency
Be an agent of change

operational data. In comparison to other industries, the health care industry has been slow to develop suitable information systems. Although evidence-based decision making should be familiar to clinicians, the concept is foreign to many health care managers and organizations (see Chapters 5 and 10).

Management decisions require information on how well the organization is functioning, and leadership decisions require information on how well the organization is staying on its planned course. Information on performance is likely to be more quantitative and complete than information on direction. Vital decisions made by leaders are often based on softer and more incomplete information than that used by managers in their decision making.

Managers and leaders use information in different ways. Managers use information for control and problem solving. When the organization is not performing as expected—as when efficiency in the OR suite has decreased—the OR manager must (1) determine why the deviation has occurred, (2) organize people to understand the problem, and (3) implement solutions. Managers use information to fine-tune the direction of an organization, keeping it on course.

Leaders, in contrast with managers, must look at a broader range of data to make strategic decisions on direction and then must align the workers in new directions. Leaders use information to convince a wide circle of people that the organization should change course for everyone's benefit.

ORs have large numbers of experienced and competent teams. The basic team of surgeon, anesthesiologist, circulating nurse, and scrub person—fundamental to providing effective patient care in the OR—is usually well seasoned. This team has clearly defined roles and strong problem-solving relationships. In fact, the team usually functions so effectively that problem solving is not obvious. Problems related to patient care constantly occur but are quickly addressed by a highly communicative team.

In the administrative realm, novice teams often need to develop new working relationships as they approach problems associated with running the OR suite. Although surgeons, anesthesiologists, and nurses traditionally work well together when dealing with clinical tasks, this sometimes is not true when administrative problems are tackled. Teams of OR personnel established to solve efficiency problems and to improve health care processes often are working together in that capacity for the first time. This is particularly true in large health care organizations; in smaller surgical centers problem-solving teams may be quite natural. When setting up a team to solve a specific problem, all interested parties must be appropriately represented, so that the true problem can be identified; any group that is not represented is likely to be inappropriately blamed for the difficulty. In addition, having all parties participate in decisions helps all groups "buy in" to the changes when they are implemented.

Teams and Teamwork

A group of people working together for a common goal requires a high degree of coordination to be effective, and this coordination requires varying degrees of communication. A team regularly and effectively performing a routine task may seem to have very little ongoing communication. In contrast, a group of people put together on an ad hoc basis to solve a new problem may struggle to develop lines of communication, even a new vocabulary, to become an effective team. The management literature is replete with discussions about teams and team building, because the process is fundamental to good management. The OR manager must select the right teams, the right team leaders, and the right goals when pursuing process improvement.

Operating Room Management

OR managers must continually make decisions in the context of the vision and strategic plan of the organization. Factors that must be considered include core strengths of the organization, customers' needs, activities of competitors, and the changing health care marketplace (see Chapter 3). For example, implementing a Saturday OR schedule may involve many operational decisions, but they must all be made within a larger strategic context. Whenever changes are made, the reactions of competitors and allies should be anticipated and monitored. Alliances often shift as the environment changes.

Inability to change rapidly is a major liability for organizations in today's health care environment. The OR manager must create an organization that anticipates customers' needs and aggressively sets targets. Decisions must be made quickly and close to the point of change. This requires empowerment at all levels in the hierarchy of workers, creating a so-called flat organization. The OR manager must continually look at the whole OR system and make system-wide changes instead of simple, small process changes. The benefits of incremental process changes are usually not realized unless the system of which they are a part is ideally designed.

Performance of the OR suite should be judged by quantitatively measuring results. This outcomes orientation should be evident throughout the organization. Objectives should be defined and communicated, the owners of critical processes identified, and barriers to progress removed. The OR manager must always measure, as quantitatively as possible, the results of change. The quantification should primarily be oriented toward what is important to the OR suite's customers. Such an orientation ultimately benefits the organization. (For an example of identifying and correcting a problem and then measuring improved performance, see Appendix 11-2 on page 165.)

Medical care delivered in OR suites is changing rapidly and profoundly. New surgical techniques and equipment, as well as improved anesthetic drugs and equipment, are continuously and aggressively being introduced. Replacing outmoded habits in the OR suite with effective methods for improving quality of patient care and efficiency in delivering that care should carry a similar urgency. Just as physicians are always looking for new ways to cure disease, OR personnel should continually be looking for improved ways to deliver high-quality and cost-effective care.

OPERATING ROOM ORGANIZATIONAL STRUCTURES

Traditional Organizational Structure

The usual organizational structure of hospitals that provide surgical services is based on common skills and duties. For example, clinical departments are traditionally based on professional skills (e.g., internal medicine, surgery, anesthesiology, nursing) with suitable subdivisions for specialization (e.g., plastic surgery, pediatric anesthesia, orthopedic nursing). In many hospitals, the medical departments are composed primarily of independent physicians who are not employed by the hospital but are in private or group practice. (See details in Surgical Practice on page 86 and in Anesthesia Practice on page 88.) Nonclinical services are also likely to be organized around common duties or skills (e.g., accounting, purchasing, information systems, clinical engineering).

Organizational structures are created to facilitate the work of an organization (Figure 6-1). Traditional organizational structures are well suited for grouping common skills. To accomplish complex tasks related to patient care, however, cross-departmental cooper-

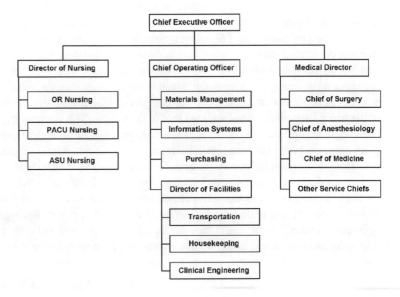

Figure 6-1. Traditional organizational structure of a hospital as it relates to the operating rooms. (OR = operating room; PACU = postanesthesia care unit; ASU = ambulatory surgery unit.)

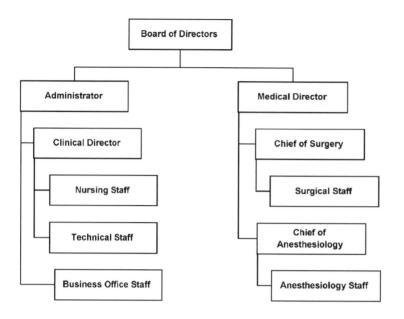

Figure 6-2. Typical organization chart for an ambulatory surgical center.

ation must occur. Such crossover tasks are usually accomplished by a variety of hospital standing committees that bring together the leadership of various departments (or their representatives) for both information sharing and problem solving. These committees often work well for information sharing but less well for problem solving, particularly when the time frame for solving a problem is short. Interdisciplinary working groups are often appointed on an ad hoc basis to address problems and to recommend quick solutions. Such working groups are sometimes called *fast-track teams* to emphasize the cooperative, time-pressured nature of the process.

To function efficiently, the OR suite requires both standing committees and short-term working groups. The basic oversight committee is often called the *operating room committee*. Membership on this committee is usually made up of the chairs (or designees) of the major surgical departments, the chief of anesthesiology, the OR manager, the OR nurse manager (who may also be the OR manager), and representatives from central hospital administration. This committee may deal with strategic and operational issues. Owing to the large constituency, OR committees are usually more effective in dealing with strategic than operational matters. Some health care organizations have supplemented the traditional OR committee with a more operationally oriented *operating room management team*, which is usually smaller and meets

more frequently (e.g., weekly rather than monthly). In this combination, the OR committee makes policy, and the OR management team monitors performance and develops methods to enforce policies.

Freestanding surgical centers typically are smaller organizations that have much flatter and more efficient organizational structures (Figure 6-2). These organizations can be more clearly focused on providing efficient surgical care, in part because less departmental hierarchy exists. Small organizations, in which everyone knows everyone else, can solve problems based on close personal relationships, which are less common in larger health care organizations. Problem-solving groups form spontaneously and dissolve naturally. In contrast to large health care organizations, upper management in small facilities can usually be less concerned about setting up formal processes for problem solving.

The contrast between large hospitals and more flexible surgical centers clearly illustrates one of the fundamental organizational issues in health care. Larger organizations can take advantage of economies of scale in delivering health care and in purchasing necessary goods and services. However, they pay the price of having more cumbersome methods for decision making and problem solving. Smaller, more focused ASCs may not enjoy economies of scale but can be much more agile in responding to environmental changes.

Figure 6-3. Typical operating room (OR) management structure for a hospital. Note that the OR suite uses the parent organization's clinical engineering and purchasing departments. However, the OR suite has its own independent transportation and housekeeping group. The materials management and the information systems units of the OR suite and of the hospital are linked. (ASU = ambulatory surgery unit; PACU = postanesthesia care unit.)

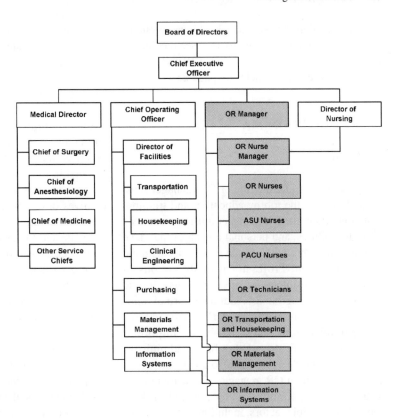

Alternative Organizational Structures

Traditional hospital OR suites can be restructured to capture some of the efficiencies inherent in smaller, freestanding centers. However, strong clinical departments are often accustomed to a large degree of autonomy, particularly in academic medical centers. Additionally, support services are usually centralized. Physically locating support services close to the OR suite results in economy of efficiency but some loss in economy of scale. An ideal structure for the OR suite may be to locate most of the support services on which the ORs depend in or adjacent to the OR suite and to have them report directly to the OR leadership (Figure 6-3). Similar reporting relationships may exist in other hospital units.

The type of structure depicted in Figure 6-3 has been termed a *hybrid organizational structure*, in which more than one line of authority is present. This structure, which seems reasonable on paper, can be problematic in practice. Problems can be minimized by not trying to push hybrid organization too far down the organizational structure. For

example, the OR nurse manager can effectively report to both the hospital nursing director and the OR director (or directly to a hospital administrator if the OR nurse manager is the chief administrator of the OR suite). However, giving second-line nursing management dual reporting relationships would be confusing. OR nursing-team leaders and staff nurses should have a clear reporting relationship only with the OR nurse manager. This type of organizational structure might be termed a *clinical service structure*.

In an even more highly integrated model, "clinical programs" combine clinical disciplines from multiple departments to coordinate care of patients who need multiple services. Cardiovascular disease programs coordinate cardiologists, cardiac surgeons, cardiac anesthesiologists, rehabilitation physicians, and specialty nurses to provide efficient services to patients referred for cardiac care. OR suites are similar to ICUs and EDs in that they provide highly specialized patient-care services and are staffed by physicians from many professional disciplines. Changing to a clinical program structure is consistent with an attempt to organize health care systems with a more patient-centered focus. (See the discussion of centers of excellence on page 19 and the discussion of core competencies on page 25.)

OPERATING ROOM MANAGER

Qualifications

The person assuming the role of OR manager must be qualified for the job by education and training. More important, the OR manager must possess a set of skills, abilities, and personal attributes that have been acquired through intimate familiarity with the OR environment. Professional qualifications in nursing, anesthesiology, or surgery are usually the most suitable backgrounds. Additional formal training in management, with a master's degree in business administration, may also be an important educational qualification. Other health administration courses and degrees may also contribute to the qualifications of an OR manager. The actual qualifications needed for a particular hospital or ASC depend on multiple factors, including the size, case volume, and relationships to support services in parent organizations. In many OR suites and surgical centers, the functions of the OR manager are assumed by the OR nurse manager. In some organizations, the OR manager's responsibilities are shared by a nursing leader and an anesthesiologist or surgeon. Because physicians in private practice outside the hospital rarely want to devote the time required to perform the duties of the OR manager, physicians holding this position are usually hospital-based (e.g., anesthesiologists).

Essential qualifications for the position of OR manager include a dedication to quality patient care and an ability to foster teamwork in a high-pressure environment. Because persuasion, rather than direct authority, is likely to be the OR manager's primary method for effecting change, the OR manager should understand how to negotiate and how to solve problems in a group setting. Such qualifications are, of course, generic attributes for any good manager and leader.

Even if the OR suite is not autonomous (as in a freestanding surgical center), the OR manager's job should encompass duties of a CEO, COO, and CFO. The OR manager should have a strong sense of ownership of the strategic plan, the daily operations, and the financial condition of the OR suite.

Strategic and Operational Responsibilities

Responsibilities for strategic planning are different from those for operational planning and implementation. Strategically, the OR manager must provide leadership to the OR and be part of the leadership of the parent health care organization. This involves developing the strategic plan for the OR suite and communicating it both to the staff of the OR suite and to the senior leadership of the institution. (See Developing a Competitive Strategy on page 25.) The strategic plan for the OR suite should be consistent with the overall strategic plan of the institution. The OR manager plays a critical role as intermediary between one of the key areas of the institution—the OR suite—and the organization's senior leadership. The OR manager must be an effective advocate for the institutional strategic plan and for the needs of the OR suite. Where conflict appears, the OR manager must seek appropriate resolution, keeping in mind that the institution's vision and goals should generally dominate.

The operational duties of the OR manager are more immediate and direct than the strategic duties. Every institution establishes a slightly different set of responsibilities and relationships for the OR manager. However, the essence of the OR manager's job is ensuring that systems are in place to provide high-quality, efficient patient care. When the number of tasks that must be accomplished is considered, it is amazing that any surgery is started on time. (See When Things Do Not Go As Planned on page 111.) Many essential tasks may not be under the immediate control of the OR manager. Thus, it is crucial that the manager develop and maintain effective liaison with all ancillary and support departments.

Much of the work of the OR manager takes place in meetings. Many of these meetings are chaired by the OR manager, and the ability to run a meeting that accomplishes its objectives is an essential skill. Problems with meetings often arise when differences regarding the goals of the meeting exist between the leader and the participants. Some meetings are for information only, as when the leader has already made the necessary decisions, and the conclusions are simply to be communicated to people attending the meeting. Another purpose for a meeting might be for a leader to seek input from the meeting participants before making a decision. The leader considers all views expressed and then arrives at a decision. In a third type of meeting, the leader expects that the participants will discuss a problem and reach a group consensus. When the leader thinks a meeting's purpose is simply to communicate a decision that has already been made, and the participants think the purpose is for them to reach a group consensus, not only confusion but perhaps even anger is likely to result. The leader must be perfectly clear about the goals of the meeting and the type of involvement (active or passive) that is expected from the participants.

Decision Making

The medical model of decision making (diagnosis, treatment, prognosis, and follow-up) and the nursing model (assessment, planning, implementation, and evaluation) also work for management decisions. First, the problem must be identified. Then it must be defined and clarified through a process similar to collecting a patient's symptoms and assessing physical signs. Collecting appropriate data from a variety of sources so that the problem can be thoroughly understood (diagnosis and assessment) is an essential step. The root causes of the problem must be diligently sought and uncovered. Fixing a readily apparent problem (treating the symptoms) without a deeper understanding of the causes (actual pathology) results in a temporary solution, at best. Only by clearly understanding the problem and its true causes can a rational and effective plan of action (treatment plan) be devised. Trying to forecast (prognosticate) how the problem and the solution are likely to change with time is helpful.

When solutions to problems are implemented, the OR manager must ensure that personnel involved in improving a faulty process fully understand the reasons for change and the goals of changes being made. Finally, follow-up must be carried out to ensure that whatever solutions are implemented have the desired effect and, if not, that the "treatment plan" is appropriately modified.

Personnel Management

Management and resolution of "people problems" are important parts of the OR manager's duties. Many personnel problems in large organizations can be dealt with by using the organization's human resources department. In small OR suites or in ASCs, however, the OR manager must be prepared to deal with many types of personnel problems. An appropriate set of personnel policies and procedures is helpful.

Some personnel problems are readily resolved by counseling about appropriate standards of conduct and productivity. Others move progressively through the disciplinary process and ultimately result in dismissal. In larger organizations, particularly those with a unionized workforce, meticulous documentation of the problem and help from the human resources department are required before an employee can be dismissed.

Many personnel issues involve people from departments outside the OR suite or nonemployee professionals who use the ORs. Here skills in negotiating are important. In fact, even in situations in which the OR manager has ultimate authority, a solution in which the other person agrees not only with the facts and their interpretation, but also with the planned course of action is usually best. OR managers must frequently deal with tense and hostile situations, because the OR suite represents a stressful environment in which life and death decisions are made regularly. William Ury, in his book on negotiating with difficult people, lists five challenges that may help in gaining an opponent's cooperation (Table 6-4). By clearly understanding an opponent's position and developing opportunities

Table 6-4. Five Negotiating Challenges

1. Control your own behavior—*don't react.*
2. Defuse your opponent's negative emotions—*disarm your opponent.*
3. Stop bargaining over positions—*change the game.*
4. Make the outcome a victory for both—*make it easy to say yes.*
5. Enhance your negotiating power—*make it hard to say no.*

Source: Excerpts from W Ury. Getting Past No: Negotiating Your Way from Confrontation to Cooperation. Copyright © 1991 by William Ury. Used by permission of Bantam Books, a division of Bantam Doubleday Dell Publishing Group Inc.

for the opponent to find it easy to accept a proposed solution, the OR manager should, in most instances, be able to achieve a desirable outcome.

SUMMARY

Managing OR suites is very difficult, because individual ORs and the OR suite itself are highly complex and often tense environments. Many personnel working in the OR suite are not under direct control of the OR manager. Similarly, the OR suite is highly dependent on many services provided by departments outside the OR manager's control. Therefore, the OR manager must understand the power of negotiation and be skilled in its application.

OR managers are leaders as well as managers. As managers, they are responsible for the day-to-day operation of the OR suite, ensuring order and efficiency. As leaders, OR managers must establish and communicate strategic goals for the OR suite that are consistent with the strategic plan of the parent organization. OR managers, as the interface between workers in the OR suite and senior leadership in the health care organization, should be advocates for the OR suite's goals to organizational leaders and advocates of the parent organization's goals to OR personnel.

OR managers must be skilled at decision making and must know how to form teams to assist in the decision-making process. Whenever possible, data should be the foundation for decisions. Work-ers who are as close as possible to the problems being solved should be included in decision making. Flat tables of organization (those having minimal hierarchy) are conducive to effective and efficient decision making. Effective implementation of solutions requires clear delineation and communication of goals and subsequent follow-up to ensure that the desired effects have been achieved.

FURTHER READING

Deming WE. Out of the Crisis. Cambridge, MA: Massachusetts Institute of Technology, Center for Advanced Engineering Study, 1982.

Fisher R, Ury W, Patton B. Getting to Yes: Negotiating Agreement without Giving In (2nd ed). New York: Houghton Mifflin, 1992.

Griffith JR, Sahney VK, Mohr RA. Reengineering Health Care. Ann Arbor, MI: Health Administration Press, 1995.

Kepner CH, Tregoe BB. The New Rational Manager. Princeton, NJ: Princeton Research Press, 1981.

Marcus LJ, Dorn BC, Kritek PB, Miller V, Wyatt J. Renegotiating Health Care: Resolving Conflict to Build Collaboration. San Francisco: Jossey-Bass Publishers, 1995.

Thompson RE. Keys to Winning Physician Support: A Guide for Executives and Managers. Tampa, FL: The American College of Physician Executives, 1992.

Ury W. Getting Past No: Negotiating Your Way from Confrontation to Cooperation (rev ed). New York: Bantam Doubleday Dell, 1993.

Chapter 7
Clinical Services

Surgeons must be very careful,
When they take the knife!
Underneath their fine incisions,
Stirs the Culprit—Life!

—Emily Dickinson (1830–1886)

Three groups of professionals must interact harmoniously in the OR—surgeons, anesthesiologists, and nurses—all supported by a variety of specialized technicians and other personnel. These professionals have in common a strong commitment to the care of patients and loyalty to their professions. Members of these groups, however, have markedly different training, tasks, and professional outlooks, as well as very different relationships with the institution. Surgeons and anesthesiologists are usually self-employed, although some may be employees of the health care organization or partners or employees of multiphysician medical groups having a variety of contractual and noncontractual relationships with the health care organization. Some of the surgeons and anesthesiologists practicing at a freestanding surgical center may be shareholders or partners in the ownership group. In contrast, OR nurses are almost always employees of the hospital or surgical center, and they may be members of a nurses' union. Hospitals occasionally employ nurses who are either independent contractors hired for limited periods or employees of contractors who supply temporary workers.

SURGICAL SPECIALTIES

General surgery, which encompasses surgery of the abdominal viscera (e.g., esophagus, stomach, intestines, colon and rectum, liver, kidneys, spleen, and pancreas) and operations on other soft tissues (e.g., the thyroid and the breasts), has historically been the most important surgical specialty in most general hospitals. General surgeons have usually performed the largest number of cases, admitted the largest number of patients, and addressed the broadest range of medical problems. A general surgeon has typically been chosen to be chief of surgery. The training of general surgeons is broader than that of most other specialized surgeons, and general surgeons are often excellent general medical diagnosticians as well as expert performers of technical procedures. Trauma surgeons usually originally train as general surgeons.

The traditional dominance of general surgery is increasingly being challenged by the rapidly increasing caseload of orthopedic surgeons. The rise of orthopedic surgery can be traced to several interacting factors. First, the population is aging, with inevitable increases in fractures and degenerative arthritis that accompany advancing age. Aggressive surgical repair of hip fractures, followed by early postoperative mobilization of the patient, substantially reduces not only medical complications but also the likelihood of death associated with these fractures. Additionally, total joint replacement has become a definitive treatment for degenerative arthritis, providing pain-free mobility for increasing numbers of patients. Second, the increasing popularity of intense exercise programs has led to a dramatic increase in sports-related musculoskeletal injuries, resulting in a new subspecialty called sports medicine that is staffed primarily by orthopedic surgeons. Third, substantial advances in the practice of anesthesia and perioperative medical care have allowed major orthopedic procedures to be performed safely on ever-sicker and -older patients. Fourth, no reasonable substitute therapy for most orthopedic surgery exists, nor is any on the medical horizon. Fifth, little or no dispute exists about the indications for or the effectiveness of most orthopedic procedures. Orthopedic surgery is likely to continue to expand well into the twenty-first century. In many hospitals, orthopedic surgeons have been organized into a separate surgical department.

Gynecologic surgery is in many ways similar to general surgery, except that the abdominal viscera of focus are the uterus, ovaries, and supporting structures, as well as the perineum and vaginal tissues. Many gynecologic surgeons also have an obstetric practice. In larger facilities, the ORs for obstetric procedures, such as cesarean deliveries, are often part of the labor and delivery suite and are staffed by obstetric nurses. In smaller hospitals, the general OR suite and its nursing staff are usually used for cesarean deliveries.

Other surgical specialties include cardiothoracic, neurologic, ophthalmologic, otorhinolaryngologic, pediatric, plastic, urologic, and vascular surgery. These specialties are largely delineated by the scope of training defined by surgical specialty boards and provided by surgical residency programs, as well as by the anatomic region or structure of primary interest. Specialty surgeons may be organized as divisions of a broadly defined department of surgery. Alternatively, if the number of surgical specialists and the number of cases performed in a given specialty are high enough, certain groups of specialists may be granted departmental status. Within each department or division, salaried physicians, group partnerships, and independent practices may be mixed.

Clear boundaries do not always exist between procedures performed by different surgical specialists. For example, most neurosurgeons, who generally deal with the brain, spinal cord, and related structures, have also been trained to treat disorders of peripheral nerves, such as carpal tunnel syndrome, as well as intervertebral disk problems.

Orthopedic surgeons are also trained to perform both of these types of surgery. The distribution of surgery between neurosurgeons and orthopedic surgeons displays wide local variation. Controversies sometimes occur when members of one specialty attempt to exclude members of other specialties from performing a particular type of operation. OR managers may be in a position to cautiously mediate interdepartmental disputes regarding surgical privileges to perform specific procedures.

Nonsurgical physicians and other medical professionals may be granted privileges to use the ORs for certain procedures. Included are dentists, podiatrists, family practitioners, and internists who perform invasive procedures. These specialists generally use ORs for procedures that require sterility, anesthesia, specialized instruments, and well-qualified nursing support.

SURGICAL PRACTICE

Surgeons in private practice have traditionally been either solo practitioners or members of single- or multispecialty group practices. This type of surgeon is a member of the hospital's medical staff and is granted privileges to perform a range of surgery appropriate to the surgeon's training and experience. For such surgeons, the hospital represents a place to practice the art of surgery, but no fiduciary relationship between the surgeon and the hospital exists. Such a surgeon is, in important ways, a customer who brings business to the hospital. This relationship encourages the hospital to cater to the demands of the surgeon, just as any successful business caters to the needs of good customers. As various forms of managed care become more common, the financial relationship between physicians and health care organizations continues to evolve. Changing financial relationships among physicians, health care organizations, and payers for health care are discussed in Chapter 2. (See Reimbursement Methods on page 9.)

Some surgeons may limit their practices to a single institution; others may have surgical privileges at multiple health care facilities. Many surgeons depend on referrals from primary care physicians and therefore operate in hospitals where referring physicians have admitting privileges. This allows the primary care physicians to conveniently participate in the postoperative care of their patients. In smaller hospitals, referring physicians sometimes assist the surgeon during operative procedures on their patients. In contrast, surgeons in large tertiary-care hospitals receive a substantial proportion of referrals from physicians who do not practice there, and the surgical assistants are either hospital employees or residents involved in postgraduate medical training.

Surgical practices are organized in many different ways. At one extreme is the model in which all surgeons or perhaps even all physicians working in one hospital are members of a single, large multi-specialty group, all of whose members are salaried. Examples of this style are the Mayo Clinic, the Kaiser-Permanente Health Plan, and many university faculty practices. At the other extreme is the model in which each individual surgeon is engaged in the independent private practice of surgery. This arrangement is most commonly found in small, relatively rural hospitals located in areas that cannot support the services of more than one practitioner in a particular surgical specialty. Between these two extremes lie a multitude of organizational arrangements. For example, there may be multiple independent practitioners in each specialty or a single incorporated group of surgeons for each surgical specialty. Larger hospitals may have two or more groups in specialties, such as general surgery or orthopedics. Additionally, lone "superspecialists" may practice in such specialties as organ transplantation surgery and pediatric surgery. The scope of practice for specialists tends to narrow as the size of the community or the health care organization increases.

Surgical practice consists of several related but quite different activities. In the office, surgeons evaluate new patients referred by primary care physicians to determine whether there is a condition amenable to surgical treatment. This evaluation may require laboratory tests, diagnostic imaging such as x-rays, and multiple visits to the surgeon's office. If a surgical condition exists, the surgeon explains to the patient the working diagnosis, the proposed surgery, and the alternatives to surgery, if any. Then, if the patient wishes to proceed, the surgeon obtains written informed consent and schedules the case at a time convenient for the patient and surgeon when OR time is available.

To use time efficiently, surgeons usually attempt to schedule several consecutive operations on the day of surgery. Operations are extraordinarily variable, requiring a wide array of instruments and ranging in duration from several minutes to more than 12 hours. The operation planned and the one actually performed may vary substantially, depending on the findings at the time of surgery and on complications that may arise. The complications themselves may be trivial or substantial, and the probability of death, although extremely low for the majority of operations, is never zero.

After an operation is completed, the patient is either admitted to the hospital or sent home. In either case, the surgeon retains responsibility for care of the patient until the end of the recovery period. For some conditions, the recovery period is never over, and the surgeon assumes follow-up responsibility for the remainder of the patient's life. Most surgeons spend considerably more time with patients during pre- and postoperative periods than during the surgical procedure itself.

ORGANIZATION OF THE SURGICAL SERVICE

To provide a comprehensive integrated surgical service, the surgeons practicing in a given health care organization, regardless of their employment status, are organized into one or more departments, each having a "chief of service" (e.g., surgeon-in-chief or orthopedist-in-chief). The department has several functions that are common to almost all types of health care organizations, and others that are specific to particular institutions.

Surgical departments provide a mechanism through which schedules can be arranged to ensure immediate availability of a qualified surgeon for consultation to inpatient medical and surgical services, the ED, and the OR suite. Such coverage is usually provided through a rotating call schedule set up by the service chief in consultation with the surgeons on that service.

OR time is sometimes allocated through surgical departments, especially in larger health care organizations. For example, a block of OR time may be allocated to the orthopedic service, with the chief of service taking responsibility for distributing the time among the various orthopedic surgeons. Alternatively, OR time may be allocated directly to individual surgeons. (See Allocation of Operating Room Time on page 102.)

Surgical departments are responsible for ensuring that surgeons perform only procedures for which they have appropriate skills. Because such a wide variety of procedures may be performed, ensuring competence for each type of case is difficult. The department must establish a set of criteria by which privileges to perform various procedures are either granted or denied. Some sort of appeal process for the surgeon who feels unfairly denied should be in place. Surgeons must produce evidence of competence to perform each procedure for which privileges are sought by providing evidence of explicit training or of experience documented in a surgical log of cases performed.

Another function of surgical departments is to try to ensure that surgical practitioners provide high-quality care. This is usually done through hospital or departmental quality improvement programs, often using the case review method. All postoperative wound infections and all intra- or postoperative deaths are traditionally reviewed. Additionally, some hospitals have a "tissue committee" that examines the reports of all tissue surgically removed from patients to ensure that the surgery performed was appropriate.

As part of the quality improvement process, minor but irritating physician behavioral problems, such as lateness, incomplete medical records, and difficulties with interpersonal relations, are referred to the service chief for resolution. Conflicts between surgeons are also usually settled by the service chief. More significant problems, such as accusations of unprofessional behavior, financial irregularities, or other serious misconduct, are usually considered to be the province of the chief of the medical staff or the CEO of the health care organization.

As managed care contracts assume more influence over costs of running the OR suite, the chief of surgery must ensure that surgeons cooperate in cost-saving measures by, for example, achieving physician consensus on standardization of supplies, instruments, and equipment. In addition, surgeons must become involved in the rapidly growing development of "clinical pathways," which are clinical guidelines on how to efficiently and effectively manage surgical cases, complete with suggested time courses.

Finally, through the surgery department and the chief of surgery, surgeons can communicate their concerns regarding how the OR suite functions.

This communication can be directed to the OR manager or to another administrator in the health care organization who has responsibility for the OR suite. Concerns are often expressed regarding perceived difficulties with scheduling operations, assignments of block time, selection and timely delivery of appropriate supplies and equipment, qualifications of nursing personnel, and availability or quality of anesthesia services. The chief of surgery should be a member of the administrative group dealing with such problems (e.g., the OR committee or the OR management team). The chief of surgery should also be a part of any group involved in long-term planning for the health care organization.

ANESTHESIA PRACTICE

Anesthesiologists in most hospitals are in fee-for-service private practice. They are sometimes independent of one another but more frequently are members of a formally constituted anesthesia group, which often has a contract with the hospital granting the group an exclusive right to practice there.

An exclusive contract offers advantages to both the hospital and the anesthesia group. From the hospital's point of view, negotiating with a single entity is far easier than negotiating with a group of unassociated individuals. An exclusive contract is a valuable concession from the hospital that groups do not wish to jeopardize. Terms of the contract can specify performance standards for the group as a whole that no single individual can deliver (e.g., 24-hour-a-day obstetric anesthesia and labor analgesia coverage, acute and chronic pain management). An exclusive contract enables an anesthesia group to screen new anesthesiologists by starting them out with time-limited employment contracts. Terminating an employment contract is far easier than dismissing a physician from the medical staff if a new anesthesiologist does not work out for one reason or another.

From the anesthesiologists' point of view, an exclusive contract offers employment security. So long as the contract is in force, no other anesthesiologist can join the hospital staff to dilute the incomes of the existing anesthesiologists. On the other hand, most exclusive contracts contain a "clean sweep" clause whereby, if the contract is lost, all anesthesiologists in the group automatically lose their medical staff privileges. This permits the hospital to negotiate an exclusive contract with another group without interference or competition from the anesthesiologists being replaced.

Many other financial arrangements are possible. In some health care organizations, typically large multispecialty clinics or university hospitals, anesthesiologists are employed by the clinic or university. In small hospitals, anesthesiologists sometimes work as independent contractors traveling from hospital to hospital or sometimes are employed by one hospital. Commercial firms are available to arrange for anesthesiology coverage on a *locum tenens* basis when regular anesthesia coverage is interrupted by illness or vacations. This service is most often used by smaller hospitals.

CRNAs are advanced-practice nurses who are qualified to administer anesthesia after graduation from special schools of nurse anesthesia after completion of nursing training. Many CRNA schools confer master's degrees to their graduates. Federal Medicare regulations and many state medical practice acts currently require nurse anesthetists to practice under the supervision of a physician, who may be the surgeon performing the operation. Most CRNAs are employees of either an anesthesia group or the hospital and work under the supervision of anesthesiologists. CRNAs, as licensed semi-independent practitioners, are subject to privileging and credentialing processes similar to those of physicians. It is important that the hospital and the anesthesia group have an explicit agreement covering not only payment of CRNAs but also billing and collecting payment for their work.

The anesthesiologist's practice in ORs is highly focused. The anesthesiologist assigned to a case must evaluate the patient before the operation and formulate an anesthesia plan based on the patient's medical condition, the surgery planned, and the preferences of the patient and the surgeon. The anesthesiologist performs a review of systems and a focused physical examination, explains the anesthetic options to the patient, and obtains the patient's informed consent. Finally, the anesthesiologist, often with the assistance of a CRNA, carries out the anesthetic plan. Because surgery is so often performed on an ambulatory basis, patients frequently arrive at the hospital for the first time on the day of surgery. Consequently, the first meeting

between anesthesiologist and patient may occur only minutes before surgery commences.

Three relatively distinct types of anesthesia may be used. The first, general anesthesia, consists of administering drugs to induce a state in which the patient is totally unconscious and pain free. The second, regional anesthesia, consists of injecting local anesthetic agents adjacent to nerves, which has the effect of rendering the anatomic territory served by those nerves numb and insensitive for the duration of the surgery. The most common types of regional anesthesia are spinal and epidural, but many others are available that anesthetize smaller portions of the body (e.g., an arm or a leg). The third type of anesthetic management has various names, including *monitored anesthesia care*, *sedation/analgesia*, and *deep sedation*. This type of anesthetic management is often used when the nature of the surgery does not demand general anesthesia but is sufficiently unpleasant that most patients will not tolerate the operative procedure without deeper sedation than the surgeon is comfortable administering personally. Monitored anesthesia care is also used for procedures in which anesthesia is not ordinarily necessary, but the patient's medical condition is so precarious that the presence of an anesthesia provider is indicated to monitor and treat complications that might arise during the procedure.

After completion of the operation, the patient may be moved to any of several locations. Historically, all patients went to the postanesthesia care unit (PACU) for a period of observation while the effects of the anesthetic wore off. After a sufficient recovery period, as determined by objective criteria, inpatients were transferred to inpatient nursing units, and ambulatory patients were transferred to a "second-stage" recovery area (ambulatory surgery unit [ASU]) before being discharged home. However, with the relatively widespread use of regional anesthesia and monitored anesthesia care, neither of which ordinarily requires close monitoring in the PACU, many patients became eligible for second-stage recovery on leaving the OR. With the introduction of general anesthetic agents that have ultrafast recovery times, even some patients who have received general anesthesia can meet PACU discharge criteria while still in the OR and may be safely sent directly to second-stage recovery. Finally, patients who do not recover consciousness or the ability to breathe on their own for hours or even days postoperatively or who have complex therapeutic and monitoring requirements are often transferred directly from the OR to the ICU after surgery, bypassing the PACU. This has the added advantage of eliminating a handoff and allows physicians managing the patient during the intraoperative period to transfer responsibility for patient care directly to the ICU physicians and nurses.

Unlike surgeons, most anesthesiologists spend the vast majority of their clinical time in the OR suite. Although anesthesia subspecialties exist (e.g., cardiac, neurosurgical, and pediatric), most anesthesiologists provide anesthesia care to patients undergoing a wide variety of surgical procedures.

ORGANIZATION OF THE ANESTHESIA SERVICE

The anesthesia service is usually a separate department, although in some (typically smaller) hospitals, anesthesiologists form a division of the department of surgery. In contrast with surgical subspecialists, anesthesiologists specializing in specific clinical areas, such as pediatric anesthesia, obstetric anesthesia, and cardiac anesthesia, are not typically organized into distinct departments. The anesthesia department must be organized in such a way as to ensure availability of a sufficient number of anesthesia providers to supply safe surgical and obstetric anesthesia for elective and emergency cases, which requires 24-hour-a-day, 7-day-a-week coverage. An anesthesia group is much more likely than a surgical group to provide professional services exclusively at one hospital. In some metropolitan communities, large anesthesia organizations may provide services at multiple facilities. When this is the case, subgroups of practitioners often routinely provide most or all of the anesthesia services at given facilities.

Many of the functions of the anesthesia department are similar to those of the surgery department—privileging, credentialing, quality assurance, cooperation with hospital departments for standardization and other cost-saving measures, and long-term planning. In larger health care organizations, the anesthesia department often provides a daily anesthesia coordinator for the OR suite. The coordinator has responsibility, usually shared with a nursing coordinator, for ensuring the smooth and efficient running of the daily OR schedule.

UNIVERSITY MEDICAL CENTERS

In teaching institutions, faculty members in both the surgery and anesthesiology departments have responsibilities beyond patient care: teaching residents and medical students and performing research. Although residents may contribute substantially to the quality of patient care in academic hospitals, the teaching mission generally slows down the running of the ORs. OR managers must support the teaching mission, but they must ensure that teaching does not become an excuse for inefficient or costly practices.

Department chairs and the OR manager must establish policies governing the privileges of surgical and anesthesiology residents. These rules should address details such as the requirement for an attending surgeon or an attending anesthesiologist to be present in the OR suite when residents are operating or administering anesthesia. Rules should also address the system established for scheduling surgical residents' cases and for ensuring quality practice by residents. The OR manager should have some familiarity with the accreditation requirements for surgery and anesthesiology residency programs and should work with the program directors to ensure that the requirements are being met.

NURSING SERVICE

Nurses are involved in every aspect of OR function, from the preoperative clinic through the postoperative period. Nurses prepare patients for surgery, assist in the induction of anesthesia, participate in the performance of the surgery itself, and care for patients recovering from anesthesia and surgery.

The surgical nursing staff is usually organized into several functional units. The largest unit is made up of nurses who work in the OR suite itself. Another group of specialized nurses works in the PACU, formerly known as the *recovery room*. Because an ever-increasing proportion of surgery is performed on an ambulatory or day-of-surgery basis, hospitals have established ASUs to care for patients in the immediate pre- and postoperative period. The nurses who work in ASUs form another large functional group. These three nursing groups can be administratively organized under a single nurse manager or, more often in larger organizations, under central nursing administration.

Operating Room Nursing

The first responsibility of perioperative RNs or of teams of RNs and surgical technologists (STs) working in the OR suite is to prepare patients, ORs, and the supplies and equipment necessary for safe, effective, and efficient performance of surgery. Then, once an operation is under way, the task shifts to ensuring the continued safety of the patient and continued delivery of necessary supplies, equipment, and assistance to the surgeon and anesthesiologist. These responsibilities are the same whether the surgery is performed in a large or small hospital or in a freestanding surgical center.

Each intraoperative nursing team typically consists of a circulating nurse and a scrub nurse or technologist. The circulating nurse—an RN—is the nursing team leader who performs the perioperative nursing assessment of the patient and has overall responsibility for the smooth running of the case. The circulator documents the perioperative nursing process, is responsible for patient safety, and provides supplies and equipment as necessary. The job of the scrub person, a role increasingly filled by STs, is to organize and deliver to the surgeon in a timely manner the many different instruments and tools used during the course of the operation.

Historically, nursing training in 3-year diploma nursing programs included clinical experience in the OR. New graduates familiar with the setting and the challenges of working there often applied to work in the OR suite immediately after graduation. However, diploma programs have slowly been replaced with 2-year associate's and 4-year bachelor's degree programs. Most of these programs do not have an OR rotation, although nursing students occasionally come to the OR to observe operations performed on patients for whom they are caring elsewhere, and baccalaureate students may take an elective in OR nursing. As a result of this fundamental change in nursing

education, the OR is no longer recognized as a place where "real" nursing takes place and where attractive career opportunities exist for new graduates. Because the average age of OR nurses is 40–50 years, many facilities are recognizing a need to develop orientation and training programs for experienced nurses and new graduates who have had no previous OR experience to replace retiring baby boomers.

A complete orientation to OR nursing takes 9–12 months in a typical community hospital. In larger facilities that have more specialties and more complex cases and equipment, orientation may take even longer. The curriculum, composed of a didactic classroom program followed by precepted clinical experience in multiple specialty areas, is designed to produce an experienced OR nurse capable of caring for patients in a competent, cost-effective manner.

Continuing education (*in-service training*) for all nursing and technical staff should be the norm in all facilities. A typical curriculum includes such issues as new policies, new equipment, basic laser and electrical safety, and OR costs. Competency training in procedures and use of equipment should be ongoing. Many continuing education programs are available from the Association of periOperative Registered Nurses* (AORN) and from commercial vendors of OR equipment and supplies. Orientation and inservice are ideally coordinated—and often taught—by one RN who, in larger organizations, may have this as a sole responsibility. Other valuable teachers include experienced staff members and invited guests. Educational time should be set aside weekly or monthly when other clinical units, such as the departments of anesthesiology and of surgery, are also meeting.

Nursing staff models in the OR vary depending on the type of setting. Some staff finish a basic orientation and decide they wish to remain generalists. This means that they are assigned to a variety of cases and have a good grasp of the basic knowledge necessary to scrub or circulate in any room. Every nursing staff needs some individuals like these who are comfortable in all settings. The second type of staff member—either RN or ST—finishes orientation and may then work primarily in a particular

---

*Name changed from Association of Operating Room Nurses in April 1999.

specialty. After further specialty orientation, these staff members are assigned either to a particular group of services (e.g., ophthalmology, gynecology, and dentistry) or, in large institutions, to a particular OR in which the same types of cases are performed day after day (e.g., cardiac surgery, joint replacements, or spine surgery). These staff members are eventually recognized by other team members for their expertise in their chosen areas and act as specialty consultants.

All large OR suites need a mix of both generalist and specialist staff members to ensure efficient service of patients whose care requires highly technical skills and equipment. Some larger facilities may group specialty staff together in clusters to foster team building and networking. Most facilities schedule call teams or evening, night, and weekend shifts that require nursing and technical staff covering those periods to be competent in performing a large variety of operations, both emergency procedures and elective cases. Large health care organizations that perform highly specialized surgery, such as organ transplantation and open-heart surgery, often have special call teams for these surgical services.

RNs who have been employed in the OR suite for at least 2 years are qualified to take the Certified Operating Room Nursing (CNOR) examination given by the Certification Board Perioperative Nursing (CBPN). Certification is one method for demonstrating competency in OR nursing. Certified RNs must recertify every 5 years either by retesting or by accruing academic credits or continuing education hours. (Information on CBPN can be found on its Web site at <http://www.certboard.org>.)

STs can demonstrate their competence by passing an examination leading to recognition as a Certified Surgical Technologist: Level I, Level II (Advanced), or Level III (Specialist). Requirements can be found at <http://www.ast.org/cert/index.html>.

The size of the health care organization and hours of operation of the OR suite determine the number of nursing and technical staff needed and the number of appropriate shifts. Shifts lasting 8, 10, or 12 hours are routine in larger facilities to cover staff breaks, lunches, late-running elective cases, and emergencies. Depending on the benefits package of the organization, 2.2–2.5 FTEs are usually needed per OR for a routine 7:00 AM to 3:30 PM day. (See Figure 10-5 on page 146.)

Setting up an OR for a surgical procedure involves accurately identifying the surgeon performing the case and the anticipated procedure. For elective cases, this information is gathered by the scheduling office when the case is booked. For add-on and emergency cases, identifying information is transmitted directly from the surgeon or the surgeon's agent (surgical resident, nurse, or secretary) to the OR desk clerk, who passes it on to the nursing staff. The combination of surgeon and procedure information is then used to look up the appropriate preference card.

Surgeon-specific preference cards have three major sections: (1) nursing care plan, (2) instruments and supplies, and (3) special equipment. (Detailed discussion of preference cards is found beginning on page 115.) Before a procedure starts, the nursing team must ascertain that the correct preference card has been selected. Then they must ensure that all items on the list have, in fact, been delivered in satisfactory condition to the OR in which the procedure is to be performed. Before opening the sterile supplies and equipment, the nursing team checks the room to be sure that it has been properly cleaned and that all equipment is present and in good working order.

Finally, the nursing team sets out the sterile work surfaces, opens and arranges the sterile instruments, and, as a last, critical step, counts the sponges, needles, and instruments to be used during surgery. These items are counted again at the end of surgery to ensure that nothing has unintentionally been left in the surgical wound. Standard recommended practices promulgated by AORN guide the practice of these components of perioperative nursing care.

Once the OR is ready for surgery, the circulating nurse locates the patient and performs a preoperative nursing assessment. After a self-introduction, the RN (1) positively identifies the patient, preferably by both identification bracelet and the patient's self-identification; (2) confirms the operation to be performed and the body part and side involved; and (3) checks the written consent form to be sure that it is filled out completely and accurately according to the written policies of the hospital. (See the discussion regarding ensuring that surgery is performed on the correct side of the body in Consent Forms on page 159.) The assessment period is brief, requiring the nurse to collect pertinent data using critical thinking skills based on perioperative clinical experience and a thorough understanding of the nursing process. The preoperative assessment allows the nurse to develop a care plan with a focus on optimal clinical outcome for the patient.

Then the patient is taken to the OR, usually by the circulating nurse and the anesthesiologist, although sometimes by the anesthesiology team (attending anesthesiologist and nurse anesthetist or resident) or by the anesthesiologist and the surgeon. The role of the circulating nurse when the patient enters the OR is to ensure patient safety and help the patient adapt to the environment by providing teaching, emotional support, and comfort measures (e.g., a warm blanket). As the anesthesiologist performs the anesthetic induction, the circulating nurse assists as appropriate. After anesthesia has been induced, the team positions the patient, prepares the skin, and drapes the sterile field before beginning the operation.

Duties of the Circulating Nurse

Certain aspects of the patient's care in the OR are the responsibility of the circulating nurse. The RN shares responsibility with the surgeon and the anesthesiologist for safely positioning the patient for surgery. This is an important part of the operative procedure, because the position of the patient is sometimes a compromise between optimal exposure for the surgery and optimal position to reduce risk of limb ischemia, joint stress, skin injury, or nerve damage.

The circulating nurse is responsible for monitoring maintenance of aseptic technique throughout the procedure. The nurse ensures that proper scrubbing technique (hand and arm washing) is followed, that proper attire is worn, and that all actions are consistent with the OR's policy on sterile technique. The RN is responsible for ensuring that proper procedures are followed by personnel when putting on gown and gloves, when opening sterile packages, and when performing all other procedures involving sterile instruments and supplies. The circulating nurse controls access to the OR during the case, paying particular attention to reducing unnecessary traffic. The RN calls attention to breaks in sterile technique. When the sterile field becomes contaminated, as occasionally happens, the operative team is responsible for ensuring that proper reprepping, redraping, or resterilization is performed.

The circulating nurse also ensures adherence to appropriate safety precautions during surgery (e.g., ensuring that personnel are wearing appropriate protective skin and eye covering when ultraviolet lights or lasers are being used) and is responsible for correctly labeling specimens collected during cases, such as tissue or cultures taken from the surgical field. The RN prepares the requisition forms that accompany specimens to the laboratory. The anesthesiologist and the circulating nurse share responsibility for correctly identifying and recording any blood or blood products administered during the course of surgery.

The circulating nurse identifies damaged or malfunctioning instruments or equipment and sends them for repair. RNs with experience and expert knowledge in particular specialties are best able to suggest modifications to surgeons' preference lists, noting instruments and supplies that are needed but not on the preference list or suggesting removal of infrequently used items.

Finally, documentation is a major responsibility of the circulating nurse, who maintains complete records of the case. Included are the names of all persons present, the operation performed, and all pertinent times (e.g., time of entry and departure from the OR and time of tourniquet inflation and deflation). This documentation also serves as a nursing care plan. When prosthetic implants such as pacemakers, heart valves, and prosthetic joints are used, the RN enters the name and lot number of the implant into a log for future tracking according to federal law. (See Medical Device Tracking on page 155.) The composite record kept by the circulating nurse is often compiled into an "OR log," which is legally required in some jurisdictions.

Part of the documentation carried out by circulating nurses is used in preparing reports for the hospital's quality improvement program. The circulating nurse reports any untoward or potentially dangerous or improper activity that occurs during the case, such as accidental damage to supplies and equipment, breaks in sterile technique, and behavioral problems displayed by personnel or by the patient. Furthermore, the circulating nurse should report delays caused by unavailability of equipment or personnel. The RN is responsible for identifying and reporting, in writing, cases in which quality of care may be an issue. This includes cases involving excessive blood loss, the occurrence of adverse events, such as cardiac arrest, and other issues that must be addressed by the quality improvement committee.

Duties of the Scrub Nurse or Technologist

The scrub nurse or technologist is an integral part of the operating team who supplies the surgeon with the correct surgical instrument on a moment-to-moment basis. Masked, gowned, and gloved exactly like the surgeon, the scrub person keeps the instruments free of tissue debris and blood and maintains them in an orderly and accessible array on the instrument table. To perform the scrub task effectively, the scrub person must be familiar with the operative procedure being performed and with the instruments required. The role of scrub person is increasingly being filled by STs, who are not trained in nursing but are trained in the technical aspects of the surgical procedure.

Other Nursing Functions

Many pieces of equipment necessary for performing surgery must be set up and operated by nurses. Examples include video equipment for minimally invasive surgery, lasers, tourniquet boxes, pumps, and insufflation equipment. These devices are often complex, expensive, and easily damaged. Although nurses usually act as equipment managers, this job may be delegated to technicians working under the supervision of nurses.

Performance of surgery frequently involves using potentially dangerous tools or techniques. The circulating nurse has a duty to ensure that all personnel are appropriately protected from exposure to x-rays emitted during intraoperative radiograms. Similarly, the RN is responsible for ensuring that all personnel are wearing appropriate eye protection when lasers are in use, that smoke-capturing equipment is functioning when virus-laden smoke is being generated, and that the eyes and skin are protected from ultraviolet light in ORs equipped with ultraviolet germicidal lamps.

Several new opportunities for RNs have been developed that differ from the traditional roles of circulating and scrub nurses. One of these is the RN first assistant (RNFA), an RN who has completed an educational program that prepares RNs to assist surgeons during operations by helping to achieve hemostasis, to handle tissue, and to tie ligatures and sutures. After completing prescribed didactic and precepted clinical work, the RNFA is eligible to sit for a certifying examination (CRNFA) that is administered by the same organization that confers CNOR status, the CBPN. (See discussion of CBPN on page 92.)

Another advanced practice opportunity is the master's-prepared nurse practitioner (NP), who not only takes part in the preoperative assessment and teaching of patients, but may also assist in the OR and participate in postoperative care. NPs can improve continuity of care and assessment of the clinical outcome. They usually go through a privileging and credentialing process similar to that undertaken by members of the medical staff, because some of their responsibilities fall outside the purview of nursing.

RNs and STs are sometimes hired as surgeon's "private scrubs." Such persons are employees of the surgeon who assist during surgery as either the scrub person or the first assistant, depending on their training and the privileging and credentialing policies of the facility in which they work.

Two other areas of specialized nursing care in the perioperative period are ASU nursing and PACU nursing (see Ambulatory Surgery Unit Nursing and Postanesthesia Care Unit Nursing on page 95). ASU and PACU nurses, as members of the perioperative team, care for patients before and after surgical procedures. In hospitals, the roles of these two groups are often well defined and separate from each other. In freestanding surgical centers, however, the staff may be cross-trained and float from one area to another, depending on patient-care needs and the census.

As traditional OR procedures move to nontraditional settings (e.g., the cardiac catheterization laboratory [cath lab], the lithotripsy suite, and the radiology department), perioperative nurses are shifting to satellite locations to facilitate safe nursing care regardless of the setting. Nurses working in satellite locations may retain close ties with the OR suite even if they become part of the unit in which they work.

Ambulatory Surgery Unit Nursing

ASU nursing is a fast-paced process that accomplishes in 2–3 hours (preoperatively and postoperatively) what formerly took place during several days for inpatients. Before surgery, ASU RNs get patients dressed in hospital gowns and perform a nursing assessment by taking a nursing history and making a risk assessment for such factors as drug and latex allergies and skin breakdown. This information is documented, and the patient's chart is reviewed for completeness (e.g., to verify the presence of an appropriate surgical consent form) before the patient is sent to the OR. Sometimes procedures such as intravenous line insertion, medication administration, and skin preparation are performed by ASU nurses. This process takes 30–60 minutes.

Postoperatively, ASU nurses provide second-stage recovery care. Beyond monitoring recovery from anesthesia, ASU RNs assess and treat pain, nausea and vomiting, and other side effects of the surgery and anesthesia. This second-stage recovery may take as little as 30 minutes or as long as several hours, depending on the surgical procedure performed, the anesthetic administered, and the patient's response to them. The ASU nurse provides the patient and a family member or other accompanying adult with discharge instructions, including information on activity, diet, pain control, and signs and symptoms of infection. The ASU nurse usually ensures that the patient has a follow-up appointment with the surgeon and knows how to contact the surgeon if problems occur.

Finally, an important function of ASU nurses is to call each patient on the first postoperative day to see how recovery is progressing and to answer questions. Problems uncovered during telephone follow-ups, if inappropriate for the RN to handle, are referred to others, such as the surgeon, the anesthesiologist, or a patient-services representative.

Postanesthesia Care Unit Nursing

The PACU is staffed with RNs and licensed practical nurses (LPNs) in a staff mix based on the severity of illness of the patients and the recommendations of the American Society of Post Anesthesia Nurses. The time a patient spends in this first stage of the recovery process depends on the anesthetic used and the surgical operation performed. Major surgery involving invasive monitoring sometimes requires ICU-type care, whereas simple surgical procedures under spinal anesthesia require simple monitoring while the spinal anesthetic wears off. Many PACUs use objective discharge criteria approved by the medical staff. Teaching facilities may use the PACU for teaching anesthesia residents, who may discharge patients according to nursing assessment and subjective assessment of patient readiness.

In freestanding surgical centers, both first-stage (*recovery room*) and second-stage (*recovery lounge*) postoperative care may be performed by the same RNs, who float between the two areas as patient census demands.

Operating Room Nursing Management

Nursing practice in the OR should be under the direction of an experienced RN—the nurse manager—who should have a history of demonstrated excellence in OR nursing. The nurse manager usually holds a bachelor's degree in nursing, and in large hospitals or university settings often has a master's degree in business administration or a related field. This individual should also be certified in OR nursing (CNOR) and in nursing administration. To qualify for the certified nursing administrator (CNA) examination, the candidate must hold a bachelor's degree and have experience as a nurse manager. To take the CNA advanced (CNAA) examination, the nurse must hold a master's degree and must be in a leadership position at the executive level.

In larger institutions, the nurse manager may share OR management responsibilities with a surgeon or an anesthesiologist. The nurse manager may report to an OR director, who may be a nurse, a physician, or an administrator. In most small and medium-sized hospitals, the nurse manager serves as the OR director and may report either directly or through the chief of nursing to an administrator such as the COO. Regardless of the reporting relationships, it is imperative that the nurse manager be part of the overall facility nursing team to ensure that the OR leadership has input into critical institutional decisions and is aware of activities of the various other nursing units.

The OR nurse manager is responsible for developing and implementing high standards of patient care. Recruitment and retention of strong staff nurses and technical personnel are critical for maintaining the highest standards of patient care. The manager sets a tone of teamwork, ensuring that quality patient care is the primary focus of the team (Case Study 7-1).

OTHER CLINICAL SERVICES

Pathology

The pathology department's two main sections, anatomic pathology and clinical pathology, are essential to the functioning of many ORs. Anatomic pathology is concerned with the identification of tissue type and the diagnosis of disease on the basis of microscopical examination of tissue excised during surgery. This service is critical during cancer surgery, because it is often difficult or impossible for surgeons to distinguish between normal tissue, which is to remain, and tumor, which is to be removed. The solution to this problem is to send specimens from the margins of the excised tissue to the pathologist for rapid identification. The speci-

men is typically flash frozen, sectioned with a microtome, stained, and examined under a microscope. If the margins are free of tumor, the surgeon is finished and closes, and if tumor is present at the margins, further excision is performed if possible. In institutions where a substantial amount of cancer surgery is performed, a satellite pathology laboratory that is equipped to perform frozen-section evaluations is usually located within the OR suite.

The presence of a satellite anatomic pathology laboratory within the OR suite dramatically reduces frozen-section turnaround time, mainly by reducing the number of handoffs a specimen must undergo. This process simplification can, in turn, sometimes substantially shorten surgical cases for which pathology support is necessary. It also allows the surgeon to review the tissue sample with the pathologist, improving diagnostic accuracy in complex cases.

Clinical pathology is the laboratory subdivision of pathology. Laboratory evaluation of blood or other specimens offers valuable help in managing complex cases in many situations in the OR. Large OR suites commonly house a small branch of the main pathology laboratory. Such satellite laborato-

---

CASE STUDY 7-1. Physician Discipline at Community Medical Center

The OR nurse manager of CMC is meeting with the president of the medical staff and the chief of surgery regarding the behavior of one of CMC's urologists. The surgeon, a past president of the medical staff, admits large numbers of patients to the hospital and always has a busy OR schedule. Two of the surgeon's neighbors are on CMC's board of directors. The nurse manager has asked for this meeting because one of her staff nurses, who insisted on anonymity, has reported that she smelled alcohol on the surgeon's breath while he was performing emergency surgery the previous Sunday. The staff nurse stated that the surgeon cursed her when she dropped an instrument during that case.

The nurse manager reminds the chief of surgery and the president of the medical staff that this is not the first time this surgeon has been reported to be abusive. Almost all the nursing staff dislike working with him. His behavior has recently seemed to have worsened, and rumor has it that several other nurses have smelled alcohol on his breath when he arrived in the OR in the morning. The nurse manager has checked the OR log for the past 6 months and found that five of the surgeon's patients have returned to the OR for postoperative bleeding. She recommends that the chief of surgery immediately suspend the surgeon's privileges. Is this a reasonable request? How could the nurse manager have prepared a better case? What should the chief of surgery and the president of the medical staff do now?

ries usually perform relatively few types of tests. Those more commonly performed include measurement of blood gases, electrolytes, and hemoglobin concentration. Some OR laboratories also measure indices of blood coagulation.

It was once possible for the OR laboratory to be supervised by an anesthesiologist or surgeon with special knowledge and experience. Because statutory requirements for quality control have become more strict, however, a qualified pathologist should supervise all diagnostic laboratories. To comply with the federal government's Clinical Laboratory Improvement Amendments (CLIA) of 1988, all health care laboratories must be accredited or certified through an approved proficiency testing program.

Whether a satellite OR laboratory will be cost-effective depends on several factors: the response time for laboratory tests within the existing system (which is influenced by the distance between the OR suite and the main clinical laboratories), the cost of developing an OR laboratory, the estimated amount of OR time to be saved if an OR laboratory were available, and the proportion of cases in which rapid results may affect clinical outcome. Rapid return of certain blood test results can be literally lifesaving in major surgery on sick patients. Local factors, however, rather than general rules, should dominate decision making. If a satellite OR laboratory is already present or a need for one has been identified, the rules of its operation must be determined through consultation with surgeons, anesthesiologists, and pathologists. Decisions must be made regarding which tests will be offered, which hours the laboratory will be open, and how specimens will be transported to the satellite laboratory from the ORs.

Blood Bank

Approximately one-half of the blood transfused in U.S. hospitals is given at the time of surgery. Therefore, close links between the blood bank and the OR are necessary.

A system for identifying patients likely to need blood during surgery must be in place so that appropriate preoperative steps may be taken, such as offering patients the opportunity, when appropriate, to donate one or more units of their own blood so that intraoperative losses may be replaced with low-risk autologous blood. This involves collecting several units of the patient's blood over several weeks before the anticipated surgery and encouraging the patient to take iron supplements to assist in restoring red blood cells.

Two systems are commonly used to determine the potential need for blood during scheduled operations. The simplest is to require the surgeon to submit a request, either through preoperative orders or when scheduling the surgery, for the blood bank to allocate appropriate units of blood through typing and cross-matching. The other method is for the blood bank to maintain a list of the usual number of units required for each type of surgery performed (sometimes called the *maximum surgical blood ordering system*) and to check each day's surgery schedule to ensure availability of the required units, if any, for each patient on the OR schedule. Each of these systems has its proponents. The surgeon is in the best position to know the full extent of the proposed surgery and the medical status of the specific patient, including such relevant information as the patient's other medical problems (e.g., anemia or lung disease) or other factors that might affect the need for transfusion. On the other hand, proponents of the maximum surgical blood ordering system have been able to demonstrate dramatic reduction in the number of banked blood units checked for compatibility without any apparent negative clinical effects.

Many state regulations require that all blood units be checked and signed by two persons before the blood is administered, one of whom must be a licensed independent practitioner. Close communication between the OR and the blood bank at the time of surgery is sometimes crucial. Anticipation of an unusually high demand for blood or blood products, such as platelets, fresh-frozen plasma, or cryoprecipitate, should immediately be communicated to the blood bank.

The OR suite should have a reliable system to ensure that when several units of blood are issued to a patient simultaneously, the oldest ones are used first. Additionally, a system should be in place to ensure that unused blood is returned to the blood bank immediately after surgery.

Finally, managers of large OR suites must decide, in consultation with representatives of the blood bank and the anesthesiology service, whether establishing a branch of the blood bank within the OR suite, similar to a satellite pathology laboratory, is worthwhile. The reasons closely parallel those for satellite pathology laboratories—rapid response, reduction in time wasted in the OR, and improvement in clinical service. A satellite blood bank requires the same attention to detail as the main blood bank. One option is to cross-train OR laboratory technicians to perform the functions of blood bank technicians.

Radiology

Many types of surgery, but particularly orthopedic and vascular operations, depend on intraoperative x-ray imaging for satisfactory results. Two systems for imaging in the OR suite are commonly used. Conventional film-based x-rays are suitable for limited functions. When the x-ray imaging must be rapidly repetitive or continuous (e.g., in correctly siting bone-fixing screws or assessing patency of vascular grafts), film technology is too slow. In these cases, an x-ray fluoroscopy system is used, which has an x-ray generator on one end of a large, C-shaped arm and an image-intensifying x-ray camera on the other end (hence the usual name for this device: the *C-arm*). Conventional, portable x-ray equipment and the C-arm are operated by licensed technicians supervised and trained by the radiology department. OR managers, in coordination with representatives of the radiology department and central administration of the health care organization, should determine the amount of equipment and technician support the OR needs. Additionally, an OR suite that performs a lot of imaging needs its own satellite x-ray film processing laboratory, unless the distance between the OR suite and the department of radiology is short.

Freestanding surgical centers, unless large, are unlikely to be able to justify the high costs of standard C-arm technology or of a full-time radiology technician. However, less powerful and smaller C-arms have become available for fluoroscoping hands, knees, or feet. The amount of radiation generated does not require monitoring of radiation exposure or the services of a radiology technician. Surgeons operate the unit with a foot pedal and can obtain permanent pictures for documentation. Freestanding surgical centers should have the capability of taking an occasional radiograph to search for lost surgical needles.

Out-of-Operating Room Procedures

Many large and medium-sized hospitals have experienced a rapid increase in the number of invasive procedures performed in settings other than the ORs (e.g., tracheostomy, wound exploration, and insertion of gastric tubes). General anesthesia or deep sedation may be required for some of these, as well as for some noninvasive procedures such as MRI or CT in children and some adults. Patients undergoing prolonged or painful procedures in cath labs or in burn units also may benefit from general anesthesia or deep sedation. Additionally, some surgical procedures formerly limited to the OR suite are now performed at the bedside in the ICU, in the ED, or in other critical care areas. The reason for not bringing critically ill patients to the OR is that transporting such patients through the hospital is often more risky than performing surgery outside the OR.

These non-OR procedures usually require the same support they would if performed in the OR suite—anesthesia and nursing personnel, supplies, and equipment. Delivering all the required pieces to an outside location requires a substantial amount of time and effort. As the size of the non-OR business increases, such cases should be integrated into the management scheme of the OR suite. In larger health care facilities, this includes scheduling, supply and equipment lists, nurses, technicians, and all other OR support functions.

OTHER PROFESSIONAL RELATIONSHIPS

Emergency Department

A busy ED, especially in a level 1 trauma center, can place significant strains on the ORs. The problem for the OR is to ensure capability of supplying surgical support—not only an available OR, but also a full complement of personnel, instruments, and supplies—on short notice. The difficulty is to determine the best way of doing this. Some hospitals keep a "trauma OR" empty and staffed at all times. However, this is extraordinarily expensive and probably not necessary. A careful analysis of the data from a university hospital with 21 ORs revealed that all 21 rooms are occupied at once during the 8 daytime hours less than 1% of the time. The ORs are never all occupied during evening and night hours. And even when all are running, the median delay until the first open room is only 10 minutes. Therefore, having an OR and appropriate nursing and anesthesia personnel readily available for emergency cases that require immediate surgery is rarely a problem for a facility having a large number of ORs. Smaller health care organizations that have fewer trauma cases and less seriously ill patients are less likely to need to perform immediate surgery.

Although delaying scheduled cases to accommodate trauma cases or other such emergencies is disruptive, the disruption is usually relatively brief. The most significant operational problem for the OR suite is to obtain accurate information from the physicians in the ED regarding the nature and urgency of the case. A clear line of communication should be open between the ED and the OR suite. The worst possible scenario occurs when a bleeding ED patient appears at the OR main door, accompanied by excited physicians and nurses, with little or no advance warning. To avoid this scenario, the hospital must have a trauma committee (required in level 1 trauma centers), with representation from OR management, to set policies specifying who has responsibility for notifying the OR suite and who in the OR suite has authority to accept the information. Many hospitals have set up a special dedicated telephone line between the ED and the OR suite. The same communication channel may be used by ED staff to request support from the OR suite for supplies, equipment, or specially trained personnel.

Cardiac Catheterization Laboratory

Issues involving the cardiac cath lab are similar to those involving the ED. The cath lab will, from time to time, need immediate surgical intervention for some of its patients—usually coronary artery bypass, but sometimes repair of a large blood vessel injured during catheterization. The system by which this requirement is met should be established well in advance of need. Clear expectations of both catheterization and OR personnel must be established. Because the cath lab, unlike the ED, is able to control the scheduling of many of its patients, coordination between the OR schedule and the cath lab schedule can markedly reduce both the risk of disruption of the OR schedule and potentially dangerous delays before rescue surgery.

Intensive Care Unit

OR personnel must appropriately communicate the OR's needs to the ICU, rather than vice versa (as with the ED and the cath lab). OR personnel must formally notify the ICU of patients scheduled for surgery who will require ICU care postoperatively and of patients who unexpectedly require postoperative transfer to the ICU. Standard protocols for these notifications should be established. Scheduled admissions are often published on the OR schedule, and unscheduled admissions are usually arranged by telephone consultation between the surgeon or the anesthesiologist and the ICU admitting physician.

In hospitals with insufficient ICU capacity, decisions about whether to proceed with elective surgery in patients requiring postoperative ICU care must be made each morning on the basis of available ICU space and predicted surgical requirements. Again, representatives of the ICU, the OR suite, and the surgical services should generate clearly understood rules that specify who is to make decisions and how decisions are to be communicated. The system must have some flexibility, because estimates occasionally are wrong. That flexibility is usually provided by the PACU. Use of the PACU as ICU overflow space entails its own problems, particularly coverage by physicians and nurses. These issues must also be addressed in clear policies established by managers of the OR suite and the ICU.

Obstetric Suite

In most hospitals, the obstetric suite is independent from the OR suite, because its main focus is on labor and delivery. This situation exists despite the fact that many procedures, supplies, equipment, and personnel are common to the two areas, as are most of the protocols regarding such issues as sterile procedure and operative consent. Because of the similarities and the fact that the obstetric suite is usually much smaller than the OR suite, the obstetric suite often relies on the main OR for backup in many areas, including personnel and supplies. To ensure a harmonious relationship, managers of the two areas should develop good communication and should establish written policies regarding the sharing of common resources.

Other Issues in Common

Many different matters (e.g., choice of monitors and transducers; choice of drugs for certain conditions; concentration, route, and method for administering vasoactive drugs; and type of intravenous access) require standardization among the OR, the ED, and the ICU. Otherwise, all conflicting items are discarded each time a patient moves from one unit to another, a practice that is expensive in wasted time, supplies, drugs, and processed equipment. Additionally, the hospital should establish a standard protocol governing the transportation of patients between units that covers matters such as who is responsible, what monitoring is required, who must accompany the patient, and who must receive the patient. Although interdepartmental standardization is not the OR manager's direct responsibility, the OR manager should be a part of the decision-making process. Lack of standardization among acute-care hospital units can have a negative affect on the smooth functioning of the ORs and can have an adverse impact on the quality of patient care.

FURTHER READING

Atkinson LJ, Fortunato NH. Berry and Kohn's Operating Room Technique (8th ed). St. Louis: Mosby–Year Book, 1996.

Comprehensive Accreditation Manual for Hospitals: The Official Handbook. Oakbrook Terrace, IL: Joint Commission on Accreditation of Healthcare Organizations, 1998.

Fairchild SS. Perioperative Nursing: Principles and Practice (2nd ed). Philadelphia: Lippincott–Raven, 1996.

Groah LK, Nicolette LH. Perioperative Nursing (3rd ed). Stamford, CT: Appleton & Lange, 1995.

Gruendemann BJ, Fernsebner B. Comprehensive Perioperative Nursing. Sudbury, MA: Jones & Bartlett, 1995.

Manual for Anesthesia Department Organization and Management. Park Ridge, IL: American Society of Anesthesiologists, 1998.

Meeker MH, Rothrock JC. Alexander's Care of the Patient in Surgery (10th ed). St. Louis: Mosby–Year Book, 1995.

Rothrock JC. Perioperative Nursing Care Planning (2nd ed). St. Louis: Mosby–Year Book, 1996.

Standards, Recommended Practices, and Guidelines. Denver: Association of Operating Room Nurses, 1999.

Chapter 8

Operations Management:
The Operating Room Schedule

A pessimist sees the difficulty in every opportunity; an optimist sees the opportunity in every difficulty.

—*Sir Winston Churchill (1874–1965)*

An efficient OR suite requires a substantial commitment of managerial effort to daily operational problems. Many long-term management decisions can be made and strategic plans developed in relative serenity. However, long-term decisions and plans succeed or fail mainly on the strength of the operational skills of the people making the OR suite actually work. A steady stream of critical decisions must be made, and compromises must be reached. That these decisions may occasionally have life-or-death implications intensifies the problem. Because ORs are not industrial production lines, uncertainty and even apparent chaos are facts of daily existence. Successful OR managers try to have systems in place that bring as much consistency as possible to crucial daily decisions that must be made in an environment that is intrinsically less orderly than desirable.

Daily management of the OR suite consists largely of controlling the flow of people—patients and staff—into and around the suite. The OR schedule sets the stage for the daily flow. Most of the fundamental trade-offs between convenience and efficiency for the different groups using the OR suite and the potential profitability of the enterprise are established through the rules that govern production of the schedule. Once the day starts, however, deviations from this schedule are frequent and expected. Emergency cases must be accommodated, cases may be longer or (rarely) shorter than scheduled, patients may be late or fail to arrive at all, and personnel may call in sick

or become ill during the course of the day. OR managers must ensure that decisions made as a consequence of unpredictable or unexpected events are perceived by the user groups (i.e., patients, surgeons, anesthesiologists, nurses) as fair and equitable while at the same time conserving institutional resources.

SCHEDULING CONSIDERATIONS

A busy, efficient OR suite normally accommodates 800–1,000 cases per OR per year, depending on case mix, case duration, and other factors. Generally, approximately 85% of these cases are elective (scheduled 2 or more days before the day of surgery), and the remainder are emergencies or urgent cases. An *emergency* is defined as a case in which the patient is in danger of loss of life or limb if the surgery is not performed within some specified time. An example is an open fracture, which needs surgical attention within 6 hours of the injury for optimal outcome. An *urgent case* is one that requires attention within roughly 24 hours, whether for improved medical outcome or medical cost savings. (A case delayed because of unavailability of OR time is more costly for the hospital, because it increases length of hospital stay.) A cholecystectomy for common duct stones performed on a patient admitted to the hospital for evaluation of abdominal pain is an example of an urgent case. Although not a true emergency, the patient's medical condition may slowly deteriorate until the operation is performed, and each day of hospitalization is costly.

The task of the OR scheduling system, whether electronic or manual, is to process elective cases into a smooth lineup that can be taken care of with minimal waste of time and effort. The OR scheduling system must attempt to achieve a satisfactory balance between several competing goals. It must meet the needs of surgeons for easy access to the OR at suitable times. Most surgeons also want to be able to conduct cases in succession rather than scattered at different times on different days; for a surgeon whose practice consists primarily of relatively short procedures, being able to schedule cases to follow each other is critical for efficient use of time. Moreover, from the institution's standpoint, allotting a block of OR time to one surgeon performing a series of operations is well known to reduce delays and minimize between-case turnover times. However, the scheduling system must also serve the institution's need to conserve resources, both people and space. This means that the scheduling system should be designed to fit as many cases as possible into the available space on busy days and to conserve resources when the ORs are less busy.

Several factors control whether surgeons perceive scheduling surgical operations to be easy or difficult. The most important factor is the number of ORs relative to the number of cases. An OR suite in which patients occupy ORs one-half of the time (50% occupancy*) almost always has OR time available, even on short notice. However, 50% use of available nursing and anesthesia personnel is not financially feasible in most hospitals. On the other hand, in hospitals that have higher rates of OR utilization, central administrators are not likely to be receptive to increasing the number of staffed ORs simply to make scheduling more convenient for surgeons, because convenience will cost the hospital money.

Further problems arise when a substantial proportion of patients belong to MCOs, because an MCO may have a contract with the hospital to perform some or all of the surgery needed by members of the plan. Because the primary goal of such a

contract is financial, most MCO administrators recognize that cost-effective OR management requires an efficient, tightly packed system that has relatively little flexibility. Although not explicitly stated, some MCO managers may even wish to use OR availability as a queue-forming or rationing system. At the same time, the hospital's largest group of patients is likely to be insured by some form of fee-for-service payment system, which inherently has weaker incentives for efficiency. Fee-for-service patients and their doctors generally want convenience and amenities and may be put off by the requirements of high-efficiency scheduling.

Ease of scheduling is facilitated when the scheduling office is available to book cases at appropriate hours. The office should be open to accept cases during the hours when the surgeons' offices are open. This means that closing at the end of the elective surgery day, often around 3:30 PM, is almost certainly unsatisfactory. The scheduling clerks should work the same hours as the surgeons' secretaries, because for a surgeon's office to call the OR at 4:30 PM to schedule a case only to find the scheduling office closed for the day is not good customer service.

A well-run scheduling office should have one-call scheduling, so that the surgeon's office secretary need not call the OR, the same-day surgery unit (SDSU), and the hospital admissions office to schedule a single operation. Similarly, patient-identifying information (demographics), such as name, address, insurance coverage, the patient's diagnosis, and the planned operation, should be requested only once.

The scheduling office is the OR's interface with the world and an important point of contact between the OR and its most immediate customers, the surgeons. For the surgeons' secretaries who book operations, the scheduling office may be the only point of contact. Therefore, it is critically important for the scheduling office to run smoothly and efficiently and for the scheduling clerks to be courteous, knowledgeable, and helpful.

ALLOCATION OF OPERATING ROOM TIME

A small OR suite may offer all its ORs on a first-come first-served basis. Such a system can work well, particularly when no single surgeon has a large, predictable case load. However, most OR

*See Appendix 1 for a standard set of definitions, specifically sections 3.7, Productivity Index, and 3.8, Raw Utilitzation, on page 196.

managers find that a system allocating repeating blocks of reserved time to a particular surgeon or surgical group works far better for the surgeons and the hospital. Allocation of blocks can be contentious or cooperative, depending on the rules used for making the block assignments and the perceived willingness of the OR manager to accommodate extra cases. Because a well-designed block allocation system generates benefits for the surgeons and the hospital, such a system is usually well received.

In a block scheduling system, one or more OR time slots are generally reserved for a particular surgeon, surgical group, or surgical service. One block is usually defined as a day's lineup of cases, approximately 8 hours, although some block time schemes allocate half-day blocks. At some academic medical centers, a set of blocks is allocated to each surgical service, and the service chief distributes the block times among the various surgeons on that service.

Many OR scheduling systems relate each block to a specific OR (Table 8-1). This is not necessary, however, because ensuring that the number of blocks allocated does not exceed the number of rooms available is all that is required.

In most OR suites that use block allocation, a cutoff time before the day of surgery specifies when unfilled OR blocks are released for use on a first-come, first-served basis by surgeons other than the assigned blockholders. The block release should be long enough before the day of surgery to provide sufficient time for the scheduling office to try to find another user for the OR time. Block release is commonly 3–5 working days before the day of surgery. If the block release time is 24 or fewer hours before surgery, the OR time usually goes unused except for emergency or urgent cases. A sophisticated scheduling system maintains a waiting list so that when the release time comes, surgeons on the waiting list can be offered the released block time.

The OR manager must decide in advance how to handle the problem of surgeons who repeatedly overbook their block time (i.e., schedule more surgery than will fit into the allocated time). The OR manager may decide to assign estimated case durations based on historical information for each surgeon, if such information exists and is reliable. Before implementing such a system, the predictions generated by it should be shown to provide significant improvements in booking accuracy. Such a

method should be used only if it is important to the smooth functioning of the OR suite, because it will almost surely be perceived as an inconvenience to any surgeon who purposely overbooked in the first place. A customer-friendly OR suite offers longer elective hours to surgeons who consistently overbook their block times.

Agreement on the rules governing the block allocation system should be secured from the surgeons at the outset. Increases or decreases in block time for a particular surgeon or group should be based on demonstrated use. Block time is commonly increased for surgical groups that demonstrate more than 80–85% utilization and decreased when utilization is less than 70–75%. Use of block time should be reported to the user (individual surgeon or service head, as appropriate) at regular intervals. Because losing or gaining block time may force the affected service to modify many other activities, such as office hours or teaching rounds, block reallocations should occur infrequently. Unless use of a block changes abruptly, as would occur with the retirement of a surgeon, block time allocations should probably be adjusted no more frequently than yearly.

Several potential problems are not addressed by a block allocation system. First, some surgical services have a relatively greater number of urgent cases than others. Cardiac surgery, for example, is frequently performed during the same hospital admission as the diagnostic workup demonstrating its necessity. Therefore, releasing the cardiac service block to other services may result in extended hospital stays while cardiac patients await OR time. Two remedies are available: (1) the service using the cardiac block may have to accept the risk of being displaced by a late-arriving cardiac case or (2) the cardiac block may be assigned a later release time or may retain the block until the day of surgery. In an optimally flexible system, OR time can be provided for all urgent cases within 24 hours of the request.

A second problem in the block system is that it does not easily accommodate emergencies, which are particularly common in trauma centers. In some medical centers, an OR block is reserved for the trauma service. In others, the surgeons generally agree that a trauma case will be offered the first available OR. Even in a busy OR suite, only on extraordinarily rare occasions are all of the available ORs occupied at the same time, except perhaps at the start of the OR day. A facility's ability to han-

Table 8-1. Block Allocation of Operating Room Time at University Medical Center*

OR No.	Monday	Tuesday	Wednesday	Thursday	Friday
1	Plastic	Plastic (Dr. 1)	Plastic (Dr. 2)	Plastic (Dr. 3)	Plastic (Dr. 1)
2	General (G1)	General (G1)	General (G1)	General (G1)	General (G1)
3	Neurosurgery (Dr. 1)	Open	Neurosurgery (Dr. 2)	Neurosurgery (Dr. 1)	Neurosurgery (Dr. 3)
4	Urology	Urology	Thoracic (Dr. 1)	Urology	Urology
5	General	General (G2)	Orthopedics (Dr. 1)	Open	Thoracic (Dr. 2)
6	Plastic	Orthopedics (Dr. 2)	Neurosurgery (Dr. 3)	Neurosurgery (Dr. 2)	Neurosurgery (Dr. 1)
7	Peripheral vascular	Peripheral vascular	Peripheral vascular	Peripheral vascular	Peripheral vascular
8	Orthopedics (Dr. 3)	Orthopedics (Dr. 4)	Orthopedics (Dr. 5)	Orthopedics (Dr. 4)	Orthopedics (Dr. 6)
9	Orthopedics (Dr. 7)	Orthopedics (Dr. 8)	Orthopedics (Dr. 6)	Orthopedics (Dr. 3)	Orthopedics (Dr. 9)
10	Orthopedics (Dr. 1)	Orthopedics (Dr. 10)	Orthopedics (Dr. 11)	Orthopedics (Dr. 12)	Orthopedics (Dr. 11)
11	Orthopedics (Dr. 13)	Orthopedics (Dr. 14)	Orthopedics (Dr. 15)	Orthopedics (Dr. 8)	Orthopedics (Dr. 16)
12	Orthopedics (Dr. 14)	Open	Open	General	Orthopedics (Dr. 17)
13	General (G2)	General	Open	Orthopedics (Dr. 18)	Peripheral vascular
14	ENT (Dr. 1)	ENT (Dr. 2)	ENT (Dr. 2)	ENT (Dr. 3)	ENT (Dr. 4)
15	Cardiac	Thoracic (Dr. 3)	Cardiac	General (G2)	Open
16	Cardiac	Cardiac	Cardiac	Cardiac	Cardiac
17	Cardiac	Cardiac	Cardiac	Cardiac	Cardiac
18	Gynecology (Dr. 1)	Dental	Oral surgery	Urology	General
19	Gynecology (G1)	Gynecology (G2)	Gynecology (G1)	Gynecology (G2)	Gynecology (G3)
20	Gynecology (G2)	Gynecology (G4)	Gynecology (G3)	Gynecology (G4)	Gynecology (G4)
21	Open	Pediatric (Dr. 1)	Ophthalmology	Ophthalmology	Pediatric (Dr. 2)

ENT = ear, nose, and throat (otorhinolaryngology).

*Some allocations are generically made to surgical services; others are made to individual surgeons or to groups within surgical services (see General and Gynecology). Some blocks are designated *open* and are not service specific. These blocks are generally available on a first-come, first-served basis. Numbers after "G" and "Dr." indicate different groups and doctors.

dle emergencies is partly determined by the overall utilization of the ORs. An OR suite that has a high rate of occupancy cannot easily absorb the sudden arrival of an emergency case without considerable disruption of the elective surgical schedule.

Finally, the block allocation system should not allocate 100% of the available OR time. If all the time is assigned, the system loses essential flexibility. Surgeons wishing to schedule cases on a day in which they have no block time will be routinely unable to do so before the block release date. The OR manager will have no ability to close an OR for a day to perform repairs or maintenance. A new surgeon will not be able to book cases except as add-ons. The decision as to how much of the overall OR schedule should be first-come, first-served is based largely on the OR's business plan. The block allocations in Table 8-1 show ORs designated as "open" that may be assigned as needed.

The block booking system, by its very nature, limits flexibility. For the system to work smoothly, with a low level of complaints by surgeons, it should be fine-tuned by the OR suite's day-to-day coordinators (often an anesthesiologist and a nurse). In particular, surgeons with high proportions of urgent cases—usually cardiac, vascular, general, and trauma surgeons—frequently rely on the OR manager or coordinators to fit the extra cases in.

Implementing a scheduling system for a large OR suite demands use of a computer database. A well-designed system is integrated with the OR suite's material and instrument processing systems. It tracks the scheduling of special ORs and limited equipment, such as lasers or operating microscopes, to ensure that the necessary resources are available. (See Operating Room Scheduling on page 148.)

AMBULATORY SURGERY SCHEDULING

When freestanding ASCs began to challenge hospital-based ORs in the early to mid-1980s, some hospitals established separate ambulatory OR suites. Ambulatory ORs are sometimes physically adjacent to existing inpatient ORs and are sometimes set in an entirely different location. The goal of a separate set of ambulatory ORs is to try to match the speed and customer-friendliness of freestanding ASCs.

Some hospitals have fully integrated the features of a freestanding ASC into the hospital's main OR suite by establishing a space, frequently called the *ambulatory surgery unit*, adjacent to the OR suite. The ASU is used for staging patients before their operations and for preparing patients for discharge after return from the PACU. The goal of such an ambulatory unit is to match the performance of the freestanding ASC while performing ambulatory cases in the same OR suite as inpatient cases. (See Special Considerations in the Design of Ambulatory Surgery Units and Freestanding Ambulatory Surgical Centers on page 187.)

An ASU as the front end of a hospital OR suite offers two advantages over a separate ambulatory surgery suite. First, it is far more convenient for surgeons (and for the OR suite as well) to be able to schedule all surgery in a single location, with a single set of rules, a single set of instruments, and a single set of procedures for preoperative visits. Ambulatory patients may be interspersed among inpatients as the surgeon prefers, except that scheduling ASU patients earlier in the day to limit the workday of the ASU staff as much as possible is preferable. A second major selling point for an ASU front end are the economies of scale and of timing associated with having surgical operations on all patients performed in one location, such as not having to wait for another surgeon to finish earlier cases, not having to assemble a large enough list of patients to fill either an ambulatory block or an inpatient block, and not having to duplicate inventories of in-suite supplies.

In addition to serving ambulatory patients, an expanded ASU is an ideal entry point for surgical patients who are to be admitted to the hospital on the day of surgery. Many MCOs mandate that preoperative preparation for most patients be carried out in an outpatient setting. Then, on the day of surgery, the path of patients admitted to the facility is the same as the path for ASU patients until departure from the PACU. The ASU patient returns to the ASU and then goes home for recovery, whereas the same-day patient is admitted to the hospital for recovery. Some health care organizations refer to such combined facilities as the *same-day surgery unit* or some other similarly descriptive phrase.

Addition of an SDSU front end to the hospital's ORs offers other advantages as well. As the practice of medicine changes, the SDSU may be an entry point to the hospital for a large number of other services, such as cardiac catheterization and other invasive diagnostic tests or procedures other than OR surgery that require general anesthesia (e.g., MRI scans in children). Such SDSU procedures can be scheduled through the OR's scheduling office, treating the extra locations like an OR or a procedure room. This maintains the cohesiveness and integrity of the OR suite complex, which extends from the entry point to the OR suite (the SDSU) through the exit point (the PACU or the SDSU).

OPERATING ROOM SCHEDULE

At some time during the last working day before the day of surgery, usually in the morning, the OR schedule is declared to be *closed*. At that point, the scheduling office ceases to accept cases, and additional cases must be placed on the standby list for the following day.

The OR manager or clinical coordinators (nurse manager and anesthesia coordinator) then review the proposed schedule for accuracy and for opportunities to improve it. For example, a surgeon may have cases scheduled sequentially in two different ORs or two cases scheduled in one OR but separated by another surgeon's case between them. Such problems can be resolved by moving cases from one OR to another and discussing proposed changes with the involved surgeons. Most surgeons attempt to comply with requests intended to make the OR run more smoothly, because they ultimately benefit. The schedule must also be checked to ensure that cases are scheduled in the most appropriate ORs. Many ORs are interchangeable, but some are more specialized. For example, cardiac ORs are usually larger, are located near a storage/supply room for bypass equipment, and often have expanded patient monitoring capabilities. Similarly, ophthalmology cases may be scheduled in designated ORs if ceiling-mounted microscopes are used.

When OR capacity is not fully scheduled for a given day, reducing the number of ORs used and assigning personnel to other activities are reasonable responses. If the cases scheduled in 14 ORs can be done in 12, the extra nursing time can be profitably used for many nonclinical nursing activities. In an OR suite that has flexible nursing staffing, the number of nurses scheduled to work on that day can be reduced.

Once the schedule is closed, the next task of the OR manager or clinical coordinators is to assign the nurses, technologists, and anesthesiologists to the various rooms. These assignments must be made by someone who is familiar with the skills of the people to whom the rooms are assigned. If the nursing service is organized into functional clusters, services, or specialties (see the discussion of nursing staff models beginning on page 91), the assignments should match the nurses and technologists to their primary services. Alternatively, nursing personnel may be assigned as generalists who assist in all types of cases or to areas in which their orientation is still incomplete or in which broadening or refreshing knowledge is worthwhile.

Assignments of anesthesiologists may also be based on the particular skills of individuals. In large medical centers, anesthesiologists may be divided into subspecialty groups concentrating on, for example, cardiac, neurosurgery, or pediatric cases. Additionally, in teaching hospitals the assignment of anesthesiologists is based on the educational needs of the residents. Not only must residents be assigned to cases that have appropriate educational value and for which the residents have adequate knowledge and skills, but their supervising attending anesthesiologists must be chosen to optimize the residents' learning experience. Furthermore, patients or surgeons occasionally request assignment of a specific anesthesiologist or nurse anesthetist to a particular case. In private practice settings in which all anesthesia personnel may be essentially interchangeable, anesthesiologists are commonly assigned to cases by a member of the anesthesia group. Alternatively, anesthesiologists may select their own rooms according to some rotation designed to distribute economically desirable cases in an equitable manner.

The interests of the OR suite and the anesthesiologists generally coincide. What is good for the OR—efficient scheduling, rapid turnover, low cancellation rate—is also good for the anesthesia group. However, one exception exists. Scheduling the ORs less densely than is possible may be to the long-term economic advantage of the OR suite (and of the health care organization). For example, the OR manager may choose to open an extra OR for a valued surgeon merely because it is less disruptive to the surgeon's office schedule, even though adding the case to another OR later in the day is also an option. This choice has the effect of forcing the anesthesia group to provide an extra anesthesiologist for that day. Just as surgeons must occasionally be willing to accommodate scheduling changes, anesthesiologists must sometimes be flexible to produce an optimal schedule. All parties benefit in the long run. However, the OR manager has the responsibility of convincing people that the short-term trade-offs are of long-term benefit to all.

After the room assignments have been optimized and nursing and anesthesia assignments made, the schedule for the following day is distributed to the various parts of the hospital in which personnel need the information. The distribution list is usually very long and includes the ASU/SDSU or ASC, PACU, admitting office, inpatient nursing units, laboratory medicine department, anatomic pathology department, radiology department, blood bank, anesthesia department, patient transportation department, central sterile supply (CSS), materials management, and anyone else whose services may be required on the day of surgery. Distribution by delivery of printed copies to each of the many users is gradually giving way to distribution through an intranet computer network. (See The Operating Room Schedule as an Electronic Report on page 149.)

Changes to the final schedule after it has been distributed must be carefully controlled because of the large number of interacting people who support the OR suite. Limiting the number of people who have the authority to modify the schedule to the smallest number possible, preferably one, is wise.

PREOPERATIVE EVALUATION

As a matter of good clinical practice, patients scheduled for surgery should have a complete medical history taken and at least a focused physical examination performed and documented. Laboratory studies, x-rays, and other diagnostic evaluations are carried out as appropriate. This preoperative workup has traditionally been the responsibility of the surgeon. For relatively healthy patients, this system may work well, whereas for patients with complicated medical problems, more extensive studies and consultations may be needed. If the preoperative evaluation is incomplete, or if certain studies have been requested but the results not yet placed in the chart, substantial and expensive delays on the day of surgery may result.

Many surgical facilities have preoperative evaluation clinics to ensure that the preoperative evaluation is complete, appropriate, and well documented. Such clinics are sometimes staffed by specially trained nurses, often supervised by an anesthesiologist. The clinic staff ensure that the paperwork is in order and that the results of ordered studies have been documented. Specially trained RNs record the patient's medical history, usually on a form designed to prompt important questions. An anesthesiologist performs a focused physical examination relating primarily to the cardiovascular and respiratory systems. The surgeon's examination, which is often limited to the part of the body destined for surgery, is usually performed outside the preoperative evaluation clinic, and the documentation is often faxed to the clinic for inclusion in the hospital/ASC record. If statutory or regulatory requirements demand that a general physical examination be performed on all preoperative patients, NPs or physician assistants are often employed to perform this function.

The preoperative clinic should have a well-documented set of guidelines for appropriate laboratory studies and a system for following up on any laboratory studies ordered. (Many health care organizations require certain screening studies before surgery, such as an electrocardiogram for men older than 40 years and for women older than 50 years.) Written protocols for managing common clinical problems, such as diabetes and hypertension, should be available, as should accepted rules for authorizing specialist consultations when indicated.

Clearly, not all patients need the services of the preoperative clinic. A clinic visit is generally advisable for patients who have long-standing or unresolved medical problems (e.g., hypertension, insulin-dependent diabetes, or recent electrocardiographic changes suggesting ischemia or infarction). Patient request is sufficient indication for scheduling a preoperative clinic visit. Deciding which patients should be scheduled for an appointment in the preoperative evaluation clinic can be difficult. Some health care organizations leave this decision to the surgeons, and others have a method of triage involving review of existing medical records and other criteria, such as the need for a preoperative electrocardiogram. In some health care organizations, particularly freestanding ASCs, patients' medical histories are obtained by telephone, and the nurse obtaining this information schedules patients for visits to the preoperative evaluation clinic when certain pre-established criteria are met.

Institutions that have preoperative clinics have discovered that the cost of running the clinic is more than offset by improvements in patient and surgeon satisfaction and by reductions in the rate of expensive case cancellations on the day of surgery.

DAY OF SURGERY

Patient Flow to the Operating Rooms

Moving inpatients through the OR suite presents some special challenges. The first problem is making sure that the patient is ready to go to the OR at the correct time. Although every patient-care unit in the hospital receives a copy of the OR schedule, misunderstandings and delays are common. It may be advisable for the OR secretary to call the inpatient unit as much as 2 hours in advance of the anticipated surgery start time and to send a transporter for the patient 1 hour before the patient is scheduled to enter the OR. (Appropriate times may vary widely, depending on the size of the hospital, proximity of the patient-care units to the OR suite, and adequacy of preoperative holding facilities in the OR suite.)

When an inpatient arrives at the preoperative holding unit (PHU), a nurse reviews the chart for completeness, including history and physical examination, required laboratory work (if any), consent, and other documents. The RN assigned to the PHU performs an initial patient assessment and reports any special needs of the patient to the circulating nurse. Before the patient enters the OR, the assigned anesthesiologist (who may not be the anesthesiologist who previously evaluated the patient) greets the patient, carries out a last-minute review of the chart, performs a brief physical examination, and answers any remaining questions. The final decision regarding anesthetic management is often made at this interview by the patient and the anesthesiologist. Informed consent for the anesthetic is obtained at this time, if it was not acquired as part of an evaluation in the preoperative clinic. (See Informed Consent on page 158.)

Intravenous infusions may be started by a nurse or technician before the patient's arrival in the OR suite or by a nurse or the anesthesiologist in the PHU. If ordered by the surgeon, a nurse or aide may clip or shave hair off the surgical site. The anesthesiologist may insert one or more invasive monitoring catheters (e.g., an arterial line, a central venous catheter, or both) or administer a regional anesthetic (e.g., axillary block or insertion of an epidural catheter) in the PHU. (Appropriate monitoring equipment—blood pressure, electrocardiogram, and pulse oximetry—should be available in the PHU when regional anesthetics are administered or invasive procedures are performed there.)

Inpatients coming from an ICU are frequently physiologically unstable and require minute-to-minute medical decision making. For such a patient to be parked in a busy PHU where the nurses have many patients to look after is undesirable. Moreover, family members may be in the holding area. Consequently, the ICU should be asked to send patients to the OR only after the anesthesiologist and circulating nurse in the patient's OR have given authorization. That way, the OR team can be ready to assume responsibility for the patient's care immediately on arrival in the OR suite. ICU patients are usually transported by ICU nurses rather than by regular transport personnel.

Most patients come to the OR suite from the ASU or SDSU and either go home postoperatively or are admitted as inpatients. When a patient arrives at the hospital on the day of surgery, many details must be attended to before the patient is ready for surgery. The chart is reviewed for completeness and any missing information is found. The patient disrobes and his or her clothing is safely stored. The patient's vital signs are determined and a nursing evaluation made of the patient's understanding of the planned procedure. If ordered or part of the preoperative protocol, an intravenous line is inserted and preoperative medicines administered. Performing these tasks when everything is in order takes approximately 30 minutes. Because patients are sometimes late in arriving, particularly during winter months in northern climates and in large cities with heavy traffic, and because the duration of operative procedures is often uncertain, most ASUs and ASCs request that patients arrive 2 hours before the start time of scheduled surgery. Patients who are scheduled for surgery late in the day are asked to be available by telephone throughout the day so they can be moved earlier on the schedule if a preceding case is canceled.

ASU and SDSU patients may come directly to the OR from the ambulatory unit, or they may be taken to the PHU in the OR suite as inpatients are. Which alternative is preferable depends on the distances and transport times involved. If the ASU or SDSU is relatively close to the ORs, patients need not be moved to the PHU first. On the other hand, some ASU and SDSU patients may require special procedures before surgery (e.g., insertion of special monitoring lines or administration of regional anesthesia). Time can often be saved between cases if these procedures are performed while the OR is being cleaned and prepared for the next case. The PHU is often better equipped and a more private place for these activities than the ASU or SDSU.

Patients meet and are identified by the circulating nurse in the ASU or SDSU or in the PHU. The circulating nurse assesses the patient and begins planning care, does a final check on the consent for the procedure, and confirms the proposed surgical site. (See the discussion of ensuring that the correct site of surgery is confirmed on page 159.) On arrival in the OR itself, the patient moves to the operating table with the assistance of the nursing and anesthesia team. After application of a safety strap and monitoring devices (blood pressure cuff, electrocardiogram pads, and pulse oximeter probe), the patient is anesthetized for surgery. Most OR suites have rules specifying where the patient's surgeon should be at the time of transport to the OR or at induction of anesthesia. These rules are intended to avoid a situation in which the patient is anesthetized but the surgeon is unavailable. Strict rules are usually observed in teaching hospitals because of Medicare reimbursement policies governing the supervision of resident physicians.

Patient Flow from the Operating Rooms

After surgery, patients may be transported to several different destinations. Most patients are taken to the PACU, where they recover from the residual effects of general or regional anesthesia under the care of specially trained PACU nurses. The PACU is similar in many ways to an ICU; patients' vital signs may be unstable, their tracheas may be intubated, and they may require mechanical ventilation. Patients in the PACU may also require continuous monitoring or medical interventions of various types (e.g., control of pain or treatment of high or low blood pressure). Most patients, though, need little more than a short period of recovery from anesthesia before they are ready to leave the PACU, either

for the ASU or ASC and home or for admission to one of the hospital's nursing units. (Recall that the ASC has its own freestanding ORs, while the ASU is the front-end ambulatory unit for a combined inpatient and ambulatory OR suite.) In the ASU or ASC, the patient goes through a second stage of recovery, lasting from 30 minutes to 2–3 hours, during which the patient becomes ready for the trip home. ASU and ASC nurses instruct patients and family members in basic postoperative management, often from a standing protocol prepared in consultation with the surgeon. Written instructions for home care are also provided.

The duration of a postoperative ASU or ASC stay depends largely on how well the patient's postoperative pain is controlled and whether nausea or vomiting is present. Some facilities and some surgeons have policies that arbitrarily prolong durations of postoperative stay in the ASU or ASC. For example, some surgeons want to see their patients before discharge, which usually means that discharge time depends on the duration of the surgeon's next operation rather than on readiness of the patient for discharge. Some facilities have discharge criteria such as the ability to urinate or to drink liquids without nausea, although neither may be necessary for safe discharge.

Some patients, usually those who have had major surgery such as cardiac or thoracic operations, may move directly from the OR to the ICU, because moving comatose patients through the hospital, often by elevator, is inherently difficult and potentially dangerous. Such patients require mobile monitoring equipment and are accompanied by teams of physicians and nurses. To make the move once is much safer than twice, and it is best if the team accompanying the patient during transfer is the same team that managed the patient during the operation. The OR team can then give its report on the course of surgery, complications, management plans, and other pertinent information directly to the ICU team.

Another group of patients may also bypass the PACU: patients ready to go directly from the OR to the ASU or ASC. This population includes patients who have had relatively minor regional anesthetics or those who have had monitored anesthesia care, which usually involves sedation that is deeper than the surgeon can safely manage alone but lighter than full general anesthesia. The advent of new anesthetic agents has added another group of patients to this list. The new agents, which are characterized by extremely short duration of action and rapid recovery, are given by continuous infusion. When the infusion stops, the patient quickly wakes up. Recovery is so rapid that the patient may satisfy PACU discharge criteria before leaving the OR. In this case, a PACU stay is a wasteful formality, and the patient can go directly from the OR to the ASU or ASC and then home. Omitting the PACU stay represents a relatively new style of patient management in most institutions and should be implemented through careful planning involving the leadership of the OR suite and the ASU or ASC.

Managing Patient Flow

As the surgical day progresses, many different people in various places must know the location and status of patients flowing through the OR suite. Given the complex interdependencies of personnel, material, and locations within the OR suite, communication becomes critical. In a small OR suite, the nursing coordinator may be able to determine the location of most patients merely by making rounds of the different areas where patients might be. This method is highly inefficient even in medium-sized OR suites with six or seven ORs. A formal system for communicating patient status to everyone who needs to know is necessary.

Several mechanisms have evolved for communicating the status of patients while they are in the OR suite. One simple method involves keeping a clipboard at the counter of the OR control desk with a copy of the day's schedule on which the progress of each patient is charted. Another is having a central control board, usually opposite the OR suite front desk, on which the day's cases and the status of each patient are listed (using erasable colored markers). Information on the board is maintained by clerical personnel at the front desk. Because the control board (or the clipboard) is in one location, the control desk clerks must individually telephone or page surgeons, anesthesiologists, nurses, and other personnel to inform them of case status. Other modes of communication include the use of alphanumeric pagers, centralized intercommunications systems (intercoms), and overhead pages. (See Design of Operating Room Communication Systems on page 188.)

The control board generally includes for each case, at a minimum, name of the patient; scheduled time of the case; OR number; operation to be performed; names of the surgical, anesthesia, and nursing personnel involved; and some indication of the status of the case. Minimum status information includes times for the arrival of the patient at the hospital (if ambulatory), arrival in the preoperative holding area, and entry to the OR. (The patient's listing on the control board is usually erased when the patient leaves the OR.) Circulating nurses keep the front desk clerks informed on the progress of cases in the ORs (e.g., when it is time to call for the surgical team, to send for the next patient scheduled in the room, or to call the housekeeping crew for cleanup at the end of cases). Front desk clerks then transmit these messages to others who need to know. The role of front desk clerks is critical to keeping the OR schedule moving.

Some hospitals and ASCs have moved from a handwritten control board to a computer monitor display of case status. Advantages of a computerized display are several. First, the information is more legible than when handwritten. Second, monitors can be scattered throughout the OR suite—in the ASU or SDSU, the PHU, the PACU, and the lounges where OR personnel congregate—so that the status of all cases is widely available. In fact, if the hospital has an intranet, the information can be maintained in real time in a database on a network computer, making it available to remote locations, such as surgeons' offices. Such a system must include security features to protect patient confidentiality. (See Data Confidentiality and Security on page 147.)

Expectations regarding the duty to keep each OR on track vary substantially from one institution to another. The same nursing and anesthesia team typically works in a given OR for an entire day. In some institutions, the circulating nurse pushes the surgeon and anesthesiologist to start the next case, and in others the anesthesiologist or the surgeon may be the prime mover. Different incentives motivate different personnel. Surgeons and anesthesiologists are usually reimbursed by the case (except in settings such as staff-model HMOs and academic medical centers) and thus have strong motivations to finish operations as rapidly as possible. On the other hand, salaried personnel may regard early completion of the OR's scheduled cases as an invitation to be assigned extra cases from the standby list. The OR manager's goal should be to motivate all personnel to get the work done expeditiously.

Some institutions have devised systems to keep incentives better aligned. For example, the OR manager might institute a policy stating that when a day's schedule is completed, the OR team may go home without loss of pay. This incentive is common in freestanding ASCs. In other institutions, the nursing staff may be divided up into specialty teams, with a team leader responsible for keeping the team on track. Some institutions are experimenting with monetary incentive programs that pay extra for work output in excess of established benchmarks. The best motivator is a personal sense of pride at having done a difficult job well, reinforced by appropriate recognition from the OR leadership.

When Things Do Not Go As Planned

The discussion so far describes how an OR suite should ideally run, and it assumes that the patients, surgeons, anesthesiologists, and nurses are all on time, that all the required paperwork and laboratory tests have been completed satisfactorily, and that the surgery lasts the predicted amount of time. It further assumes that all necessary resources, including simple disposable supplies, complex equipment, and specialized implants, as well as ORs and empty beds on postoperative nursing care units, are available. Most critically, it assumes that no emergency cases are added to an already full OR schedule.

Not one of the above is consistently true. The single constant of OR function is variation from what has been carefully planned. The patient load varies unpredictably from day to day, which is probably the most difficult problem to manage. Strategies to reduce variation in case load, such as block booking, have been shown to be of value. To completely eliminate large swings in the number and variability of cases, however, is impossible. Additionally, surgery is inherently unpredictable. Even when the best available preoperative diagnostic methodology is used, findings at surgery are a surprise in a high proportion of cases. Furthermore, even when the preoperative diagnosis is exactly correct, unexpected anatomic variations can substantially alter the expected duration of surgery.

A major role of the OR's daily coordinators is to deal with unforeseen variations in the flow of cases. Depending on the type of OR suite, running the daily schedule falls either to the charge nurse, consulting with the anesthesiologists and surgeons as necessary, or, in larger settings, to a team consisting of a nursing and an anesthesia coordinator. Teamwork and coordinated responses to the problems of the schedule are essential, and such cooperation can be realized only in a setting of mutual respect and trust.

Problems that arise tend to fall into several categories. The most spectacular event is the true life-or-death emergency. Such a case goes into the first available OR, regardless of what case had been intended for that room, and regardless of whether it is the "correct" room for the emergency case. Emergencies of this type are often related to uncontrolled bleeding or to nearly complete airway obstruction. (Complete airway obstruction must be treated outside the OR if the patient is to survive.) Supplies and instruments for such emergency cases should be assembled well in advance of their need and kept on a cart designed for emergency use.

More common is the emergency case that must be attended to within 1–2 hours to ensure the best possible outcome for the patient. If an OR is empty and sufficient anesthesia and nursing staff are available, the nursing and anesthesia coordinators assign appropriate teams and arrange for notification of all participants, and the surgery proceeds. A well-established protocol should be in place for preparing the OR; for assembling and delivering appropriate supplies, instruments, and equipment; and for notifying all involved personnel through the front desk clerks.

In many OR suites, emergency and urgent cases are classified by their relative urgency. Typically, they are divided into three levels, corresponding to cases that should be attended to immediately, within 4–6 hours, and within 24 hours. The surgeon scheduling an urgent case assigns it to the appropriate category. Requiring the surgeon to inform the anesthesia or nursing coordinator of the reason why an operation must be performed within 4 hours is a reasonable check on the validity of the assignment. For cases requiring immediate surgery, it is imperative that the surgeon speak directly with an OR coordinator to transmit vital information on the patient's condition and on special surgical requirements.

When no empty OR is or will be available within the requested time limit for a surgery, postponing (bumping) a case already scheduled but not yet started is necessary. Postponement is disruptive to OR personnel as well as to the surgeon and patient being bumped. If possible, the bumped case should be one of those scheduled to be performed by the surgeon who is caring for the emergency case. Failing that (the usual situation), the bumped case should belong to the same surgical service as the emergency case (i.e., an orthopedic emergency should bump another orthopedic case, not a general surgery case). This practice has the salutary effect of forcing surgeons scheduling emergency cases to be able to justify the action to their own colleagues, thus reducing the temptation to overstate the degree of emergency for convenience of the surgeon rather than for benefit of the patient.

Far more common than emergency or even urgent cases are delays produced by underestimation of the duration of surgery, as when a case scheduled for 3 hours actually requires 6. If the operations following are scheduled to be performed by the same surgeon, the only problem is that the OR may run well beyond the usual end of the elective OR day. If the next cases belong to another surgeon, however, the situation is different. If at all possible, these cases should be moved to another OR to mitigate the delay.

Another reason to move cases from one OR to another occurs when an unexpected opening appears in the schedule as the result of cancellation. If the surgeon is available and the patient is ready, filling the available space by moving a case scheduled later in the day into another OR may be possible. If no suitable elective case is scheduled, the space can be offered to a standby case (to be carried out within 24 hours). Because standby cases may amount to 10% or more of the day's caseload, fitting them into the schedule is highly cost effective for the hospital as well as beneficial to patients and surgeons.

A substantial potential for conflict arises in assigning priority to standby cases and cases considered for moving up in the schedule. A good way to reduce conflict is to have explicit rules, developed jointly by surgeons, anesthesiologists, and nurses, that specify who gets bumped under what circumstances. These rules may include a provision that an emergency case should preferentially bump another case from the same service, that an extreme emergency takes the first open OR, and that if an elective case cannot be started within 30 minutes after the OR is ready for the patient (because of a late patient or a late surgeon), the case may be converted to standby status and the next case moved up. Whatever the exact rules, it is critical that the nursing and anesthesia leadership be perceived as fair and evenhanded in making impromptu assignments.

Chapter 9
Materials Management

The world is moving so fast these days, that the man who says it can't be done is generally interrupted by someone doing it.

—Elbert Hubbard (1856–1915)

To perform surgery in a safe, efficient, and economical manner, all necessary instruments, supplies, and equipment must be reliably brought together at the correct time and in the correct place, case after case, day after day. Even a simple, routine case typically requires more than 100 instruments and a lengthy list of supplies such as sutures, scalpel blades, drapes, dressings, and drains. Tables 9-1 and 9-2 list the contents of a general surgery "minor" pan (instruments) and custom pack (supplies) intended for use in a wide variety of relatively simple cases. Additionally, large pieces of equipment may be needed, such as an electrocautery or a video system. The instruments, supplies, and equipment needed for one type of surgical operation often are not suitable for other types of operations (Case Study 9-1).

For many surgical procedures, several techniques may be acceptable, each of which has its proponents and its critics. Consequently, the specific instruments and supplies one surgeon uses for a given procedure may vary substantially from those preferred by a colleague performing the same operation. The OR suite has historically provided supplies and equipment specific not only to the type of operation but also to the surgeon performing it. Variation from one surgeon to another is based on many factors, including the institution at which the surgeon was trained, the mentors who influenced the surgeon's style, personal preferences, and even such things as whether the surgeon is left- or right-handed, tall or short.

With increasing emphasis on constraining the cost of health care, many OR suites are now working with surgeons to standardize instrument sets and supplies to help reduce the costs of procedures (and sometimes to facilitate cost comparisons among practitioners performing similar procedures). Some medical centers use cost of supplies and personnel, coupled with patient outcomes, to measure whether the financial and clinical goals of the ORs are being achieved (see Financial Performance on page 39 and Operational Performance on page 42).

As new procedures are devised, the list of operations performed changes. In addition, new instruments and techniques are invented for existing operations. For a variety of reasons, some procedures gradually or suddenly disappear. For example, surgical treatment of gastric ulcers nearly vanished after the discovery that many ulcers are amenable to treatment with antibiotics.

Ensuring reliable and timely availability of the requisite instruments, supplies, equipment, and personnel in every OR to facilitate the performance of surgery is one of the three major problems at the heart of the day-to-day management of an OR suite (the other two being scheduling cases and managing personnel). The logistics of supplying and staffing ORs is far more complex than the comparable task in a manufacturing environment. The same procedure is not usually performed many times consecutively in an OR. Rather, the procedures vary from case to case, from surgeon

Table 9-1. Contents of General Surgery Minor Pan

Item File Number	Quantity	Description	Catalog Number
Clamps			
109572	6	Curved mosquito	334001
102066	10	Curved Crile	344031
102067	2	Straight Crile	344030
117926	4	Regular Kelly	344071
116376	4	Allis	347000
3627	4	Grab hook	304088
3615	1	Fine right angle	304494
100066	1	Right angle	195580
102242	6	Cystic duct	304291
101911	2	Kocher	344130
3620	2	Sponge stick	326030
101908	4	Towel clip	325000
Needle holders			
102561	2	Ryder	363001
116559	2	Crile Wood	362002
Forceps			
5507	2	Toothed Cushing	301186
5508	2	Toothed	304152
102341	2	DeBakey	371011
102340	2	Long DeBakey	371012
2327	2	Bonney	301129
Retractors			
102326	2	Vein	501020
102369	2	Right angle	504121
9877	2	Thyroid	504130
102359	1	Small self-retainer	501197
2316	1	Large self-retainer	511714
3590	2	Sharp rakes	504222
102346	2	Small Richardson	504110
113850	2	Medium Richardson	504116
113852	2	Large Richardson	504117
1354	1	Narrow ribbon	504210
119546	2	Small springs	488151
Scissors			
101001	1	Metz, 7 in.	365016
100304	1	Lillie	MO1620
102604	1	Nurse	365051
4447	1	Mayo	365061
Miscellaneous			
5509	2	No. 3 Knife handle	115530
3415	1	No. 4 Knife handle	115531
3586	2	Double skin hooks	386647
3587	2	Single skin hooks	386642
109578	1	Probe	494033
2394	2	Facelift retractors	P509

to surgeon, and from day to day. It has been estimated that an OR must stock at least 10 times as many different items of inventory as a manufacturing firm that has the same dollar volume. (UMC keeps more than 8,000 different inventory items in stock, ranging in price from less than $0.01 for gauze sponges to thousands of dollars for items such as pacemakers, artificial heart valves, and orthopedic joint implants.)

Table 9-2. Contents of General Surgery Minor Custom Pack

Quantity	Description
1	Syringe, Asepto bulb, 50 cc
2	Towel, absorbent, 13 in. × 19 in., Polysorb
1	Blade, surgical, stainless steel, no. 10
1	Blade, surgical, stainless steel, no. 15
1	Blade, surgical, stainless steel, no. 20
1 package	Needle counter, foam, plastic box
2 pair	Glove, surgeons, 7½, latex
1 pair	Glove, surgeons, 8, latex
1 pair	Glove, surgeons, 8½, latex
1	Cautery, pencil, pushbutton, blade and holster
1 package	Sponge, gauze, 8 in. × 4 in., 12-ply
1	Tubing, suction, nonconductive, 5 mm × 12 ft
1	Handle, suction, Yankauer, bulb tip
1	Cautery tip cleaner
1	Cover, back table, 65 in. × 90 in.
1	Cover, Mayo stand
1	Drape, half, 44 in. × 57 in.
1	Skin marker
10	Towel, fluff, 17 in. × 27 in.
1	Ruler, 6 in., polyvinylchloride
1	Tray, organizer, 9 in. × 4¾ in. × 2 in.
1	Bag, bedside
1	Tray, Mayo stand, polypropylene, 13 in. × 19 in.
3	Tray, soaking, 5 in. × 5 in. × 2 in.
2	Applicator, cotton-tipped, 3 in., plastic
4	Sponge, winged, small, 3½ in. × 1¾ in. × 1 in.
1	Label, sheet of six, blank
1	Pouch, sterilization, 26 in. × 24 in.
1	Bag, glassine, 2¾ in. × 3¾ in.
2 packages	Sponge, lap, 12 in. × 12 in.
2	Handle, light, green
3	Gown, fabric reinforced, extra large

Additionally, an OR suite must have all supplies and instruments on hand before the start of a case. Unavailability of a single essential item in the midst of surgery may force the surgeon to perform the case less than optimally, or may even cause the surgery to be discontinued and completed at a later date. The attendant increase in anesthetic and surgical risks, costs, and patient and surgeon dissatisfaction, along with potential legal liability, are clearly unacceptable.

PREFERENCE AND PROCEDURE CARDS

Because of the large variety of procedures and of surgeon preferences, every OR suite maintains a record for each operation that lists the instruments, supplies, and equipment needed and the preferences of each surgeon who may perform the operation, as well as any special requirements the surgeon might have. In some hospitals and surgical centers, this list may take the form of an actual card, the surgeon's "preference card," which may be kept in a card file box. When an operation is scheduled, the nursing staff consults the card, draws the required items from storage, and prepares the OR for the case. The handwritten preference card is rapidly being replaced by electronic database systems. The computerized preference card system should ideally be integrated with the OR suite's electronic system for scheduling, billing, and inventory management. Surgery at large medical centers would be nearly impossible without a computerized case management system.

Generating Preference Cards

A preference card for a new type of surgery or for a new surgeon is usually generated by a member of the OR nursing staff in consultation with the surgeon. New surgeons just beginning at a hospital are asked for a list of procedures they plan to perform. To generate the new preference cards, the nurse may print out sample preference cards of other surgeons who perform the same procedures. Then the new surgeon and the nurse jointly review the printouts and modify them as required to fit the preferences of the surgeon. If no preference card already exists, or if the existing cards are unsatisfactory, new cards may be generated from scratch. If the surgeon is transferring from one hospital to another, attempting to obtain copies of the surgeon's preference cards from the former hospital is worthwhile.

Some surgeons have little idea of the exact supplies that they use in a given operation and ask the nurses to generate a preference card for them. This has the potential for creating conflict the first time the surgeon operates, because many of the surgeon's favorite items may be slow to arrive or may even be unavailable. It is far better to walk surgeons through planned procedures in advance and to create preference cards through simulation.

CASE STUDY 9-1. Materials Management at University Medical Center

In a large hospital like UMC, with its 200 academic surgeons in 12 different specialties and its 25 ORs, an enormous number of different procedures are performed over the course of a year. A review of the *CPT* codes of the 16,438 cases performed in a 12-month period reveals that 1,375 different procedures were performed, 567 of which were performed only once. The most frequently performed procedure (knee arthroscopy) accounted for only 3.6% of the overall volume. The following table lists the procedures that were performed 50 times or more and the number of times each was performed. Every procedure listed requires a unique set of supplies, instruments, and equipment.

Rank	Procedure	Number of cases	Percentage
1	Knee arthroscopy	603	3.6
2	Lumbar laminectomy	505	3.0
3	Coronary artery bypass graft	450	2.7
4	Dilation and curettage	416	2.5
5	Tonsillectomy and adenoidectomy	391	2.3
6	Dental restorations and extractions	374	2.2
7	Total abdominal hysterectomy	320	1.9
8	Laparoscopic bilateral tubal ligation	279	1.7
9	Repair inguinal hernia	240	1.4
10	Laparoscopic cholecystectomy	235	1.4
11	Insertion of pressure equalizing tubes	221	1.3
12	Incision and drainage of wound	208	1.2
13	Appendectomy	201	1.2
14	Hardware removal	197	1.2
15	Breast biopsy	195	1.2
16	Diagnostic laparoscopy	185	1.1
17	Total hip replacement	181	1.1
18	Carotid endarterectomy	176	1.0
19	Carpal tunnel release	172	1.0
20	Exploratory laparotomy	166	1.0
21	Colectomy	151	0.9
22	Bronchoscopy, thoracotomy, wedge resection	150	0.9
23	Extracapsular cataract extraction with insertion of intraocular lens	146	0.9
24	Hysteroscopy for biopsy	142	0.8
25	Shoulder arthroscopy	142	0.8
26	Cervical laminectomy	140	0.8
27	Craniotomy for tumor	132	0.8
28	Cystoscopic biopsy and fulguration of bladder tumor	130	0.8
29	Femoral-tibial bypass graft	129	0.8
30	Total knee replacement	118	0.7
31	Open reduction and internal fixation of hip	110	0.7
32	Excision of varicose veins	109	0.6
33	Reduction mammoplasty	102	0.6
34	Direct laryngoscopy with CO_2 laser excision	98	0.6
35	Insertion of arteriovenous fistula	93	0.6
36	Insertion of ventriculoperitoneal shunt	91	0.5
37	Septoplasty	89	0.5
38	Mitral valve replacement	89	0.5
39	Hysteroscopy for diagnosis	84	0.5
40	Posterior spine fusion	81	0.5

(continued)

CASE STUDY 9-1. (*continued*)

Rank	Procedure	Number of cases	Percentage
41	Ventral hernia repair	80	0.5
42	Tracheostomy	79	0.5
43	Port-A-Cath insertion	78	0.5
44	Split-thickness skin graft	77	0.5
45	Laparoscopic oophorectomy	75	0.4
46	Open reduction and internal fixation of ankle	73	0.4
47	Open cholecystectomy	69	0.4
48	Kidney transplant	68	0.4
49	Resection of abdominal aortic aneurysm	63	0.4
50	Peritoneal dialysis catheter removal	62	0.4
51	Transurethral resection of bladder tumor	61	0.4
52	Laparoscopic-assisted vaginal hysterectomy	60	0.4
53	Transurethral resection of prostate	57	0.3
54	Intramedullary nailing of femur	56	0.3
55	Bronchoscopy and mediastinoscopy	55	0.3
56	Arch bar removal	53	0.3
57	Percutaneous endoscopic gastrostomy	53	0.3
58	Endoscopic ethmoidectomy	52	0.3
59	Hickman catheter insertion	51	0.3
60	Neuroplasty of forearm	50	0.3
Total		**9,313**	

Structure of Preference Cards

A typical preference card has three major sections: (1) nursing plan, (2) disposable supplies, and (3) instruments and small equipment (Figure 9-1).

Nursing Plan

The first section of the preference card contains the nursing plan, which includes such information as method of skin preparation, initial electrocautery settings, patient position, and devices used to aid in positioning. The need for special support staff, such as x-ray technicians, laser safety personnel, and special monitoring personnel (e.g., electroencephalography technicians), is usually listed in the nursing plan. Also included is a list of the large pieces of required equipment: devices specific to the particular operation (e.g., special orthopedic operating tables, specialized laser devices, and high-speed cement-removal tools for joint replacement revisions) and common items that may be used in many different types of surgery (e.g., electrocautery devices, operating microscopes, and tourniquet boxes).

Sometimes listed in the nursing plan is the fact that the procedure is performed only in certain ORs. For example, some orthopedic procedures are performed in ORs that have laminar-flow air circulation or ultraviolet lights. Similarly, cardiac surgery, liver transplant surgery, and neurosurgery cases are usually assigned to larger ORs because of the extra space required for equipment such as the heart-lung bypass machine and particularly large sterile tables for instruments.

Disposable Supplies

The second section of the preference card lists the quantity of each single-use supply item needed for the operation. These items must be identified accurately and unambiguously to avoid errors when they are assembled for surgery by a stock-keeper who may not be familiar with how they will be used. The preference list should include the name of the item, the quantity desired, and the manufacturer's catalog number (see example in Figure 9-1). The card should also include a hospital-specific inventory number, because identical supplies may be obtained from several different suppliers. For many items, size and configuration should also be specified. Many supply items have several common names that do not closely match the manufacturer's nomenclature. The most commonly used name may be a trademark that has become, through familiarity, the only name by which an item is known, regardless of

---

University Medical Center
Preference List: 951
Preference List Procedure: Thyroidectomy
Surgeon: Dr. General   Gloves: 8.0 NLTX Right-Handed
Nursing Plan
Patient position:
    Supine with both arms tucked
    Thyroid pillow covered and beneath shoulders before induction of anesthesia
    Gel headring under head after induction of anesthesia
Room setup:
    Room temperature 80° F at start, 70° F after patient draped
    Have slush available, but may not use; kidney basin in slush with small amount NS in it
    IV poles ×2
Prep: Betadine solution after placement of drip towels
Draping:
    6 towels
    4 towel clips
    Lap sheet with sticky tabs exposed
Routine:
    Uses DeBakey forceps on all cases
    Bovie set to 26 cutting, 30 coagulation; 30 bipolar
Dressings:
    If no drain used—2 packs fluffs
    If Penrose drain used—3 in. × 4 in. gauze, fluffs, abdominal pad, towel folded in thirds, 3-in. paper tape

Item File Number	Quantity	Description	Catalog Number
Dressings			
65008	2 packages	Sponge, sterile, 3 in. × 4 in.	3157
35010	4 packages	Dressing, fluff, 6 in.	2585
35001	1	Dressing, abdominal pad	9190
Supplies			
20	1	Cord, bipolar	S2050B
761	1	Pad, magnetic	20020
65071	5 packages	Sponge, x-ray, 4 in. × 8 in., sterile	7318
7218	1	Drape, slush machine	ORS100
116904	1	Electrode, adult dispersive	4002100
43146	1	Stapler, skin, 35 W	528235
65021	1 package	Sponge, K dissector	V7102
73050	1	Drain, Penrose, ½ in. × 12 in.	513002
			(*continued*)

Figure 9-1. Typical preference card (thyroidectomy). (IV = intravenous; NS = normal saline; W = wide; XL = extra large; NLTX = nonlatex; sh, blk, pop, ct, x-1, rb-1 = proprietary information on suture pack to identify contents.)

Item File Number	Quantity	Description	Catalog Number
Drapes			
76023	1	Sheet, pediatric lap, 74 in. × 124 in.	66886
76003	1	Gown, XL, ultra reinforced	95221
Gloves			
100261	1 pair	Glove, NLTX, size 8	8506
Sutures			
522	1	Suture, silk, 2-0 sh blk 30 in.	K833H
2480	1	Suture, silk, 4-0 tie blk 30 in.	A303H
114667	1	Suture, silk, 2-0 tie blk 30 in.	A305H
2486	1	Suture, silk, 3-0 sh pop blk 18 in.	C013D
513	1	Suture, silk, 3-0 tie blk 30 in.	A304H
527	1	Suture, silk, 2-0 x-1 blk 18 in.	737G
569	1	Suture, Vicryl, 4-0 reel ct 54 in.	J204G
2501	4	Suture, Vicryl, 2-0 sh ct 27 in.	J317H
2506	2	Suture, Vicryl, 3-0 sh ct 27 in.	J316H
2508	2	Suture, Vicryl, 4-0 rb-1 ct 27 in.	J304H
Basins			

1573	1	Basin set:
		  Kidney basin (1)
		  Round basin (2)
			1573

Instruments			
119694	1	Pan, general surgery, minor (See Table 9-1 for contents of pan.)	119694
Custom Pack			
108855	1	Pack, custom, general surgery, minor (See Table 9-2 for contents of pack.)	SBA14MLSMD

Figure 9-1. (*continued*)

manufacturer. If an item has several common names, such as *Kitner, peanut, dissector,* or *d-sponge,* using the manufacturer's name on the preference card, rather than local slang that may vary from surgeon to surgeon, is advisable.

It is crucial for every item entered onto a preference card to be in the hospital's inventory. If a preference card calls for items that are not stocked, the result will be frustration or anger. Rarely does it make sense to specify a particular brand of an item, because the vast majority of supplies are manufactured by many different companies and are, in effect, commodities. For some items, though, the surgeon may claim superiority for one brand. Dealing with this issue is discussed in Standardization of Supplies starting on page 124.

Certain other items of information should be specified on the preference card for each supply item. The most important of these, given the pressure to control costs, is price. The purpose of recording price is to continuously remind staff of the often extraordinarily high cost of supplies used in the OR. Heightened awareness of cost may help to reduce waste. Prices recorded on preference cards should be acquisition costs paid by the hospital, not "charges" generated for third-party payers. The actual cost of each item is relatively easy to determine, because it comes from the purchasing component of the OR suite's electronic database. On the other hand, the amount that the patient or the patient's insurance company is charged is determined by a host of factors, such as details of the hospital's contract with the insurance company and government regulations for patients on Medicare or Medicaid.

Most supply items on the preference card appear as a generic OR charge on the patient's bill. Some, however, are specifically tracked and later billed separately (if allowed by the terms of the insurance contract); these items should be so identified. Under current federal regulations, implantable items must be separately tracked. (See Medical Device Tracking on page 155.) This is one reason why a comprehensive ORDB is helpful, if not imperative. (See Operating Room Database on page 136.) Finally, every item should be identified by the hospital's inventory number, so that when there is a change of supplier, the preference cards can be easily updated.

Instruments and Equipment

The third section of the preference card lists the basic (e.g., general surgery minor, orthopedic major) and special instrument sets required for the surgery. Like supplies, instruments must be positively identified by descriptive names and by manufacturer and catalog number. To an even greater extent than supplies, surgical instruments may have several different names that vary from institution to institution and from surgeon to surgeon. The most common hemostatic clamp is variously called a *Crile*, *hemostat*, *snap*, and even just *clamp*. In many ORs, the instruments are assembled into sets designed for certain operations or types of operation. In this case, only the name of the set is included on the preference card. Separate lists with complete information are included with the sets to permit checking for completeness and counting before and after the operation.

The best way to determine how many of a particular instrument should be included in the instrument set for a given operation is through experience. This variable is influenced by the style of the surgeon. Some surgeons rarely deploy more than one or two instruments at a time; others fill the operative field with clamps and retractors, so that several dozen instruments may all be in action at once. This sort of variation makes standardization of instrument sets difficult.

The supply of resources needed for certain types of surgery is often limited. For example, the OR suite may have only one laser of a particular type, or only two ORs may be suitable for cardiac surgery. The number of sets of certain types of instruments (e.g., total hip sets, spine sets) may also be limited. All such resource limitations should be assembled in a single, central file (sometimes called the *common resources file*) so that the OR schedule can be created to ensure that requirements of the scheduled operations do not exceed the capabilities of the OR suite. The need for resources on the common resource list must be identified on the preference cards, so that potential conflicts can be identified and eliminated at the time of scheduling. If only two ORs are suitable for open heart surgery, scheduling three such cases simultaneously is pointless. Maintenance of the common resources list is time consuming but must not be neglected if the OR suite is to run smoothly.

Some operations require that certain items be specially ordered. Such items include supplies not routinely kept in inventory, such as pacemakers or custom-made orthopedic implants. A patient may be scheduled for revision of an orthopedic implant of a type that the hospital's surgeons do not routinely use. Additionally, certain equipment may not be used often enough to justify its purchase but may be available on a 1-day lease. These requirements not only must be flagged on the preference card, but also require direct communication between the surgeon and the appropriate OR nurse or the OR suite's materials manager.

Maintaining Preference Cards

Nurses who regularly work with specific surgeons should be responsible for modifications and updates to their preference cards. Because much of the information leading to changes in preference cards is generated in an OR at the time of surgery, the circulating nurse should note when items that are needed are not on the preference card and when items on the card are not used. This information can be passed on to the nurse in charge of the surgeon's preference list once the case has been completed. In addition, the nursing plan should be modified based on actual experience. Modifications in the card should be limited to permanent changes in the manner of performing the case, as confirmed through discussion with the surgeon, rather than based on observation alone.

Spending most of the maintenance effort on the most commonly used preference cards is one way to minimize maintenance time. When the preference card system is computerized, determining which cards have a high use rate is possible. In large institutions, 15–20% of the preference cards usually cover approximately 80% of the cases. These commonly used cards deserve the closest scrutiny.

Computerization of preference cards permits changes in the supplier or description of a particular item to be automatically updated on all preference cards at once. Similarly, changes to the common resources list can be made globally.

Preference Cards in Action

Preference cards are useful only if the information they contain is transmitted to the people responsible for drawing the materials from inventory and delivering them to the correct OR at the correct time. The first step in this process is to identify the appropriate preference card for a particular surgeon, procedure, date of surgery, and OR. In some hospitals, identification of the appropriate preference card is made in the OR scheduling office when the surgery is booked. The selection can be made by the surgeon's agent or by the scheduling clerk through matching the description of the case, as given by the surgeon's agent, with a case description on one of the surgeon's preference cards. Sometimes an RN supervisor in the scheduling office assists in choosing appropriate preference cards. Some institutions schedule operations and select preference cards according to *CPT* codes. (See Procedure Codes on page 146.) Alternatively, appropriate preference cards can be selected by OR nurses or technologists or by well-trained materials stock-keepers responsible for preparing case carts (see Delivery of Instruments and Supplies to the Operating Room, starting on page 123), based on narrative descriptions of the scheduled case or on *CPT* codes (preferably the latter).

Errors in selection of preference cards are among the most common time- and money-wasting problems in the OR suite. First, human errors are inevitable, such as a misunderstanding by the OR scheduling clerk or the surgeon's office clerk of the case description (e.g., substituting "esophagoscopy" for "esophagectomy"). A lack of standardization of names for various procedures can lead to serious systems problems; as a result, the scheduling clerk may be forced to select from a list of preference cards, none of which exactly matches the case description submitted by the surgeon's agent. When the stock-keeper makes the selection, the problem may be compounded, because selection is sometimes based on a case description that has been truncated to fit into a small field on the printed OR

schedule. Complicating matters further, supply requests are often filled during evening or night shifts, when calls for clarification are not possible.

Because of the rapid introduction of new procedures and the consequent difficulty in keeping preference cards up to date, sometimes no preference card is available for a particular combination of surgeon and procedure. Under these circumstances, the scheduling clerk, stock-keeper, or nurse may choose the closest approximation and hope for the best. If sufficient time permits, the surgeon should be consulted to ensure that appropriate supplies and equipment are available at the time of surgery.

Minimizing the error rate is important because of the high cost in time and materials related to incomplete or nonexistent preference cards or inaccurate assignments. One way to reduce scheduling errors is for the surgeon's office to schedule cases by code numbers (e.g., *CPT* codes) or by preference card name or number. This type of scheduling minimizes ambiguity about the exact procedure to be performed and the setup required. For the system to work, the OR staff should generate a list of the various preference cards used by each surgeon, review the list with the surgeon to ensure accuracy and completeness, and send a copy to the surgeon's office staff, who then use the list when scheduling cases. This system can dramatically reduce errors and minimize the problem of nonexistent preference cards. It also requires a well-established method for keeping the preference card lists in surgeons' offices up to date.

Another (more cumbersome) way to reduce scheduling errors is to fax a list of cases scheduled for the following day, along with copies of the associated preference cards, to each surgeon's office on the day before surgery. The surgeon can then review this list for errors, which can be brought to the attention of the OR staff far enough in advance to avoid delays on the day of surgery. A more sophisticated electronic system would allow surgeons read-only electronic access to the OR schedule and to the content of relevant preference cards via modem, local area network (LAN), or the Internet. (See The Operating Room Schedule as an Electronic Report on page 149.) However, to assume that most surgeons will regularly use this method for reducing errors is probably unrealistic.

One useful check is to have a nurse specialist for each surgical service review the cases and associated preference cards on the day before surgery. Obvious misassignments are usually easily recognized, and the problem of nonexistent preference cards can be immediately addressed. New preference cards are often created when nurse specialists call surgeons to determine the setup required for scheduled cases that have no suitable preference cards. This additional step has the advantage of directly involving nurse specialists in the process of selecting and delivering the correct supplies. Because these nurses are responsible for problem solving in the event of error, giving them an early sense of ownership in the process is important.

Procedure Cards

Some health care organizations are moving toward greater standardization by replacing surgeons' preference cards with procedure cards, which are not specific to any surgeon. By following a process similar to that used to standardize supplies and instruments, a consensus is arrived at on patient positioning, draping, and prepping for each operation. Only a few surgeon-specific details, such as size and type of glove and size of gown, are added as supplemental information.

Picking and Storing Supplies and Instruments

On the day before the planned surgery, the contents of the relevant preference or procedure cards should be printed and transmitted to the personnel picking supplies, instruments, and equipment. Another copy of the preference card may be printed and delivered to the nursing team assigned to each case. Some OR suites may be computerized to the extent that this information is available on computer screens in the materials management area and in the ORs. In this situation, copies of the preference cards need not be printed.

Cases requiring special treatment should be appropriately flagged. For example, if a case requires supplies not kept in inventory or equipment that must be rented, this information should be directly transmitted to the manager of supplies and equipment to arrange for delivery in time for the operation.

In small OR suites and ASCs with a relatively short list of procedures performed, necessary supplies are often kept in a storeroom immediately adjacent to or even within the OR suite (e.g., in a "center core" storage area; see discussion starting on page 181). On the day before surgery, the circulating and scrub nurses pull the preference cards for the next day's cases and assemble the supplies on a case cart or back table. If an item has been omitted, or if the surgery turns out to be different from what was anticipated, the circulating nurse can easily walk to the supply area or call for assistance in procuring missing items. Instruments are kept in sterile containers on the shelves in the supply area. Large pieces of equipment that stay in ORs where they are most often used can, if necessary, be moved the night before surgery. Other pieces of equipment (e.g., electrocoagulators) are common to all ORs. Because of the scale of small OR suites, members of the nursing staff are usually familiar with the needs of the surgeons and the location of all items in inventory.

Supplies at freestanding ASCs may be maintained by a stock clerk or purchasing agent, who passes through the supply area daily with an order sheet, checking for supply bins that are running low. The stock clerk should also regularly check with the nursing staff to determine whether use of any particular item seems to be increasing or decreasing. Because the number of surgeons, cases, and ORs in an ASC is small, the resupply system can be casual and friendly as well as businesslike and efficient. Elaborate inventory tracking systems are not necessary. The clerk or purchasing agent can look over upcoming OR schedules to see whether, for example, an unusually large number of a particular type of operation requires ordering extra inventory.

Because freestanding surgical centers usually have consistent case loads of relatively routine surgery, few of their supply items require long lead times to acquire. In large cities, medical supply distributors can usually be counted on to deliver commodity items on short notice. If the distributor has an item on back order, the stock clerk can call the manufacturer directly to have an item shipped by overnight delivery, but to do so is expensive and should be avoided as much as possible. Borrowing urgently needed supplies from a nearby hospital may be possible. In highly competitive environments, however, freestanding surgical centers may discover that hospitals are not eager to support their competition.

Simple systems of supply have several positive features. First, most personnel are familiar with the surgeons' needs and the locations of supplies. The number of individuals necessary to run the system is low. Problems with accountability of the person "picking the case" do not exist, because that person is an OR nurse or ST. Although extra cost is involved in having relatively high-salary nurses pick supplies, it may well be less than the personnel costs associated with a complex inventory system. Additionally, implementing complex administrative procedures to manage the flow of supplies is unnecessary.

Such a simple system is still in place at many larger facilities. When the number of inventory items becomes large and resupply lead times are long, however, a casual system may lead to shortages and even absence of crucial items. To avoid empty supply bins and consequent problems, the purchaser may gradually increase inventory holdings to extraordinary levels. Because a larger inventory requires more storage space, the ability of OR nurses to know the location of the entire inventory is reduced. Time-consuming searches of the supply room may be necessary to find a rare item. The time required to collect all the supplies necessary for a particular case rises rapidly as the number of different items in inventory increases. Because supply picking in simple systems is based on preference lists, which are not optimized for ease of finding the items in the supply room, searches may be disorganized and may require inefficient retracing of steps. The proportion of time devoted to gathering supplies by OR nurses rapidly increases as size of the inventory and complexity of the operations grow. At some point, this method for picking supplies should be replaced by a more efficient one.

One way to increase efficiency of picking is to electronically create a "pick ticket" for each case. The pick ticket contains much of the same information that is on the preference card, except that the information is organized according to the order in which inventory items are located in the storage area rather than according to the logic of preference cards.

In large OR suites, the inventory, no matter how carefully managed, takes up several thousand square feet of storage space. Hence, the inventory often cannot be accommodated within the surgical suite itself. Because of the inventory's large dollar value, professional management becomes necessary. Senior staff knowledgeable in this area must be carefully developed and retained. Recruiting a fully trained specialist certified by The National Institute for the Certification of Healthcare Sterile Processing and Distribution Personnel <http://www.njcc.com/~multico/nichspdp.htm> may be cost effective.

A large medical center's OR supply area can occupy more than 10,000 square feet of floor space, with supplies scattered among more than 100 wire racks, cabinets, and other storage facilities. Size and distance make it impossible for the supplies to be retrieved on an ad hoc basis. The picking of supplies must be formal and efficient. There must be a single, exhaustive database that contains information about all supply items, with the location of each item clearly identified. The inventory system should interface with the preference card system so that pick lists are generated for the stock clerks from preference cards. Different names for the same item should be cross-referenced. Supply areas of large OR suites are staffed 24 hours per day with technicians whose only job is to maintain the surgical inventory.

Delivery of Instruments and Supplies to the Operating Room

Many large hospitals use a case cart system for delivering instruments and supplies to the ORs. Case carts are enclosed rolling carts stocked with all the supplies and instruments required for a specific operation (as identified on the preference card). Filling of case carts is carried out by full-time stock clerks working under the supervision of materials management personnel. Fully stocked case carts for the first cases of the day are delivered to the OR suite before the start of the OR day, usually between midnight and 6:00 AM. When several short cases are scheduled sequentially, case carts for all of them may be delivered at the same time. This system requires that adequate case cart storage space be available near each OR.

The supplies in case carts must be supplemented by backup supplies in the OR suite. Accidental contamination of supplies is not uncommon. When any doubt about the sterility of surgical goods exists, prudent practice is to discard and replace. Sometimes there simply is not enough of an item to meet the needs of a particular operation. To avoid inordinate delays, a small inventory of commonly used supplies, such as gowns, gloves, sutures, and dressings, is stored in or immediately adjacent to each OR. Development of inventory lists for specialty supplies (e.g., orthopedic, cardiothoracic, or neurosurgical) kept in the OR suite falls to nurses familiar with the services involved—sometimes team leaders. Stock clerks usually keep these extra stocks replenished.

The case cart system, when well implemented, has the advantage of consistently delivering the required supplies to the right place at the right time. However, some supply problems must be solved through other means, because, for certain types of surgery, specifying in advance exactly what will be required is not possible. For example, in certain orthopedic cases, several hundred different screws might need to be available so that appropriate screws can be chosen at the time of surgery. The full selection cannot be packed into the case cart; rather, a separate specialty cart for this type of surgery is developed.

Surgery is inherently unpredictable. A case may turn out to be very different from what was originally intended, which means that the supplies required may be very different as well. The supply system must have a way to rapidly fill a surgeon's unanticipated needs. A central dispatch station in the supply area, staffed by individuals familiar with the nomenclature of supplies and instruments, can serve this purpose. Satisfactory and timely delivery of additional materials is one of the most difficult problems for a large OR supply system.

The case cart system has a few inherent drawbacks. Because the supplies for a particular operation are fixed in advance, and securing additional supplies during the course of a procedure may be tedious, a built-in tendency to overstock the cart exists, with the consequence that a large set of supplies is left to discard or to return to stock if not opened. Second, the case cart system requires a substantial commitment to organization and maintenance. Finally, the OR nurses, who may be accustomed to and more comfortable with selecting their own supplies, lose some control.

MANAGING MATERIALS

Management of a multimillion-dollar, dynamically changing materials supply system demands an energetic, highly motivated individual. That person should ideally be part of both the OR's management team and the hospital's purchasing and materials group. In some hospitals, the OR supply room is part of a larger warehouse that supports the supply needs of the entire hospital. This cuts down on duplication of supply inventory and eliminates the need for supervisory personnel required for an OR suite that has its own independent supply area. On the other hand, important differences exist between supplying the OR suite and supplying other parts of the hospital. The OR suite cannot easily tolerate supplies out of stock and generally demands more rapid delivery times than the rest of the hospital.

The most fundamental challenge for the OR materials manager is to run as efficient and low-cost a program as possible without ever allowing the absence of critical items at the time of surgery. These are, of course, competing goals—low cost means small standing inventory, and never running out is most easily achieved with a large inventory.

Several reasons exist for keeping as small an inventory on hand as possible. First, a small inventory ties up fewer dollars and therefore frees up capital. Second, a smaller inventory requires less space, fewer employees to maintain it, and easier retrieval of needed items. Third, a smaller inventory has more rapid turnover of its contents. Because some sterile items have limited shelf life, a more rapid turnover reduces the risk of outdating. Finally, a smaller inventory is less vulnerable to swings in medical practice. When a surgeon retires or moves to another hospital, fewer items specific to that surgeon's practice become useless. When a newly introduced device proves to be an improvement over the previous design, surgeons often wish to change immediately; a smaller inventory makes such a change much less expensive, because the stock of supplies specific to the previous technique is smaller.

Standardization of Supplies

Probably the most important method for minimizing size of the inventory is standardizing supplies as much as possible. Standardization means that the hospital does not carry several different types of a particular item from several different suppliers just to satisfy the personal preferences of various surgeons. For many commodity items, such as dressings or drapes, standardization is relatively painless. For others, such as gloves, it is more difficult, because personnel tend to have strong preferences. The reasons offered range from subtle differences between brands in fit and feel to idiosyncratic skin reactions. Having different types of gloves available—standard, non-powdered, non-latex, orthopedic—is reasonable. It should not be necessary, however, to have different brands of the same type of glove. Brands of supplies are increasingly being determined by group purchasing organizations (GPOs) with which hospitals contract for commodity items to obtain low prices. (See the discussion of GPOs in Purchasing on page 127.)

Certain supplies, particularly expensive ones, are difficult to stock according to consensus. Items such as joint implants or cardiac valves usually have powerful and highly vocal adherents. In addition to real issues of performance, surgeons may offer familiarity with an established product as a reason to continue its use. Institutional reasons to embrace the status quo, such as a vendor's superior record of customer service or staff familiarity with the product in question, may also exist. When a new surgical implant is introduced, a learning curve must be ascended, which can adversely affect patient outcomes and short-term costs. Finally, unstated but powerful personal incentives may induce a surgeon to favor one brand or another, such as financial involvement with a particular manufacturer, personal relationships with the supplier's employees, and a host of other conflicts of interest.

Standardization has advantages beyond reducing volume of inventory. Once a single supplier has been selected for an item, the purchasing department can be much more aggressive in pursuing discounts. In the case of orthopedic implants, the discount from list price, once a single manufacturer has been selected, may be as high as 40–50%. Standardization dramatically reduces the amount of training required for the nurses and technologists assigned to work on cases involving specialized equipment. Standardization of equipment also reduces the complexity of scheduling personnel, because tracking which individuals

have been trained on different manufacturer's products is no longer necessary.

Custom Packs

Another strategy for reducing inventory is to combine supplies that are common to several different procedures and surgeons into a single custom pack, which then becomes a single inventory item. A custom pack is a bundle of supplies (e.g., drapes, sponges, prep kit, knife blades, basic sutures) that is sterilized as a unit. Individual items are not individually packaged and therefore do not need to be individually opened, thus substantially reducing setup time. Custom packs also reduce inventory maintenance and minimize the need to pick many small items. This system could reduce acquisition costs as well, because an aggressive purchaser may be able to obtain a custom pack at a lower price than the total cost of the individual items making it up. Although developing the list of contents of various custom packs can be difficult, the necessary information can be obtained from nurses who are familiar with the different surgical services. A sophisticated software package for managing preference cards can scan the different preference lists looking for commonalties to suggest custom packs.

Perpetual Inventory

Inventory reduction can be achieved in ways other than standardizing supplies and using custom packs. The most far-reaching inventory controls require establishing a reliable and accurate method of tracking changes in inventory on a case-to-case basis. When the materials manager has reliable and up-to-the-minute information about actual on-shelf inventory, stocking excess to ensure adequacy is no longer necessary. The perpetual inventory is established by setting up a database of all supplies in inventory and decrementing the count each time an item is issued to the OR for a procedure. Similarly, the count is incremented when supplies are returned unused after a procedure or when fresh supplies are delivered. In a well-designed system, the risk of running out of an item can be decreased by using the scheduling system to warn of an impending increase in volume of a particular procedure so that the inventory can be augmented in anticipation. The scheduling system can advise the inventory system of special-order items that should be on hand for certain cases.

Additionally, a perpetual inventory system permits routine collection of data on rates of use of various inventory items. It also allows the materials manager to track lead times for the delivery of various supplies and to design an inventory reorder system that takes into account variations in use and differences in resupply times. The goal is to minimize standing inventory while keeping out-of-stock items to a minimum. Well-designed materials management software assists in these tasks.

To generate an accurate record of the supplies actually used during a procedure, the circulating nurse must have a way of communicating to the inventory system the items opened during an operation and the items remaining unused at the end. The supplies used during a procedure are delivered through four different routes, each of which requires a different approach for cost and inventory tracking. First, a well-implemented preference card system captures most of the items used in the majority of cases. This information may be used to decrement the central supply inventory and to attribute use of specific supplies to a particular procedure. Second, additional items requested during an operation can be entered into the system by the materials management personnel as the items are delivered to the OR. Third, some procedures require access to an expensive set of items of which only a few are actually used (e.g., orthopedic screws). The number used may be recorded by the circulating nurse at the time of use, or the number in the set may be counted by a stock clerk before delivery to the OR and again afterwards. Fourth, generic items stocked in the OR area, such as gloves, gowns, and extra sutures, need not be charged to individual cases. Their use is probably best attributed by estimate. Finally, items returned unopened on the case cart should be returned to inventory and this transaction tracked. With this system, the use of expensive items drives reordering, while small commodity items need only be inventoried and restocked on a regular basis.

Such an elaborate system of inventory management requires a computerized inventory database with seamless links to the scheduling and preference card systems. Implementing such a system requires a large amount of work, a sophisticated computer system, and a materials manager committed to making the system work. All these things cost money, and the key question is whether the effort is worth the return.

Other benefits accrue from computerizing the OR suite's materials management department. Because supply use is traceable to individual cases, a much more precise accounting of the costs associated with different types of surgery or with different surgeons can be made. Because the preference card system and the supply inventory are integrated, current cost of the items on each preference card may be directly identified. Knowledge of the items used during a particular procedure allows a sophisticated software system to suggest modifications to the preference card based on actual use.

Outsourcing Management of Supplies

An alternative approach to inventory reduction that doesn't require development of in-house managerial skills, as perpetual inventory management does, is to "outsource" inventory management. By contract, a distributor agrees to maintain the hospital's supply inventory, usually at an off-site location, and to deliver supplies to the hospital in a timely fashion. In exchange, the distributor receives a markup over the purchase cost of the supplies. This system can dramatically simplify the hospital's purchasing paperwork. Orders can be transferred directly to the distributor's computer from the OR suite's computer, eliminating the expensive and time-consuming steps of generating purchase orders and checking invoices and packing slips. This system can extend as far as having the outside company deliver supplies already packaged for insertion into case carts.

When contemplating an outsourcing supply agreement, it is critical that details be clearly spelled out. First, the agreement should specify the maximum allowed interval between placing an order and its delivery to the hospital. Second, the form in which the supplies are delivered should be specified. Ideally, supplies should be unpacked from their original shipping containers and delivered to the hospital in clean, plastic tote boxes. The locations for delivery within the hospital should also be specified. A system should be in place for identifying items that the hospital should never be without. Determining which items are on this must-have list should be the sole prerogative of the hospital. A clearly specified backup system should be in place for securing items on manufacturers' back order. The backup system should probably involve notification of the hospital by the distributor when back ordering is necessary, so that the materials manager can immediately identify a satisfactory substitute. Finally, the agreement should specify that the distributor will identify a manager to supervise the hospital's account and that the manager must be acceptable to the hospital. Such an agreement can be valuable to the distributor and to the hospital.

PURCHASING

The OR suite's materials management division may be intimately related to the hospital's purchasing department. Alternatively, the surgical suite may have its own, separate purchasing function. Having the OR suite do its own purchasing carries two advantages. First, OR personnel are much more familiar with the technical details of surgical supply items than buyers in the central purchasing office. Second, adding the central purchasing office to the supply-delivery loop adds one extra step to the process and with it one extra delay and one extra place for errors to occur.

On the other hand, OR materials managers may not have access to some of the more sophisticated purchasing techniques available to institutional purchasing agents. The price of hospital supplies is often determined through negotiation between purchasing departments and vendors. For a vendor dealing with a large-volume purchaser, list prices often represent just the opening offer. Negotiations may become complex, with offers of rebates based on use. Rebates are often in the form of products, educational materials, or other items of value to the hospital. Some vendors offer a large discount on one product if the hospital agrees to exclusively use another product. This practice, known as *tying*, requires careful analysis by the purchasing department.

In an attempt to further leverage volume purchasing, many hospitals join GPOs. Large GPOs representing scores or even hundreds of hospitals claim to use the high aggregate volume represented by the member hospitals to extract the deepest possible price cuts from suppliers. Evaluating the claims of any GPO without considerable investigation, however, is difficult. The problem is even more difficult when the GPO requires, as a condition of membership, adherence to all contracts it negotiates with its preferred suppliers. To assess this situation, hospitals must weigh the overall cost of the entire market basket of supplies covered by the GPO contract against the cost they could negotiate outside the contract. Moreover, when the GPO's preferred vendors are not those in widespread use in the hospital—or, worse, when they were the less-preferred vendors in previous trials within the hospital—convincing the nurses and medical staff of the need for change may be difficult.

Another issue demanding expert appraisal is the choice between purchasing supplies and stocking them on consignment. Vendors of expensive items, such as orthopedic joint implants, may offer to place an inventory of their product in the hospital to be paid for if and when it is used. Such an arrangement brings considerable advantages. The hospital does not need to deal with the difficult trade-off between having items readily available and tying up a large amount of money in slow-moving items, and, if a change in the preferred implant occurs, the excess inventory can often simply be returned to the vendor without financial loss.

The ethics of purchasing is included in the proper training of purchasing agents, because some salespeople make unethical offers of one sort or another to induce purchasing agents or others to select their products. These inducements may be crude (e.g., a cash offer) or more subtle (e.g., a midwinter "business trip" to the vendor's sales headquarters in Florida). When unethical offers are made, consulting with a colleague on how best to deal with the situation is wise. Under some circumstances, a polite "no thank you" is in order. In other instances, it may be appropriate to report the incident to someone higher in the administrative hierarchy of the health care organization.

Many aids are available to help those responsible for purchasing supplies, instruments, and equipment for the OR suite. For example, ECRI is an internationally recognized nonprofit organization that independently evaluates health-care technologies. ECRI publishes many helpful manuals, technical journals, newsletters, and electronic databases. Some of them provide direct comparisons of the features and costs of similar products produced by different manufacturers. (See page 198 for information on how to contact ECRI.)

Whatever the health care organization's formal methods for purchasing, they should interface with the OR's data management system. Purchase orders, back orders, invoices, packing slips, and other sources of data should pass smoothly from one department to the other. The hospital's receiving department should also be integrated with the purchasing function. A well-designed materials purchasing, inventory, and delivery system forms the data-collection foundation for a sophisticated cost-accounting system.

INSTRUMENTS

As many as 200 or more stainless steel surgical instruments, such as clamps, scalpels, and retractors, may be used during the course of a surgical operation. Problems in managing these instruments are similar to problems in dealing with OR supplies. The most important difference is that instruments, unlike supplies, are durable—they are repeatedly reused over their life cycle. The supply system must not only deliver the correct instruments for procedures to the OR, but also recover them after completion of the procedures and process them for reuse. The instrument processing system must be able to convert bloody instruments, perhaps contaminated with pathogenic bacteria and viruses, into clean, fully functional sterile ones. It must also detect and divert for repair or replacement any instruments that become defective.

Instrument processing and management in large and medium-sized hospitals occur in an area often called *central sterile supply*. The function of this part of the hospital is to maintain a supply of sterile instruments used throughout the hospital. The province of CSS includes decontamination and sterilization. When OR instruments are processed centrally, the managers of CSS and of

the OR suite are jointly responsible for controlling the size and composition of the surgical instrument supply.

Instrument Standardization

As with supplies, most facilities standardize surgical instruments into sets that include the items necessary to do different types of cases (e.g., a minor basic set, a major basic set, a major orthopedic set). (See Table 9-1 on page 114.) These sets are developed by OR and materials management staff based on years of experience in picking instruments for cases. Exceptions can be made when necessary by separately wrapping a few idiosyncratic items used by specific surgeons and adding them to the case cart when those surgeons operate. Savings from standardizing instrument sets are large. The cost of a typical surgical instrument set may range from $100 to $10,000 or more. If each surgeon were to have a personalized set of instruments for each operation, the number of instrument sets in stock would be huge, and most of the instruments would sit on the shelves unused on most operating days.

Lists of sample instrument sets are available from instrument manufacturers. Vendors will send consulting teams to hospitals to assist instrument managers with standardization. Such consultations often involve performing an inventory of existing instruments and developing sets based on local needs. New facilities can use the expertise of vendors from the outset and can purchase basic sets rather than individual instruments.

Instrument Processing

From the point of view of CSS, instrument processing begins when the surgical procedure ends. The first step is to decontaminate the instruments to make them safe for further handling. Ideally, the instruments are put back into their pans and run through a washer to disperse tissue and blood. (Some facilities wash the instruments by hand before placing them in the washer.) The automatic washing typically includes a pre-rinse cycle using enzyme treatment, a standard wash followed by a wash using sonic energy, a standard rinse followed by a rinse using an instrument lubricant, and, finally, a drying phase.

The decontaminated instruments must then be inspected for cleanliness and rewashed if necessary. This step is important, because eliminating residual tissue trapped in instruments may be difficult. Next, the functional properties of the instruments must be checked. Scissors should be smooth and nonbinding. Cutting edges must be sharp and free of nicks. Tips of forceps must precisely meet. All components of multi-part instruments, such as complex retractors, must be present. Joints of instruments with moving parts should be lubricated. Finally, the instruments must be reassembled into instrument sets, ensuring that no components are missing. Instrument technicians must have the knowledge and experience to identify defects within a wide range of instrument types.

Instrument Sterilization

Once inspection and assembly are complete, the instrument sets are placed in container systems or in pans that are wrapped in muslin before terminal sterilization. The containers, usually specifically designed for this function, are sterilized with an inner instrument tray that can be pulled out and placed on the sterile back table. Individual instruments are often placed in disposable peel-pack paper wrappers. Stainless steel instruments and their containers are usually sterilized by high-pressure steam. Some facilities use ethylene oxide (EtO) sterilization (see following paragraphs) for delicate instruments or for instruments with lenses.

During the course of surgery, instruments occasionally become contaminated. When this happens, two options are available. If a substitute instrument is available, it may be used and the contaminated instrument taken out of service. If no backup is available, the contaminated instrument may be flash sterilized. Flash sterilization consists of placing an instrument into an open pan and exposing it to high-pressure, high-temperature steam for 3–10 minutes in an autoclave. Flash sterilization is carried out without wrapping the instrument, and the flashed instrument is immediately placed back into service. The autoclave for performing flash sterilization should be immediately adjacent to the OR, because

carrying an unwrapped sterile item through an area in which personnel are not gowned and masked is not consistent with standard sterile technique. (See Substerile Areas on page 186.)

Some types of instruments cannot withstand the extreme heat and humidity of steam sterilization. Most electronic instruments and many instruments containing plastic parts are damaged or destroyed by steam. Several options exist for dealing with such instruments. The most common and oldest approach is to expose these instruments to the toxic gas EtO. Special sterilization chambers are used to perform EtO sterilization safely and economically. However, using EtO has significant drawbacks. The gas is mutagenic, teratogenic, and carcinogenic. Consequently, EtO sterilizers require elaborate safety systems, including a separate room for the sterilizer, a special venting apparatus with vent-failure alarms, and atmospheric EtO detectors located throughout the sterilizing area. Furthermore, personnel working in areas where EtO is used need special training about actions to take should an EtO accident occur. Additionally, locations in which EtO is used are subject to special scrutiny by the Occupational Safety and Health Administration (OSHA).

EtO sterilization has other environmental drawbacks as well. Because of the high flammability of pure EtO, it has traditionally been mixed with Freon 12 to reduce the risk of fire. Research has now shown Freon 12 to be a major contributor to destruction of the earth's ozone layer, and the production of Freon 12 has been dramatically reduced. Some new EtO systems take one of two different approaches: (1) substituting either a different chlorofluorohydrocarbon or carbon dioxide for Freon 12 or (2) mechanically modulating the risk of fire and using pure EtO as the sterilant gas. Each of these options requires extensive (and expensive) retrofitting of existing equipment.

EtO has another drawback that is particularly unfortunate for the attempt to minimize instrument inventory. Because of the toxicity of EtO, it is essential that all the gas be removed from instrument sets before they can be returned to service. The only cost-effective way to remove EtO is through aeration, a process that takes approximately 12 hours. When this delay is added to the 2–3 hours it takes for processing, instruments requiring EtO sterilization can, in effect, be used only once per day.

A newer sterilization technology that relies on the bactericidal and virucidal properties of certain gas plasmas has been introduced by several manufacturers. The instruments to be sterilized are bathed in a plasma generated by exposing relatively nontoxic chemicals, such as hydrogen peroxide, to a high-frequency transmitter similar to that in a microwave oven. Plasma sterilization is relatively inexpensive, has few or no dangerous by-products, requires little or no venting of the sterilizer, and has a 1–3 hour turnaround time. However, some drawbacks exist. Current plasma sterilizers have relatively small sterilization chambers. Although most of the materials used in manufacturing surgical instruments tolerate exposure to the plasma without damage, manufacturers' data sheets may not state that plasma sterilization is acceptable. No generally reliable and nondestructive method exists to determine in advance whether a particular item will be harmed by the plasma. Additionally, the gas may react with a metal in some instruments.

Another, more significant drawback to plasma sterilizers exists. According to the U.S. Food and Drug Administration (FDA), they should not be used to sterilize instruments that have long, narrow lumens. The instruments most affected by this limitation are rigid and flexible endoscopes, such as bronchoscopes, arthroscopes, and urologic instruments. After use, these instruments have traditionally been cleaned and put through a high-level disinfection process by soaking in glutaraldehyde (which is not equivalent to sterilization). Changes in FDA rules require sterilization. In response, yet another device has been introduced: the STERIS system (STERIS Corporation, Mentor, Ohio, <http://www.steris.com>). This device pumps a sterilant through the lumens of properly cleaned endoscopes at a controlled temperature for a prescribed duration, thus meeting the requirement for sterilization. The STERIS cycle takes 25–30 minutes and is performed immediately before the endoscope is used.

Discussion of sterilization technology should not end without briefly mentioning yet another system for sterilizing instruments that can be used with almost any surgical device: gamma radiation. Radiation sterilization is rapid and highly effective. It has two principal drawbacks. First, the gamma source, with its shielding, is large and expensive. Consequently, this method is useful only in high-volume sterilization facilities. Second, radiation sterilization is politically sensitive. Proposals to use gamma radiation to sterilize foodstuffs, while perfectly sound scientifically, have faced substantial political opposition.

The entire field of sterile processing is subject to extensive regulation, both state and federal. Requirements for record-keeping, sterility testing, and training extend beyond the scope of this discussion. The person in charge of CSS must be knowledgeable and up to date about this rapidly changing field. Continuing education and familiarity with current literature is essential.

EQUIPMENT

In addition to supplies and instruments, modern surgery depends on a considerable amount of sophisticated electronic and optical equipment. Modern surgical equipment is complex to operate and to maintain. Consequently, it is generally wise for an OR suite to employ technicians to store, maintain, set up, and operate major pieces of equipment. In most facilities, however, staff nurses set up and operate specialized equipment and arrange for its repair through outside vendors. Some facilities have a department of biomedical engineering to maintain electronic equipment.

Because of the high cost of surgical equipment, availability is usually limited, and systems to ensure equitable sharing are necessary. The equipment required for each case is entered on the preference card and on the common resources list. The scheduling system should communicate equipment requirements to the technicians in the same way that the supply and instrument requirements are communicated to supply and CSS areas.

Some pieces of equipment are not used often enough to justify purchase but are occasionally required for certain complex operations. It may be financially advantageous for the hospital to rent this equipment for single procedures, if possible. To avoid cancellations and delays, requiring delivery of special items before the end of the workday before surgery is a good policy. The manufacturer's representative and the biomedical engineering or OR equipment technician are thus allowed sufficient time to ensure that all required components and supplies have been delivered, that the device is in good working condition, and that the technician understands the setup and operation of the device.

The OR suite's equipment may be maintained either by an in-house biomedical engineering department or by service contracts purchased from manufacturers or distributors. For equipment in widespread use, sending hospital technicians to the manufacturer's maintenance school is probably worthwhile, particularly if the manufacturer offers different levels of maintenance under the service contract. Trained local technicians may permit the selection of more limited maintenance coverage, with consequent cost savings. Complex or unique equipment is almost always best maintained through service contracts with the manufacturer or distributor.

ANESTHESIA SUPPLIES AND EQUIPMENT

The anesthesiology department has supply and equipment needs similar to the OR suite's, but on a smaller scale, because far fewer inventory items are needed. The anesthesiology department has a large amount of equipment requiring technician support, ranging from anesthesia machines to many different types of physiologic monitors. Standardizing anesthesia supplies is usually less of a problem than standardizing surgical supplies because of the smaller number of individuals whose needs must be satisfied. Additionally, less variability exists among the various types of anesthesia than among the various types of surgery. Inventory management can be integrated with the OR's inventory system or operated as a freestanding unit. The problems of supply stocking, inventory management, and cost control are common to surgical and anesthesia supplies. Therefore, both functions may reasonably be managed by the OR suite's materials management personnel.

Because of the similarity between surgical and anesthesia equipment and the difficulty in hiring and retaining suitable technical personnel, having a single group of technicians manage the routine maintenance and setup of both anesthesia and sur-

gical equipment is usually cost-effective. Nevertheless, it is common for the anesthesia department in larger health care organizations to maintain a fully separate and distinct purchasing, inventory, and equipment maintenance system.

PERFORMANCE STANDARDS

Efficient and effective provision of all supplies, instruments, and equipment needed for a multitude of surgical operations day in and day out is a formidable task. Developing a strategy to determine whether the system devised is actually working as intended is essential. To accomplish this, performance indicators must be collected and tracked at critical points in the system.

No fixed rule exists for determining which index of performance is best to monitor. However, it is critical that data collection be ongoing and that the data be monitored regularly to enable delivery of feedback to responsible individuals. At least three variables should be tracked: (1) procedures that were incorrectly scheduled, (2) procedures in which an error in preference card assignment was made, and (3) procedures in which a preference card did not exist. Tracking these three variables identifies most of the communication problems interfering with delivery of correct supplies and instruments to the OR.

Errors in picking instruments or in selecting equipment should also be tracked. When the preference list is correct but the wrong supplies arrive, the problem is in the supply chain, not in the scheduling process. Similarly, the rate at which nonfunctional equipment or instruments are sent to the OR should be tracked. This information may direct attention to systems for identifying defective instruments and equipment or to the performance of technicians who have this responsibility. The rate of returns of unused supplies from the OR should be monitored as a check on the adequacy of the updating of the preference cards.

Finally, the true bottom line, cost per procedure, should be carefully monitored as a gauge of the overall efficiency and effectiveness of OR management. This value should be determined in the aggregate and categorized according to type of operation. (See Costing Methods for Patient Care Services on page

61.) Cost per procedure may also be calculated for different surgeons performing the same operation and can be used for cost-containment purposes.

FURTHER READING

1998 Health Devices Sourcebook. Plymouth Meeting, PA: ECRI, 1998.

PriceGuide. Plymouth Meeting, PA: ECRI, 1998.

Reichert M, Young J. Sterilization Technology for the Health Care Facility (2nd ed). Gaithersburg, MD: Aspen Publishers, 1997.

Smith EJ, Smith YR. Smiths' Reference and Illustrated Guide to Surgical Instruments. Philadelphia: Lippincott, 1983.

Starr M. Materials Management in the Operating Room/ C142901. Chicago: American Hospital Association, 1993.

Steichen FM, Welter R. Minimally Invasive Surgery and New Technology. St. Louis: Quality Medical Publishing, 1994.

Training Manual for Central Service Technicians. Chicago: American Society for Healthcare Central Service Professionals (ASHCSP) of the American Hospital Association, 1997.

Chapter 10

Information Management: Evidence-Based Operating Room Management

It is better to have less thunder in the mouth and more lightning in the hand.

—Apache proverb

ORs have often been managed according to anec-
dotes and to the desires of special interest groups.
In a competitive environment, however, OR management must be based on evidence, and that evidence can be effectively compiled only by using
computerized information systems.

Information management is needed to ensure
appropriate scheduling of operations and efficient
staffing of anesthesiologists, nurses, and support personnel. It is needed to ensure reasonable use of facilities, to facilitate implementation of cost-effective
practices, and to prepare mandatory reports for the
parent health care organization and for accrediting
and regulatory bodies.

Data must be collected and analyzed to identify
opportunities for improvement, to monitor existing
practices for variance from acceptable standards, and
to decrease uncertainty in the process of managerial
decision making. In the medical marketplace, data
are required to document excellence in clinical care
for marketing purposes and to attain and retain managed care contracts. All of these jobs are too complex
and too data intense to be carried out manually. ORs
today cannot be optimally managed without an integrated electronic method for managing information.

INFORMATION SYSTEMS DESIGN

OR information systems are made up of three major
components: (1) computer hardware and an operating system, (2) a database containing the required
information, and (3) the software needed to carry
out various functions (e.g., OR scheduling and cost
accounting). The computer software and hardware
are often collectively called the *operating room
information system* (ORIS), while the database may
be referred to as the *operating room database*
(ORDB).

The ORIS software and the ORDB can reside on
a mainframe computer, on a LAN of personal computers, or on a combination of the two. The system
can be developed uniquely to meet the needs of a
single institution or of a health care system. Alternatively, an ORIS can be purchased from software
vendors who develop electronic management tools
and sell them to health care organizations. An ORIS
is sometimes a component of a comprehensive
medical information system (MIS) installed to meet
the information needs of a hospital or of an entire
health care network.

MEDICAL INFORMATION SYSTEM

The term *medical information system* is applied to many different types of computerized MISs. Historically, most hospitals entered the era of computerized information management by installing an MIS for financial record keeping. The accounting was usually charge based, because payment for hospital services during the early years of computerized information management was based on charges (see the historical background on page 55). Charges for various aspects of patient care were entered into the MIS by data-entry clerks, and the data were aggregated in the financial office to generate patient bills.

With time, MISs gradually began to encompass clinical as well as financial data. A bare-bones clinical information system (CIS) provides for computerized order entry and results reporting. *Order entry* refers to the entry of physicians' orders for patient care (e.g., medications and laboratory studies). Orders can be either entered directly by physicians or transcribed into the computer by clerks from paper-based orders. *Results reporting* refers to the electronic reporting of laboratory or diagnostic results. These reports are often transmitted electronically to the patient-care units and then printed for insertion into the patient's paper-based medical record. The ultimate CIS is a fully electronic medical record, a reality in only a few medical centers, although many others are laying the groundwork for implementing such systems.

Electronic medical records facilitate the keeping of a longitudinal medical record (LMR). An LMR is a comprehensive medical record in which all facets of a patient's medical care—both inpatient and ambulatory—are documented by all providers. Therefore, an LMR is essentially a patient's universal medical record, containing documentation of all encounters with health care providers, no matter where the visit occurred geographically. In practice, LMRs are most likely to be implemented in managed care settings in which integration of each patient's health care is relatively tight and in which a well-defined group of health care providers work within a single organizational structure.

MISs often include satellite systems to meet the specialized information management needs of clinical departments. Early in the evolution of MISs, satellite systems for pharmacies, clinical laboratories, and radiology departments were developed. ORs have more recently begun to receive the atten-

tion they deserve for their intense information needs. MIS-satellite ORISs are becoming more common and are beginning to replace older freestanding and often "home-grown" systems.

A major problem has resulted from the piecemeal manner in which CISs have developed within health care organizations. Purchasers of satellite systems usually selected the "best of breed," without considering the bigger picture, and the satellites were often incompatible with each other. To avoid this problem, newer CISs are designed to comply with Health Level Seven, which is a set of internationally recognized standards for transferring health care information among different computer applications. (See page 199 for information on the organization that sets the Health Level Seven standards.)

OPERATING ROOM INFORMATION SYSTEM

An ORIS is usually a hybrid of financial, management, and clinical information systems. Whatever its exact configuration or origins, the ORIS and the ORDB should possess certain general characteristics (Table 10-1). First, if the ORDB is not a component of the health care organization's MIS, it should be electronically linked to the MIS. Such a link permits bidirectional exchange of information. This means, for example, that patient demographic data from the MIS are readily available when operations are scheduled or reports from the ORDB are prepared. Similarly, the MIS has online access to all of the information in the ORDB. For this bidirectional information exchange to occur, unique identifiers for patients and episodes of patient care are needed in each of the component systems.

Second, an ORDB should be perceived as belonging to the institution as a whole, rather than to any special interest group. Specifically, the ORDB should not be viewed as belonging to the nurses, the anesthesiologists, or (less likely) the surgeons. Perceived ownership is established early in the development of an ORIS, and substantial effort must sometimes be expended to try to assure that the ORDB is not considered to be a resource developed by one professional group or another to achieve or retain power. Nurses and anesthesiologists are often the first to recognize the need to develop an ORIS to achieve efficient OR management; they become

Table 10-1. Essential Characteristics of an Operating Room Information System (ORIS)

The ORIS should be directly linked to the parent health care organization's medical information system.

The ORIS should be perceived as belonging to the institution as a whole, rather than to any special interest group.

The ORDB must have credibility.

Data in the operating room database (ORDB) should be primarily quantitative and amenable to graphical display and statistical analysis.

The ORIS should comprehensively meet the information needs of the OR suite.

All functions in the ORIS should be integrated.

Table 10-2. Functions of an Operating Room Information System (ORIS)

Scheduling
  Patients
    For procedures in the OR suite
    For preoperative clinic visits
    For preoperative diagnostic studies and procedures
      Electrocardiograms
      Laboratory studies
      Autologous blood donations
  Facilities
    ORs
    Procedure rooms
    Ambulatory surgical staging units
    Preoperative clinic facilities
  Personnel
    Work schedules
    Call schedules
    Vacations
Management
  Cost accounting
  Materials management
    Inventory control
    Purchasing
Analysis
  Use of facilities
  Use of other resources
  Costs
Clinical Care
  Surgeons' preference cards
  The OR record (maintained by the circulating nurse)
  The anesthesia record
Communication
  Distribution of the OR schedule
  Tracking cases progressing through the OR suite
  Automatic transmission of digital pages when certain events occur

---

champions for the cause, and others sometimes feel disenfranchised. This conflict can lead to substantial discontent and even disruption.

Third, an ORDB must have credibility. When resources are being allocated or attempts made to modify behavior, those with vested interest in the status quo are likely to try to discredit the data supporting change. Surgeons often believe that they have the most to lose from change (e.g., reallocation of OR time and standardization of supplies and equipment). Anesthesiologists and nurses can also feel threatened by operational changes suggested by data (e.g., extending length of the elective OR day). Methods to ensure that the ORDB contains credible data are discussed in Data Integrity on page 147.

Fourth, as much as possible, data in the ORDB should be quantitative and amenable to graphical display and statistical analysis. Statistical process control (discussed on page 158) is a powerful tool in health care management. Data for analyzing OR processes by this method should come from the ORDB. Although most of the data should be quantitative, explanatory information does have a role. For example, recording delays in the OR schedule from a standard list sometimes excludes important extenuating circumstances. For such situations, a text field in which explanatory information may be entered is helpful.

Fifth, the ORIS should comprehensively meet the management information needs of the OR suite. It should at least be able to perform the functions listed in Table 10-2.

Finally, all of these functions should be integrated. For example, when an operation is scheduled, the OR inventory should be checked to ensure that necessary equipment and supplies are or will be available.

Additionally, equipment and major supply items (e.g., a hip prosthesis) should be earmarked during the scheduling process for use during the operation being scheduled. An order can then be generated to replace major items scheduled for use, or those items can be added to an order that is continuously generated but only periodically transmitted.

Electronic Medical Records

The amount of clinical (as opposed to management) information generated with the ORIS and retained in the ORDB need not be extensive for effective OR management. Only basic information about surgical operations and the anesthetics under which they are performed is necessary for management purposes. On the other hand, to the extent that the health care organization is moving toward a fully electronic medical record, the ORIS should be designed to include the anesthesia record, the operative note by the surgeon, and the information traditionally recorded by nurses (sometimes called the *surgical registry* or the *operating room record*).

Several products for electronically generating an anesthesia record are commercially available. Values are automatically captured from electronic monitoring equipment, such as pulse oximeters, capnographs, and automated blood pressure monitors. Other information, such as concentrations or doses of anesthetic agents, is manually entered by the anesthesia care provider, through either a keypad or a touch screen. The introduction of fully electronic anesthesia machines may eliminate some of this manual data entry. Although speech recognition may become an important method for entering information into electronic anesthesia records, this technology is not yet commonly used.

Those contemplating the purchase of an electronic system for maintaining the anesthesia record should keep one major concept in mind: The most important component of the electronic anesthesia record is the database from which the record is generated, not the anesthesia record itself. The printed or electronic anesthesia record is simply a clinical report from the anesthesia clinical database, prepared according to a conventional format for the anesthesia record. Additionally, information in the anesthesia database should be readily available for inventory control and for generating nonclinical reports on such information as resource use, cost containment, and quality improvement. Data in the anesthesia clinical database should also be used to bill for the professional services of the anesthesia care providers.

To round out the electronic perioperative medical record, the following are needed: the patient's preoperative evaluation (history and physical examination); laboratory data and reports of diagnostic procedures (e.g., electrocardiograms* and pulmonary function studies); the patient's medical condition in the imme-

diate preoperative period; patient consent; preoperative, intraoperative, and postoperative nursing notes (including vital signs and medications administered); and postoperative follow-up information (including patient satisfaction). This collection of information might constitute a complete electronic medical record for a freestanding ASC.

OPERATING ROOM DATABASE

The ORDB, broadly defined, includes several databases that are related to each other (i.e., relational databases). One of them contains information on cases scheduled and performed in the ORs; others are associated with inventory and surgeons' preference lists. (See Preference and Procedure Cards on page 115.) Still others have to do with costs and with scheduling of personnel. For practical reasons, these databases may appear to some users to be separate, although they should function seamlessly with one another, either as components of a single comprehensive database or as separate databases linked through common architecture.

Every database contains records, each of which represents a set of data for a single episode or category. For example, each record in the "operations scheduled/performed" database contains information on one operation scheduled or performed. Included in each record are multiple fields into which specific information is placed. For example, one field contains the patient's last name, another the patient's first name, and another the patient's medical record number. More than a hundred fields may be recorded for each operation scheduled and performed, including such information as the date and time the operation was scheduled; times of the patient's entry to and exit from the OR; names of surgeons, surgical assistants, anesthesiologists, nurses, and STs; *CPT* code(s) for the operation(s) performed; needle and sponge counts; and details on the administration of blood or blood products.

Appendix 1 on page 193 contains a detailed glossary of management data prepared by the Association of Anesthesia Clinical Directors that might be captured for every operation. If this glossary were to be made the foundation for an ORDB, each item in the list would represent a field in the ORDB or could be calculated from primary data fields. This glossary has been heralded as offering a degree of standardization that is required to provide national benchmarks for

---

*As the cost of technology falls, digital renderings of electrocardiograms and information that is viewed and stored in the form of images (e.g., radiographs) may be included directly in the electronic medical record.

efficiency of OR use. Some would argue, however, that highly effective OR management can be achieved without so complex a database. Furthermore, although extensive, the glossary does not include all procedural times that are useful for quantifying OR utilization and efficiency. For example, no entries are related to the timing of activities of support personnel, such as the time at which the case cart is delivered to the OR. Similarly, the arrival times of special items, such as organs to be transplanted or custom prostheses to be implanted, are not included.

In addition to procedural times, a comprehensive ORDB should capture data regarding the scheduling of operations (e.g., size of the backlog of cases to be done, details of all cancellations, and the number of times a surgeon is unable to schedule a case at the preferred time). The ORDB should also contain entries needed for controlling supply costs, such as the specific supplies, instruments, and equipment used in each case. This information could be obtained by linking the ORDB containing details of each case performed with the computer program used for materials management, or by using a comprehensive ORIS that serves both functions.

A list of fields included in the ORDB of UMC appears in Case Study 10-1.

DATA ENTRY

The method by which data are entered into the ORDB depends on the degree to which the availability of computer terminals becomes widespread within the OR suite. When a computer terminal is readily available for every worker in the OR suite (including nonprofessional support personnel), virtually all data entry is performed by the person generating the information. For example, the clerk at the front desk records directly into the ORDB the time the patient transporter is asked to bring the patient to the OR suite and the time the patient arrives. (Alternatively, the transporter could enter these data.) Information traditionally recorded by the circulating nurse, such as the time the patient enters the OR, the instrument count, and estimated blood loss at various times during the operation, is directly entered into the database by the RN documenting the patient's perioperative course. For real-time entry, the computer provides the time the data are entered. Similarly, if an electronic anesthesia record is part of the system, the moment-to-moment physiologic condition of the

patient is automatically entered into the patient's perioperative electronic medical record.

Such a degree of automation is unlikely to be feasible in many of today's OR suites. Therefore, a hybrid of direct and batch data entry is the most commonly used method, at least until higher-level technology becomes more readily available in the OR suite. In batch data entry, a clerk transcribes information into the ORDB from standard paper forms filled out by the people who collect the data. For example, the time the patient is sent for and arrives from the inpatient unit might be taken from the front desk log, the time the patient enters and leaves a specific OR might be taken from the circulating nurse's record, and the time the patient enters and leaves the PACU might be taken from the PACU record. One or more data entry clerks may be needed, depending on how large the OR suite is and how it is administratively organized. In a large suite, a PACU clerk might enter the PACU data and an anesthesia clerk might enter information required for anesthesia billing. In a small OR suite, one clerk is likely to be responsible for batch entry of all relevant data into the ORDB. The importance of having the ORDB on a LAN or on terminals linked to a central computer should be evident, because many persons are likely to be responsible for entering data, and data must be entered at various times—before, during, and after a patient's perioperative course.

An ORDB record for a given case is usually initiated by the scheduling module—that is, a new record in the database is created for a patient at the time the patient's operation is scheduled by the surgeon or the surgeon's agent. Thereafter, various fields in the record are filled in as the information becomes available. At some point, perhaps on the first working day after the day of surgery, all records for a given day of surgery should be evaluated for completeness. The data manager is then responsible for ensuring that incomplete fields in the database are filled in or that an exception is warranted.

REPORT GENERATION

All reports from the ORDB should be generated for a specific purpose, not simply as a matter of routine or for archiving. The principal purpose for reports is decision making. Some progressive organizations periodically apply a decision-making test to determine whether routine reports should continue to be generated. If no management changes

CASE STUDY 10-1. Typical Fields in the Home-Grown Operating Room Database of University Medical Center

This ORDB contains fields serving many functions. When the ORDB was developed, all potential users were invited to submit their recommendations for fields they wished to have included. The only condition was that the groups had to pledge to make resources available for entering the data into all the fields they specified. Making this gesture was not really magnanimous, because storing data is relatively inexpensive. The major expenses are for entering data and ensuring the integrity of the data.

What additional data fields would be useful? How would the data be entered? What data in this list would not be useful in your health care organization?

Last name	Other personnel
First name	Pathology specimen
Medical record number	Microbiology specimen
Account number	Urgency status
Sex	Date of request
Date of birth	Time of request
Date admitted	Date of surgery requested
Time admitted	Estimated duration
Admitting physician	Scheduled date
Preoperative location	Scheduled time
Date of surgery	Time patient called
OR suite	Time transport requested
OR number	Time transport left
Surgical service	Time patient arrived
Preoperative diagnosis	Time surgeon available
Preoperative diagnosis code A	Time anesthesiologist available
Preoperative diagnosis code B	Time nurses available
Surgical procedure	Time anesthesia care started
Surgical procedure code A	Time patient in OR
Surgical procedure code B	Time anesthesia induced
Postoperative diagnosis	Time surgeon in OR
Postoperative diagnosis code A	Time surgical care started
Postoperative diagnosis code B	Time operation started
DRG	Time surgical care ended
Anesthesia procedure	Time surgeon out of OR
Anesthesia procedure code	Time patient out of OR
Anesthesia special monitoring	Time anesthesia care ended
Anesthesia physical status	Time patient out of OR suite
Surgeon	Time into PACU
Assistant surgeon	PACU nurse
Anesthesiologist	PACU code
Anesthetist	PACU patient class
Circulating nurse	Time out of PACU
Scrub nurse or technologist	Discharge destination
Perfusionist	Complications

have been made as a result of a given report during some fixed period (e.g., 1 year), the report is no longer generated.

Reports are valuable not only to suggest changes that ought to be made, but also to determine the effectiveness of changes that have been made. Changes in process should always be reassessed to determine whether they have accomplished what they were designed to accomplish. The decision then becomes whether to retain a change in process because an improvement in efficiency or cost-effectiveness has occurred or to reverse or modify the change because its benefits do not justify the cost.

Many reports generated from the ORDB are standard and are produced on a weekly or monthly basis for routine management purposes. Others are produced irregularly, in response to special requests from within and outside the OR management team. During the first year or so after the development of an ORDB, requests for information usually increase progressively, as people in other parts of the health care organization (e.g., blood bank, laboratories, and residency training programs) realize that the ORDB contains information of value to them in carrying out their jobs on behalf of the organization.

To maximize ease of analysis, most reports from the ORDB should be graphical, reserving the tabular format to provide details when necessary. Most of the necessary graphical reports can be generated using off-the-shelf software packages. Additionally, commercial ORISs are likely to provide methods for generating standard graphical OR management reports. However, some of the more specialized reports may require either in-house or outsourced computer programming. For guidance on designing graphical displays, Edward R. Tufte is a widely acclaimed expert (see Further Reading). Smaller health care facilities are more likely to use standard commercial software.

Reports generally fall into two classes: utilization analysis and cost analysis. These are discussed separately.

OPERATING ROOM UTILIZATION ANALYSIS

OR utilization can be plotted for various time periods, from 1 day to several years. The independent variables can be identifiers of specific ORs; surgical specialty groups; individual surgeons; months, quarters, or years; or times of the day. (The examples that follow should help make this clear.) The dependent variables can be hours of OR occupancy, number of operations, or other units of productivity. In measuring OR utilization, duration of OR occupancy is generally superior to number of operations. An even more powerful dependent variable for measuring productivity is revenues derived from surgical operations performed, if that information is available.

An example of a utilization report is shown in Figure 10-1. Hours of OR occupancy (the dependent variable) are plotted for 17 ORs to display inpatient and ambulatory use month-by-month for an 18-month period. The independent variables are the 17 individual ORs, the classification of patients (inpatient or ambulatory), and the months of the year (not labeled, but identifiable by counting across the bars). These data represent all operations performed during 8-hour OR days. No correction was made for the variable number of working days occurring in various months of the year (owing to holidays and natural variations in the calendar).

The graphs in Figure 10-1 demonstrate that well-used ORs, such as ORs 7, 8, and 9, are occupied nearly 120 hours per month, or approximately 6 hours for each of the nominal 20 working days per month. It can be seen at a glance that considerable OR time is available for increasing surgical volume in rooms 4, 6, and 13. Furthermore, it looks as if improved utilization should be possible in several other ORs. A clear upward trend is visible in the use of OR number 13. Graphs such as these can help identify opportunities for increasing surgical volume or for consolidating operations from two or more ORs into one, thereby reducing fixed (primarily personnel) costs (Case Study 10-2).

Figure 10-2A and 10-2B provide examples of OR utilization for one surgical service by quarter year. For this type of graphical report, plotting both absolute use in terms of hours of OR occupancy (see Figure 10-2A) and relative use as a percentage of the amount of OR time allocated through block booking (see Figure 10-2B) is helpful. The plots showing absolute numbers of OR hours demonstrate trends in use by the surgical service. The plots showing percentage of allocated time used are helpful in determining when allocations of OR time to surgical services need modification (either increase or decrease).

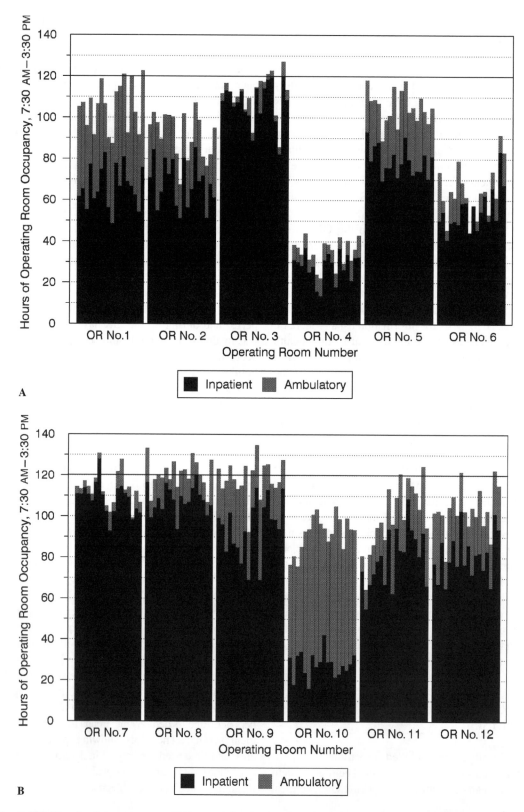

Figure 10-1. Use of each operating room (OR) over 18 months. **A.** Hours of occupancy for ORs 1–6. **B.** Hours of occupancy for ORs 7–12. **C.** Hours of occupancy for ORs 13–17. (See the text for further explanation. Historical data are displayed here to illustrate points discussed in the text.)

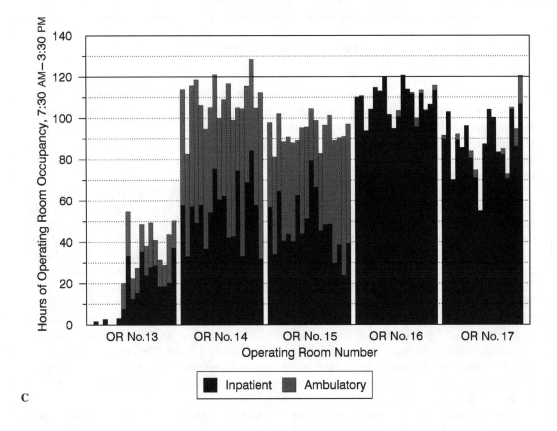

C

Data depicted in the figure show a progressive increase in surgical volume of one surgical service at the hypothetical UMC over a 3-year period. Allocated OR time was increased 25% in year 3, which resulted in some interesting changes in utilization. In the first quarter of year 3, the number of hours of elective cases performed outside allocated time decreased by approximately one-half. Some of this time shifting may have been financially beneficial to UMC, because more realistic elective scheduling tends to minimize overruns of the elective clinical day into overtime hours. Similarly, the number of hours of nonelective procedures performed within allocated time increased by approximately one-third in the first quarter of year 3, with the same potential for financial benefit to the health care organization. Of course, these potential benefits could be offset if the surgical service's unused time cannot be effectively used by other surgical services on an ad hoc basis.

Plots similar to those shown in Figure 10-2A and 10-2B can also be prepared in which OR utilization by all surgical services for a given period (e.g., 1 year) is shown on a single graph. These plots provide side-by-side comparisons of patterns of OR use by the various surgical services. When absolute hours of OR utilization by multiple surgical services are plotted on the same graph, the graph clearly distinguishes high-use from low-use services. A similar graph that shows utilization by multiple services relative to allocated hours can be used to justify reallocation of block time from surgical services that are underutilizing to those that are overutilizing their allocated time. If all services are using a large proportion of their allocated time, the length of the elective OR day may have to be increased or new facilities may have to be built (or, in a health care system encompassing more than one facility, cases may have to be moved to a facility with lower rates of OR utilization).

A particularly useful graphical report is the day picture, which shows the activity in each OR during each hour of the day. This report is produced daily on the morning after the OR day (or call period) being sum-

CASE STUDY 10-2. Evidence-Based Allocation of Operating Room Time at University Medical Center

The CEO of UMC recently contacted the newly hired OR director regarding a complaint received from the chair of the Department of Orthopedics. The chair complained that orthopedic surgeons have been unable to schedule operations in a timely fashion because they are allocated insufficient OR time. His recommendation was that the length of the OR day for his surgical service be increased from 8 hours to 10 hours. The ORs are currently staffed from 7:00 AM to 3:00 PM, and he recommended that they be staffed until 5:00 PM.

The new OR director scouted around the OR utilization files on the computer in his office and found the graph in Figure 10-1. He saw that OR number 4, number 6, and number 13, although fully staffed, are substantially underutilized. He also reviewed the OR allocations and utilization of the orthopedic surgeons and found that some of them were assigned half days of OR time on days when ORs 4, 6, and 13 were underutilized. Therefore, he wrote to the CEO with an analysis of the costs of solving the orthopedic surgeons' scheduling problems by two methods that would accommodate the chair's request: (1) rearranging a number of OR nurses' schedules into 10-hour days or (2) paying overtime when necessary to staff the Department of Orthopedics' ORs until 5:00 PM. Both options increased the OR suite's personnel costs. He also proposed several scenarios through which the needs of the orthopedic surgeons could be met by reallocating their OR time into currently underutilized OR space, at no additional cost to the medical center. The OR director then met with the chair of orthopedics to discuss the options available and their relative merits in solving the orthopedic surgeons' scheduling problems, taking into consideration the perspective of the medical center as well as of the surgeons.

How should the final decision be made regarding how to increase the amount of OR time allocated to the orthopedic surgeons? How should the OR director proceed if the orthopedic chair insists on choosing an option that would increase the OR suite's personnel costs?

marized. The version shown in Figure 10-3 documents the surgical service occupying each OR. Another version of the day picture (not shown) substitutes names of the surgeon and anesthesiologist for name of the surgical service involved with each operation. From this graphical representation, one can readily approximate overall degree of utilization as well as durations of turnover times (time between operations) and how efficiently standby cases were handled. Although the example shown depicts only the hours from 6:00 AM to 8:00 PM, a larger-format day picture can depict activity in each OR during a full 24-hour period.

On the bottom of the day picture, listed at frequent intervals, are the numbers of standby procedures waiting to be performed. One can see from this listing in Figure 10-3 that all of the existing standby cases in this example were accommodated by 5:00 PM. (Standby data should be interpreted with the understanding that an occasional standby procedure is scheduled and then canceled by the surgeon before the case is performed.) Also included at the bottom of the day picture is a running tally of the number of ORs occupied.

Figure 10-4 shows a plot of the numbers of ORs occupied during hour-long periods between 6:00 AM and 6:00 PM. The data cover 13 Mondays over a 3-month period. (Isolating data for specific days of the week is sometimes advisable when considerable day-to-day variability occurs, as when different surgical services have block time on different days of the week.) These graphs are "box-and-whisker" plots in which the median is represented by a horizontal line in the box (bar), the box from bottom to top spans from the 75th to the 25th percentile, the bottom of the lower whisker represents the 95th

Figure 10-2. A. Operating room utilization by one surgical service by quarter year: absolute number of operating room hours used. **B.** Operating room utilization by one surgical service by quarter year: relative number of operating room hours used, normalized according to the number of allocated hours.

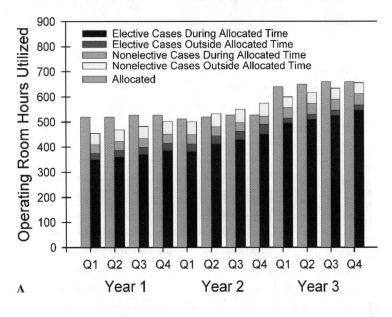

A

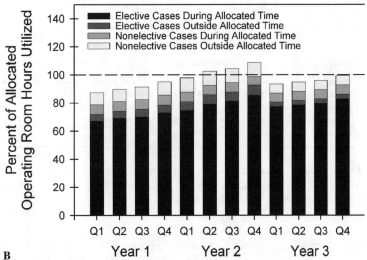

B

percentile, and the top of the upper whisker represents the fifth percentile.

Box-and-whisker plots like the one shown in Figure 10-4 can be used to plan appropriate staffing. For example, if the 13 days plotted are representative of all Mondays, nursing staffing for 14 ORs at 3:00 PM and for 12 ORs at 4:00 PM should be sufficient 100% of the time. With this degree of staffing, however, on average an excess of staff can be expected on 12 of every 13 days. This report provides strong support for introducing a flexible nursing schedule that permits some nurses to leave early

and others to stay late on a voluntary basis. (Usually some personnel want time off, even if unpaid, and others want opportunities to earn supplementary income.) If such a program is implemented equitably, the workers and the business enterprise both can gain substantial benefits.

One useful measure of resource use is the ratio between number of OR teams and number of ORs functioning at any given time of day. With few exceptions, each case requires at least one circulating nurse and one scrub person (together constituting an OR team). Under certain circumstances (e.g., when start-

```
                        Operating Room Day Picture

TIME   6---|---7---|---8---|---9---|--10---|--11---|--12---|--13---|--14---|--15---|--16---|--17---|--18---|--19---|--20   TIME
OR#1   |            PL                      PL                       PL
       |            <****************>      <******************>     <****************************>                   |   OR#1
OR#2   |            G1                      G1                       G1                    G1
       |            <****************>      <****************>       <*************>        <4444444>                 |   OR#2
OR#3   |            NE                       NE                      NE
       |            <****************> <****************> <****************************>                              |   OR#3
OR#4   |            UR                                              G1                    G1
       |            <**********************************>            <111111111111>        <22222222>                 |   OR#4
OR#5   |1111111111>  G1                      G1
       |            <****************>      <***********************************************************************>|   OR#5
OR#6   |            NE            NE                     NE                          NE
       |            <**********> <1111111111111111>      <4444444444444444>          <333333333333>                 |   OR#6
OR#7   |            PV                                   G1
       |            <************************>           <*********************>                                     |   OR#7
OR#8   |            OR
       |            <*******************************************>                                                    |   OR#8
OR#9   |            OR         OR        OR          OR                          OR
       |            <**********> <******> <**********> <**********************> <***********>                        |   OR#9
OR#10  |            OR                OR
       |            <****************> <************************************************>                             |   OR#10
OR#11  |            OR        OR         OR                       OR
       |            <********> <********> <******************************> <***********>                             |   OR#11
OR#12  |            G1        G1                OR
       |            <********> <********>       <33333333333333333333333333333333333333333333333333333333333333333|   OR#12
OR#13  |            G1        G1        G1                       G1
       |            <********> <********> <**********************> <********>                                        |   OR#13
OR#14  |          EN  EN  EN   EN              EN                 EN
       |          <**><**><**> <**************> <***********>     <444444444>                                        |   OR#14
OR#15  |            CT                      EN
       |            <****************>      <2222222222222>                                                          |   OR#15
OR#16  |            CT                              CT
       |            <******************************> <44444444444444>                                               |   OR#16
OR#17  |            CT                              CT
       |            <4444444444444444444444444> <4444444444444444444444444>                                          |   OR#17

TIME   6---|---7---|---8---|---9---|--10---|--11---|--12---|--13---|--14---|--15---|--16---|--17---|--18---|--19---|--20   TIME
STANDBY 6 6 6 6 6 6 5 7 7 7 7 7 8 7 7 7 7 6 6 6 7 6 7 7 6 3 3 4 3 2 2 2 2 2 3 2 2 1 1 0 0 0 0 0 0 0 0 1   STANDBY
ACTIVE  1   1   1   4  16  17  14  17  16  11  16  12  11  12  11  13  14  14  12  10  10   8   8   4   3   3   2   2   ACTIVE

                        Standby Urgency:   1 = Immediate      3 = Within 6 hours
                                           2 = Within 3 hours  4 = Within 24 hours
```

Figure 10-3. Day picture showing the activity in each operating room during each hour of the day. (PL = plastic; G1 = general; NE = neurosurgery; UR = urology; PV = peripheral vascular; OR = orthopedics; OR# = operating room number; EN = otolaryngology; CT = cardiothoracic.)

ing a complex or difficult case), a third person (RN or OR technologist) may be added to the OR team. Although OR teams serve many functions beyond staffing cases, a lower ratio generally reflects more efficient use of labor (Figure 10-5).

OPERATING ROOM COST ANALYSIS

All information used to perform cost analysis should be in the ORDB except payroll information and global institutional information for estimating overhead. Overhead costs must be obtained through the finance department of the health care organization. (See Direct versus Indirect Costs on page 60 and simplified examples of cost analyses on page 65 and page 68.)

Personnel costs are a large portion of the direct costs of running the OR enterprise. To meet reasonable standards of confidentiality, however, salaries of individuals should not be made part of the ORDB. Salary information can be incorporated into OR cost analyses in two ways. The first is to obtain from the payroll department an electronic listing of the pay grades and related salaries and benefits of all OR employees, devoid of information that would identify individuals. The second is to use average or median salaries and benefits for each pay grade, along with the actual pay grade of each OR employee, to account for the costs of personnel. Cost analyses using this information would, of course, not include the professional fees of physicians or others who are not employed by the health care organization.

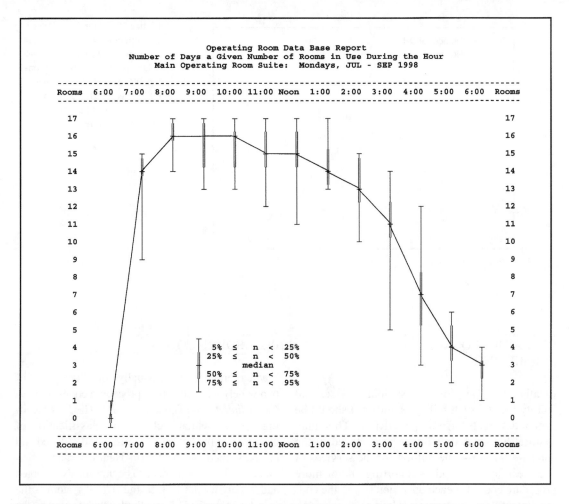

Figure 10-4. Numbers of operating rooms (ORs) occupied during hour-long periods between 6:00 AM and 6:00 PM on Monday between July and September of 1998. On 95% of the days, more ORs were occupied than the number represented by the lower end of the bottom whisker; on 75% of the days, more ORs were occupied than the number represented by the lower end of the box; on 50% of the days, more ORs were occupied than the number represented by the median line; on 25% of the days, more ORs were occupied than the number represented by the upper end of the box; and on 5% of the days, more ORs were occupied than the number represented by the upper end of the top whisker.

MISCELLANEOUS REPORTS FROM THE OPERATING ROOM DATABASE

The types of reports that can be generated from the ORDB are virtually limitless (e.g., reports to central administration of the health care organization, to clinical departments, to accrediting organizations, to regulatory agencies, to residency program directors). As availability of data becomes known throughout the institution, requests for reports usually flow to the ORDB data manager. As mentioned in Data Confidentiality and Security (page 147), the rules set up to govern the ORDB may require approval of an appropriate individual for the release of data.

Not all reports from the ORDB have to be generated in printed form. Some departments or agencies are likely to request raw data (perhaps formatted in some standard way). These reports can be transmitted either on some transportable medium (such as floppy discs, removable hard drives, or CD-ROM) or via LAN, modem, or the Internet. Other agencies and departments will request printed reports, which may require that the data manager or a designee be skilled in preparing printed database reports.

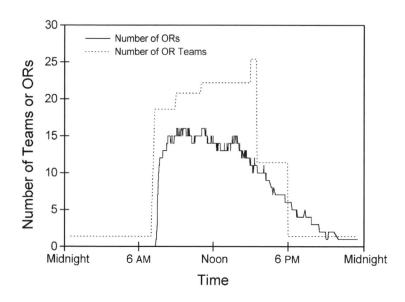

Figure 10-5. Number of scheduled operating room (OR) teams and number of functioning ORs. Where the number of functioning ORs exceeds the number of OR teams scheduled, the personnel deficit is made up through overtime.

OPERATING ROOM DATABASE FOR BILLING

Ideally, all billing for professional services and facility fees (if such billing is allowed) should be initiated directly from the ORDB. This may require that specialized data be captured in the database. For example, billing for the services of anesthesiologists requires reporting one or more procedure codes for each operation (using the coding system in an appropriate relative value guide), the times administration of the anesthetic began and ended, and codes to represent allowable modifiers (such as for extremes of age or for certain procedures). Likewise, the ORDB can be designed to facilitate billing for the professional services of the surgeons.

Using the database for professional billing is appropriate whether the physicians are employees of the health care organization or not. Such an arrangement helps foster physician loyalty while costing the institution little. Data can be made available to anesthesiologists or surgeons who are independent practitioners either by providing direct database access via LAN or modem (using appropriate safeguards for data security) or by issuing periodic electronic reports containing the relevant data on some type of portable storage medium.

PROCEDURE CODES

Medical procedures are usually coded using one of two widely adopted sets of procedure codes: *ICD-9-CM* (*Clinical Modification*) or *CPT*. The *ICD-9* coding system, which includes the classification of diseases and medical procedures, was developed and is maintained by the World Health Organization (WHO). Therefore, it tends to be universally accepted and widely used.* In fact, the *ICD-9* system is the foundation for the DRG method, which is used by the U.S. Federal Government to reimburse hospitals for the care of Medicare beneficiaries. Almost all hospitals use the *ICD-9* system to code discharge diagnoses and procedures performed during a hospitalization.

The *CPT* system was developed and is revised annually by the American Medical Association. Many third-party payers require physicians to code

---

*WHO has revised the *International Classification of Diseases* approximately every 10 years since 1948. A modified version has usually been adopted in the United States 1–3 years after each WHO publication. Based on this schedule, *ICD-10* would have been released in 1987; the first volume of *ICD-10*, however, was not published until June 1992. Before being implemented in the United States, *ICD-10* must be approved by a variety of private and government committees, agencies, and organizations. HCFA has announced that *ICD-10* will not be mandated for Medicare claims until "at least the year 2000."

their bills using the *CPT* system. Some payers require the code number under which an anesthesiologist bills for professional services to match the *CPT* code under which the surgeon bills for the operation. Under these circumstances, the incentive for maintaining a single electronic site for all *CPT* codes relevant to each patient's surgical operation is strong. *CPT* coding done by a trained coder using the surgeon's dictated operative note ensures that the documentation supports the code. This may be required when audits are performed by payers.

Entry into the ORDB of the *CPT* code for every operation performed in an OR suite serves several purposes. First, for utilization analysis *CPT* coding definitively identifies the operation (or operations) performed. Simply entering a set of words into the ORDB to describe an operation (e.g., "sigmoid colon resection") makes precise data analysis virtually impossible, because different words are often used to describe the same operation (e.g., "sigmoid resection"). The importance of using precise data amenable to graphical and statistical analysis was previously emphasized as one of the important characteristics of ORDBs. If historical data are ever to be used to assign estimated durations of operations for scheduling purposes, procedures must be coded in the historical database (see Operating Room Scheduling on page 148). Entering procedure codes into the ORDB also facilitates direct electronic billing from the ORDB for the professional services of surgeons and anesthesiologists.

DATA INTEGRITY

Having accurate data with which to manage the OR suite, as well as for appropriate reporting to outside agencies, is extremely important. Therefore, systematic methods must be incorporated into the ORIS to ensure accuracy.

Some checking for data integrity can be automated. For example, the computer can flag errors in the recording of times of sequential activities—when an OR departure time is earlier than the time recorded for a patient's arrival in the OR, one of the entries is usually incorrect. (An exception, of course, occurs when an operation begins on one day and is completed on the next. Even short operations that start just before midnight are subject to this exception. Having

a database field to indicate that an operation spanned midnight is one way to deal with this exception. A more cumbersome method is to specify date as well as time of completing the operation.) Similarly, an orthopedic prosthesis would not normally be debited from inventory when the operation performed is an appendectomy, and this discrepancy should create an error flag to be investigated by the OR data manager.

Some human review is essential to ensure accuracy of the data in the ORDB. One common method for systematically subjecting the data to human consideration is to generate threshold reports. One threshold report might list all operations with OR occupancy less than 30 minutes or greater than 8 hours for a given week. Some trained individual should review reports of this kind to determine whether the data appear reasonable. If not, additional information should be sought to ascertain whether the suspect data resulted from an unusual circumstance or from inaccurate data recording or data entry. Another useful way to help ensure data integrity is to periodically submit physician-specific data to the physicians themselves for review. Surgeons are usually quick to identify errors in the durations of their operations, and anesthesiologists are almost certain to speak up if they believe that their anesthetic inductions take less time than the durations recorded in the ORDB. Again, the data manager or a designee must look into the suspect data and seek supplementary information with which the suspect data can be either confirmed or corrected.

DATA CONFIDENTIALITY AND SECURITY

Confidentiality of information in a patient's medical record is of utmost importance. When information is recorded and stored electronically, the problems associated with ensuring confidentiality are somewhat different than when a traditional medical record is used. However, the basic principles remain the same. People who have a need to know should have access, and safeguards should be in place to prohibit others from having access to the data.

Although details of electronic data security are beyond the scope of this discussion, a few principles can be mentioned. Well-designed MISs have high levels of built-in data security. They require that electronic signatures (passwords or personal identification numbers) be used to identify not only all persons recording data in the medical record but all persons accessing the record as well. Altering the medical record (through addition, deletion, or other modification) requires a higher level of security clearance than simply reading the record. MISs with the highest level of security retain an archived copy of the record before and after editing and a record of who did the editing. With such systems, not only can the person responsible for making any changes be identified (assuming that a password has not been fraudulently used), but the changes that person made in the record can be reviewed. If electronic medical records are being used in the OR suite, data security is likely to be provided by the parent MIS rather than by the local or satellite ORIS.

Management data in the ORDB, similar to clinical data, must be carefully controlled. At the very least, some responsible person should approve release of reports generated from the ORDB. In smaller facilities, that person is likely to be the OR manager, whereas in larger facilities the responsibility may be delegated to a data manager.

OPERATING ROOM SCHEDULING

In OR scheduling, the ORIS usually functions as an aid to a scheduling clerk rather than as a fully automated scheduling system. In this supporting role, the ORIS provides convenient displays of available future times and dates during which operations can be scheduled in various ORs. The scheduling clerk manually enters the operation to be scheduled into a time slot requested by the surgeon or the surgeon's agent. When a block booking system is used, only time slots allocated to the surgeon being scheduled should be shown on the computer screen. Additionally, the computer program should prohibit scheduling conflicts by locking out conflicting options or at least by reporting conflicts. For example, a surgeon should not be simultaneously scheduled in two ORs (except in teaching hospitals, where this may be permissible), and an operation should not be scheduled for a time at which essential equipment is unavailable. When options are locked out, the system must be flexible enough to permit manual override. Annotation should be included to inform the scheduling clerk why certain options are not being permitted.

Nothing inherent to the scheduling process prohibits surgeons or their agents from directly interacting with an ORIS scheduling system via LAN, modem, or the Internet. The computer program can restrict available choices to block time assigned to the surgeon or to the surgeon's specialty service and can lock out times at which conflicts appear, such as unavailability of necessary equipment or requested personnel (e.g., a particular anesthesiologist). Although the technology reflected in today's state-of-the-art commercial ORISs does not permit bypassing a scheduling clerk, the additional degree of automation needed for surgeons to schedule operations electronically will be a natural step forward as the technology of computerized scheduling matures. (Electronic scheduling of airline travel by customers is already commonplace.)

Patient identification is an important issue when an operation is being scheduled. Ideally, relevant demographic information about the patient will already be recorded in the health care organization's master MIS. If not, ORISs that are linked to the institution's MIS sometimes permit a temporary medical record number to be assigned. Subsequently, when the patient who has been scheduled for an operation makes initial personal contact with the health care organization, such as at a preoperative evaluation (see Preoperative Evaluation on page 107), essential demographics can be obtained and a permanent medical record number assigned through a standard registration process.

Admitting departments are very careful about the assignment of medical record numbers. They usually try to maintain tight control because of the importance of ensuring that one and only one medical record number is assigned to each patient. Furthermore, the admitting department does not want to "waste" medical record numbers by assigning a number to a potential patient that is never actually used because of cancellation of surgery. This is justification for using temporary identification numbers. The need to link the identifying information and other demographics obtained at registration to the OR scheduling module illustrates the importance of direct communication between the ORIS and the institutional MIS.

The OR scheduling module of the ORIS should not discard information on operations that have been canceled before being performed. Rather, the scheduling module should require entry of the date and time a case is canceled, and this information should be retained in the ORDB. Valuable management information is available in these data. Late cancellations sometimes prohibit efficient use of the OR time freed up by the cancellations. Hospital systems may have to be analyzed to identify reasons for cancellations, and policies regarding the timing or performance of preoperative evaluations may have to be changed to minimize cancellations. In some instances, surgeon behavior may have to be modified.

THE OPERATING ROOM SCHEDULE AS AN ELECTRONIC REPORT

The principal report generated by the scheduling module of the ORIS is the OR schedule, which is usually printed. When the technology becomes more mature, printed schedules are likely to be replaced by electronic renditions of the OR schedule, which can be made electronically accessible to all persons or locations currently on the distribution list for daily printed copies, such as surgeons, anesthesiologists, the blood bank, the pathology department, the hospital director's office, instrument processing, and patient transporters. (The list is usually very long.) In this case, the distribution of information in electronic rather than printed form is likely to help preserve patient confidentiality, because printed OR schedules are all too frequently posted in prominent places where people who do not need to know have ready access to them.

When the OR schedule is perceived as an electronic report, "limited editions" that are filtered for certain fields in the ORDB can be "published." For example, the blood bank's edition of the OR can be limited to cases that require action by the blood bank. In some hospitals, the surgeon indicates at the time an operation is scheduled that a certain number of units of blood should be cross-matched for possible use during the operation. In other hospitals, this determination is made automatically, according to an algorithm that factors in characteristics of the operation, the patient, or both (see Blood Bank on page 97). Such an algorithm can be incorporated into the scheduling module.

Similar filters can be applied for other purposes. For example, nurses, surgeons, and anesthesiologists should be able to access information limited to the cases for which they are going to be personally responsible. The PACU should be able to limit the schedule from which it works to patients scheduled for recovery in the PACU (excluding, for example, patients scheduled to have operations performed under local anesthesia or regional block, who normally bypass the PACU). Similarly, the ASU or SDSU and inpatient nursing units should be able to work from schedules that show only those patients for whom they will be responsible. (In each instance, the full OR schedule can be made available for reference.)

When the OR schedule is published electronically, surgeons, anesthesiologists, and others who may not be in the hospital when they need to know should be able to gain access to the schedule from their offices or homes via LAN, modem, or the Internet. Using the same methods of access, surgeons should also be able to electronically review the relevant preference cards for operations they are scheduled to perform (see Preference and Procedure Cards on page 115).

Yet another benefit of using an electronic report for the OR schedule is the ability to update the report in real time. The OR schedule for a given day is forever changing as operations are completed, canceled, or added. The ability to electronically track the progressive and continuous changes throughout the day holds considerable value. Most people are familiar with the real-time displays of airline schedules that are posted on large screens at airports. Similar displays can be located at the front desk of the OR suite, in the doctors' and nurses' lounges, in the PACU, and in other key locations. As with the electronic version of the standard (proposed) OR schedule, physicians and others should be able to access the real-time, continuously updated OR schedule from their offices via modem, LAN, or the Internet. Communication of this type can substantially reduce the need for telephone calls to and from the OR control desk. In fact, a decrease in delays waiting for key personnel may result, because such personnel will have a ready means for estimating when their presence will be required in the OR suite.

SCHEDULING WORK HOURS OF PERSONNEL

The ORIS should be used to schedule all persons who work in the OR suite on a regular basis: anesthesiologists, nurses, and support personnel. These schedules should be integrated and should reflect historical utilization patterns of the OR suite. (See the discussion of Figure 10-4 on page 143.) It is clearly inefficient to have sufficient anesthesia personnel to run four ORs from 3:30 PM to 7:30 PM but only enough nurses to run two ORs, or vice versa. Yet this is often the case in the real world. Such unbalanced staffing can be disruptive, because surgeons often probe to identify the factors limiting their ability to schedule or perform operations. It is unpleasant to hear the complaint—which is often justified—"Why isn't there an anesthesiologist to do my case? A nursing team is available" or "The anesthesiologist is ready. Where are the nurses?"

The working hours of transportation and housekeeping personnel should also be congruent with professional staffing patterns. The easiest way to assure this is by scheduling the working hours of these personnel through the same ORIS staff-scheduling module as is used for professional personnel.

SCHEDULING PATIENT FLOW: PREOPERATIVE USE OF THE FACILITY

The ORs are not the only institutional facilities that should be scheduled through the ORIS. Preoperative and postoperative facilities should be scheduled in concert with the ORs to ensure smooth patient flow. For example, the time of in-house preoperative evaluation, if such evaluation before the day of surgery is thought to be necessary, should be scheduled far enough in advance of the surgical operation that necessary laboratory and diagnostic tests and specialty consultations can be carried out. Failure to provide enough lead time is a common reason for canceled (postponed) operations.

Scheduling the preoperative evaluation at least 2 weeks before the surgical operation usually provides sufficient lead time. If, during the preoperative evaluation, 2 weeks is found to be insufficient time to ensure patient readiness, as when a hypertensive patient has to be referred to the primary care physician for adjustment of an antihypertensive regimen, the previously allocated OR can be freed up in plenty of time to be used for another patient.

Patients should be scheduled for preoperative evaluation by appointment for several reasons: (1) to minimize waiting time for the patient, (2) to ensure availability of sufficient interview and examining space in the preoperative clinic, and (3) to ensure availability of appropriate personnel (e.g., nurses, anesthesiologists, electrocardiography technicians, phlebotomists) to carry out the preoperative evaluation in a timely fashion. Integrated scheduling of the preoperative interview with scheduling of the necessary space and personnel is important.

Some health care facilities may wish to sacrifice efficiency for the sake of user friendliness and provide open hours for walk-in preoperative evaluation. It is still important to ensure that the preoperative evaluation is performed sufficiently far in advance of the operation to permit appropriate additional workup, if necessary, between the preoperative evaluation and the operation.

Scheduling of postoperative facilities should also be integrated with the scheduling of surgical operations. For example, certain types of operations are known to require postoperative admission to the surgical ICU (SICU). Those responsible for SICU admissions must be notified at least 24 hours before anticipated postoperative admissions. Sometimes other patients have to be transferred out of the SICU to accommodate new postoperative patients. Space in the SICU occasionally cannot be made available for elective admissions, requiring surgical operations to be postponed. Early notification of postponement is less disruptive for everyone.

It is likely that not all functions—scheduling operations, scheduling preoperative visits, and scheduling health care personnel for preoperative visits and duty in the OR suite—will be available in most commercial ORISs. Therefore, OR managers may need to request that vendors of OR management software supply the type of integrated scheduling system previously described. Alternatively, and less desirably, individual scheduling software can be purchased (with an eye toward integration) and then integrated by in-house or outside software developers.

FURTHER READING

Bourke MK. Strategy and Architecture of Health Care Information Systems. New York: Springer, 1994.
International Classification of Diseases, Ninth Revision, Clinical Modification (5th ed). Los Angeles: Practice Management Information Corporation, 1999.
Johns ML. Information Management for Health Professionals. Albany, NY: Delmar Publishers, 1996.
Current Procedural Terminology (4th ed). Chicago: American Medical Association, 1999.
Tufte ER. Envisioning Information: Pictures of Nouns. Cheshire, CT: Graphics Press, 1990.
Tufte ER. The Visual Display of Quantitative Information: Pictures of Numbers. Cheshire, CT: Graphics Press, 1992.
Tufte ER. Visual Explanations: Pictures of Verbs. Cheshire, CT: Graphics Press, 1997.

Chapter 11
Standards, Quality, and Consent

We arrive at truth, not by reason only, but also by the heart.

—Blaise Pascal (1623–1662)

In this chapter, we do not attempt to discuss or even to list the myriad of standards that must be known, understood, and applied by the leadership of the OR suite. Rather, in the available space, we identify the major standards-setting organizations and provide an overview of their influence. Additionally, we broadly discuss quality improvement and dedicate considerable attention to informed consent.

STANDARDS

Standards lay at the heart of quality-driven organizations. The OR enterprise is subject to a large number of externally imposed standards covering several key areas. The organizations that have promulgated OR standards are a combination of voluntary and governmental agencies functioning on a national, state, and local level. Some of the key players are listed in Table 11-1.

OPERATING ROOM SAFETY AND OCCUPATIONAL HEALTH

Standards for safety and occupational health involve (1) physical safety, (2) electrical safety, (3) fire safety, and (4) safety with respect to infectious diseases and carcinogens.

Physical, Electrical, and Fire Safety

The National Fire Protection Association (NFPA) is considered by most health care professionals to be the domestic pacesetter for establishing voluntary standards for physical, electrical, and fire safety in health care facilities. NFPA's involvement historically evolved from fire safety to electrical safety to physical safety. NFPA's standards for fire safety are voluntary only to the extent that health care facilities desire eligibility to purchase fire insurance, because adherence to NFPA standards is a virtual requirement for the purchase of fire insurance by health care facilities. Likewise, adherence to NFPA's Standard for Health Care Facilities (NFPA 99), its *National Electrical Code*®*, and its *Life Safety Code*®* are widely imposed requirements for accreditation of health care facilities by accrediting agencies.

The Joint Commission on Accreditation of Healthcare Organizations (JCAHO) makes the following statement in the glossary of its *Comprehensive Accreditation Manual for Hospitals: The Official Handbook* (*CAMH*):

> **Life Safety Code**® A set of standards for the construction and operation of buildings, intended to provide a reasonable degree of safety to life during fires; prepared,

---

*National Electrical Code® and Life Safety Code® are registered trademarks of the National Fire Protection Association, Quincy, MA 02269.

Table 11-1. Organizations That Promulgate Operating Room Standards in the United States[a]

Accreditation Association for Ambulatory Health Care
American Association for Accreditation of Ambulatory
  Surgery Facilities
American Society of Anesthesiologists
Association for the Advancement of Medical Instrumentation
Association of periOperative Registered Nurses[b]
U.S. Food and Drug Administration
Health Level Seven
Joint Commission on Accreditation of Healthcare
  Organizations
National Committee for Quality Assurance
National Fire Protection Association
Occupational Safety & Health Administration
State health codes
State, county, and local building codes

[a]Telephone and fax numbers and mailing and Internet addresses are listed in Appendix 2 (page 197).
[b]Name changed from Association of Operating Room Nurses in April 1999.

published, and periodically revised by the National Fire Protection Association and adopted by the Joint Commission to evaluate health care organizations under its life safety management program.

Detailing the multitude of standards for physical, electrical, and fire safety is beyond the scope of this book. However, an idea of the range of standards is available in Appendices 3, 4, and 5, which present the tables of contents of the NFPA's *Life Safety Code*® (page 203), *National Electrical Code*® (page 205), and Standard for Health Care Facilities (page 207).

Every OR suite should have an evacuation plan for use in the event of fire; Appendix 11-1 (page 163) contains a model evacuation plan for the OR suite.

Bloodborne Infectious Diseases

The gold standard for OR personnel safety with respect to bloodborne infectious diseases is Universal Precautions. These standards were established by OSHA in 1991 in response to increasing concerns about the exposure of health care workers to the hepatitis B virus and the human immunodeficiency virus. Universal precautions are described in a document titled "Occupational Exposure to Bloodborne Pathogens; Final Rule" (standard number 1910.1030), which was published in the *Fed-*

eral Register (#56:64004) on December 6, 1991. "Occupational Exposure to Bloodborne Pathogens; Final Rule" is available from OSHA at the address listed in Appendix 2. It is also available on OSHA's Web site <http://www.osha.gov> and at <http://www.oshaslc.gov:80/OshStd_data/1910_1030.html>.

As with many standards of this type, the federal government's standard number 1910.1030 leaves considerable discretion to the employer in its interpretation. Three citations from the standard illustrate this point:

(b)
According to the concept of Universal Precautions, all human blood and certain human body fluids are treated as if known to be infectious for human immunodeficiency virus, hepatitis B virus, and other bloodborne pathogens.

(d)(3)(ii)
The employer shall ensure that the employee uses appropriate personal protective equipment unless the employer shows that the employee temporarily and briefly declined to use personal protective equipment when, under rare and extraordinary circumstances, it was the employee's professional judgment that in the specific instance its use would have prevented the delivery of health care or public safety services or would have posed an increased hazard to the safety of the worker or coworker.

(d)(3)(ix)
Gloves shall be worn when it can be reasonably anticipated that the employee may have hand contact with blood, other potentially infectious materials, mucous membranes, and non-intact skin; when performing vascular access procedures except as specified in paragraph (d)(3)(ix)(D) [applicable to blood donation centers]; and when handling or touching contaminated items or surfaces.

Similarly, the Recommended Practices for Standard and Transmission-Based Precautions in the Perioperative Practice Setting, published by AORN in its *Standards, Recommended Practices, and Guidelines*, are quite general (Table 11-2). Therefore, each health care organization may want to establish specific policies and procedures for applying these general tenets to individual environments of care.

Airborne Infectious Diseases

Concern about potential for the spread of tuberculosis (TB) within health care facilities has had a resurgence. This heightened concern resulted from several outbreaks of TB in health care facilities, some

Table 11-2. Association of Operating Room Nurses Recommended Practices for Standard and Transmission-Based Precautions in the Perioperative Practice Setting

I.   Standard precautions to prevent pathogen transmission should be used during all invasive procedures.
II. Standard precautions should include use of protective barriers and prompt and frequent hand washing to reduce the risk of exposure to potentially infectious materials.
III. Personnel should take precautions to prevent injuries caused by scalpels and other sharp instruments.
IV. Personnel should handle specimens as potentially infectious material.
V.   Work practices should be designed to minimize risk of occupational exposure to bloodborne and other potentially infectious pathogens.
VI. Personnel who have exudative lesions or weeping dermatitis should refrain from providing direct patient care or handling medical devices used in performing invasive procedures.
VII. Personnel who participate in invasive procedures are encouraged to voluntarily know their HIV and HBV antibody status and disclose a positive status to the appropriate facility authority.
VIII. Guidelines of the CDC Advisory Committee on Immunization Practices regarding HBV immunization should be followed.
IX. Transmission-based precautions should be used in addition to standard precautions for patients who are known or suspected to be infected with epidemiologically important and highly transmissible pathogens. Types of transmission-based precautions include airborne, droplet, and contact precautions.
X.   Policies and procedures that address occupational exposure to blood and body fluids and epidemiologically important microorganisms should be written, reviewed periodically, and readily available within the practice setting.

HIV = human immunodeficiency virus; HBV = hepatitis B virus; CDC = Centers for Disease Control and Prevention.
Source: Reprinted with permission from AORN Standards, Recommended Practices, and Guidelines. Denver: Association of Operating Room Nurses, 1999. (Copyright © AORN, Inc., 2170 South Parker Road, Suite 300, Denver, CO 80231.)

involving multidrug-resistant *Mycobacterium tuberculosis*. Consequently, extensive guidelines have been developed by the Centers for Disease Control and Prevention that include specific recommendations for preventing the transmission of TB from hospitalized patients to other patients or to health care workers. Guidelines specifically directed toward ORs

are listed in Table 11-3. Additionally, a full copy of the guidelines can be found on the Internet at <ftp://ftp.cdc.gov/pub/publications/mmwr/rr/rr4313.pdf>. OSHA's enforcement directive can be found at <http://www.osha-slc.gov/OshDoc/Directive_data/CPL_2_106.html>.

Carcinogens

Concern about potential carcinogens in the OR environment is directed mainly toward smoke emitted during the application of either lasers or electrocautery to malignant tumors or virus-laden tissues. No universal agreement exists regarding the degree to which inhaling this smoke might be harmful to the health of OR personnel. It is generally agreed, however, that several precautions should be taken, including evacuation of the smoke into a vacuum system of the health care facility or into devices manufactured for the purpose of filtering such emissions. Additionally, it is sometimes recommended that OR personnel wear masks that are designed to filter out smaller particles than standard OR masks, including potentially dangerous smoke particles discharged from the ablation of tumors or virus-laden tissues by lasers or electrocautery.

JOINT COMMISSION ON ACCREDITATION OF HEALTHCARE ORGANIZATIONS

The JCAHO deserves special mention because it has the power to determine the destiny of hospitals and many other types of health care organizations. Accreditation by the JCAHO is required for all hospitals receiving reimbursement for the care of Medicare beneficiaries, which makes JCAHO accreditation virtually mandatory. Whether the JCAHO is held in awe, fear, or disdain, its standards must be taken seriously.

The *CAMH* contains not only all of the JCAHO's standards for hospitals, but also a description of its methods for scoring health care organizations to determine whether they should be accredited. The major categories into which the standards are divided are enumerated in Table 11-4. During the 1990s, the standards have been integrated into broader and broader categories. Standards applying to surgery and anesthesia are currently spread throughout the *CAMH*.

JCAHO standards have traditionally focused on health care processes, based on the assumption that

Table 11-3. Centers for Disease Control and Prevention Guidelines for Preventing the Transmission of *Mycobacterium tuberculosis* in Health Care Facilities, 1994

Section II.M: Considerations for Selected Areas in Health-Care Facilities: Operating Rooms
- Elective operative procedures on patients who have TB should be delayed until the patient is no longer infectious.
- If operative procedures must be performed, they should be done, if possible, in operating rooms that have anterooms. For operating rooms without anterooms, the doors to the operating room should be closed, and traffic into and out of the room should be minimal to reduce the frequency of opening and closing the door. Attempts should be made to perform the procedure at a time when other patients are not present in the operative suite and when a minimum number of personnel are present (e.g., at the end of the day).
- Placing a bacterial filter on the patient's endotracheal tube (or at the expiratory side of the breathing circuit of a ventilator or anesthesia machine if these are used) when operating on a patient who has confirmed or suspected TB may help reduce the risk for contaminating anesthesia equipment or discharging tubercle bacilli into the ambient air.
- During postoperative recovery, the patient should be monitored and should be placed in a private room that meets recommended standards for ventilating TB isolation rooms.
- When operative procedures (or other procedures requiring a sterile field) are performed on patients who may have infectious TB, respiratory protection worn by the HCW must protect the field from the respiratory secretions of the HCW and protect the HCW from the infectious droplet nuclei generated by the patient. Valved or positive-pressure respirators do not protect the sterile field; therefore, a respirator that does not have a valve and that meets the criteria in Section II.G should be used.

Section II.G: Respiratory protective devices used in health-care settings for protection against *M. tuberculosis* should meet the following standard performance criteria:
- The ability to filter particles 1 µm in size in the unloaded* state with a filter efficiency of ≥95% (i.e., filter leakage of ≤5%), given flow rates of up to 50 L per minute.
- The ability to be qualitatively or quantitatively fit tested in a reliable way to obtain a face-seal leakage of ≤10%.
- The ability to fit the different facial sizes and characteristics of HCWs, which can usually be met by making the respirators available in at least three sizes.
- The ability to be checked for facepiece fit, in accordance with standards established by the Occupational Safety and Health Administration (OSHA) and good industrial hygiene practice, by HCWs each time they put on their respirators.

TB = tuberculosis; HCW = health care worker.
*Some filters become more efficient as they become loaded with dust. Health care settings do not have enough dust in the air to load a filter on a respirator. Therefore, the filter efficiency for respirators used in health care settings must be determined in the unloaded state.
Source: Adapted from Centers for Disease Control and Prevention. Guidelines for preventing the transmission of *Mycobacterium tuberculosis* in health-care facilities, 1994. MMWR Morb Mortal Wkly Rep 1994;43(RR-13):1-132. Available at <http://www.cdc.gov/epo/mmwr/preview/mmwrhtml/0035909.htm> and at <ftp://ftp.cdc.gov/pub/publications/mmwr/rr4313.pdf>.

certain processes are essential to maintaining high quality patient care. Although never scientifically validated, this premise is widely accepted. The JCAHO generally does not dictate how specific processes should be carried out. Rather, it requires health care organizations to establish policies that ensure appropriate processes in clearly defined realms and to document or otherwise demonstrate that those policies are upheld. For example, the intent of the first standard in the *CAMH* ("The hospital addresses ethical issues in providing patient care") is explained as follows:

A mere listing of patient rights cannot guarantee that those rights are respected. Rather a hospital demonstrates its support of patient rights through the processes by which staff members interact with and care for

patients. These day-to-day interactions reflect a fundamental concern with and respect for patients' rights. All staff members are aware of the ethical issues surrounding patient care, the hospital's policies governing these issues, and the structures available to support ethical decision making.

Expanding beyond processes, the JCAHO has begun to formally recognize the importance of considering outcomes of health care. Consequently, JCAHO standards are evolving toward judging performance of health care organizations through outcomes measurement. Requirements for performance measurement are gradually being increased and are elaborated in recent revisions of the *CAMH*.

Performance measurement assesses both processes and outcomes. The JCAHO has no intention of abandoning the assessment of process, largely because it recognizes that measuring outcomes is more difficult than evaluating processes. Good reason exists to believe that outcomes are strongly linked to processes—at least, it seems obvious that good processes are more likely to lead to good outcomes than bad processes. A hybrid approach to measuring quality is probably superior to assessing only processes or only outcomes.

That virtually every JCAHO category has relevance to the care of patients in the OR suite is evident from the classification of standards shown in Table 11-4. Therefore, well-informed OR managers should have a copy of the *CAMH* at arm's reach in their offices and should familiarize themselves with its contents. If the OR manager knows the standards, and if the policies and procedures of the OR suite are designed to reflect the broad intent of the JCAHO standards, the traditional flurry of activity preceding a JCAHO survey should be unnecessary. Instead, the JCAHO's visit should be viewed as an opportunity to receive external validation of the quality of the OR enterprise and to learn where opportunities exist to improve structure, function, and outcomes.

Table 11-4. Classification of Standards of the Joint Commission on Accreditation of Healthcare Organizations

Patient-focused functions
    Patients' rights and organization ethics
    Assessment of patients
    Care of patients
    Education
    Continuum of care
Organization-focused functions
    Improving organization performance
    Leadership
    Management of the environment of care
    Management of human resources
    Management of information
    Surveillance, prevention, and control of infection
Structures and functions
    Governance
    Management
    Medical staff
    Nursing

Source: Adapted from Comprehensive Accreditation Manual for Hospitals: The Official Handbook. Oakbrook Terrace, IL: Joint Commission on Accreditation of Healthcare Organizations, 1999.

MEDICAL DEVICE TRACKING

In 1990, Congress enacted the Safe Medical Devices Act (SMDA), which requires health care facilities to notify manufacturers of the "receipt, distribution, and permanent disposal" of certain medical devices. The purpose of medical device tracking is to enable manufacturers to identify, locate, and notify patients if a medical device is found to have a serious defect requiring some action. Under SMDA, the FDA regulates "FDA-designated devices" and "permanently implantable devices whose failure would be reasonably likely to have serious adverse health consequences." A permanently implantable device is defined as "a device that is intended to be placed into a surgically or naturally formed cavity of the human body to continuously assist, restore, or replace the function of an organ system or structure of the human body throughout the useful life of the device." Table 11-5 offers examples of permanently implantable devices.

According to regulations issued by the FDA under SMDA, "implanting facilities" (final distributors) are required to provide information to the manufacturer three times: on receipt of the device, on implantation, and on explanation or permanent disposal of the device (e.g., patient death or permanent discarding). The information that must be sent to the manufacturer at these times is listed in Table 11-6. Failure to comply with these reporting requirements can lead to penalties as high as $1 million.

Table 11-5. Permanently Implantable Medical Devices That Require Tracking Under the Safe Medical Devices Act of 1990, as Revised

Temporomandibular joint prosthesis
Glenoid fossa prosthesis
Mandibular condyle prosthesis
Implantable pacemaker pulse generator
Cardiovascular permanent pacemaker electrode
Replacement heart valve
Automatic implantable cardioverter/defibrillator
Implanted cerebellar stimulator
Implanted diaphragmatic/phrenic nerve stimulator
Implantable infusion pumps

Source: Adapted from Guidance on Medical Device Tracking. <http://www.fda.gov:80/cdrh/modact/tracking.html>. Document issued Feb. 12, 1999.

Table 11-6. Information That Must Be Provided to the Manufacturer of Permanently Implantable Devices According to U.S. Food and Drug Administration Regulations

On purchase or acquisition
  Facility's name and address
  Lot, batch, model, and serial number or other device identifier
  Date the device was received
  Person from whom the device was received
On implantation
  Facility's name and address
  Lot, batch, model, and serial number or other device identifier
  Name, address, telephone number, and Social Security number (if available) of the patient receiving the device
  Date the device was provided to the patient
  Name, address, and telephone number of the prescribing physician
  Name, address, and telephone number of the physician who regularly follows the patient
On explantation or permanent disposal
  Facility's name and address
  Lot, batch, model, and serial number or other device identifier
  Name, address, telephone number, and Social Security number (if available) of the patient from whom the device was explanted
  Date the device was explanted
  Name, address, and telephone number of the explanting physician
  Date of the patient's death (if applicable)
  Date the device was returned to the manufacturer or distributor, permanently retired from use, or otherwise permanently disposed of (if applicable)

Source: Adapted from Guidance on Medical Device Tracking. <http://www.fda.gov:80/cdrh/modact/tracking.html>. Document issued Feb. 12, 1999.

QUALITY IMPROVEMENT

For an introduction to the role of the OR leadership in establishing a program of quality improvement in the OR suite, see Total Quality Management on page 75.

Quality improvement is based on the following premises:

1. The workers in a workplace are doing their best to do their jobs as they understand them.
2. The system under which everyone is working is the principal factor controlling quality.
3. "The system" is under the control of management.
4. The workers are in the best position to identify problems in quality and to recommend changes

in the system to permit them to do their jobs more effectively.
5. The system is largely made up of interactions between all workers, both professional and support.
6. Each worker (professional and support) is sometimes a "supplier" and sometimes a "customer" in an interaction with a coworker. All transactions between workers involve an "internal supplier" and an "internal customer."
7. Clear communication between internal customers and internal suppliers is key to ensuring that the system works. Internal customers should ensure that their needs and expectations are clearly communicated to internal suppliers, and internal suppliers are responsible for ensuring that they clearly understand the needs and expectations of their internal customers.
8. Trade-offs of responsibility for patient care are key locations for communication problems between internal customers and internal suppliers and, consequently, are important points at which to identify opportunities for quality improvement.
9. *High quality* is defined as "meeting or exceeding the needs and expectations of the customer." This definition applies equally to the internal customer within a health care system and to the ultimate customer of health services, the patient.

In an environment such as the one described, in which quality is explicitly defined and the system, rather than the performance of individual workers, is considered the principal target for improving quality, a formal mechanism for quality improvement assumes the following characteristics:

1. The mechanism for quality improvement is multidisciplinary, involving workers at all levels in the hierarchy: physicians, nurses, administrators, direct support personnel (e.g., transportation and housekeeping), and indirect support personnel (e.g., laboratory, pharmacy, and blood bank).
2. It focuses on failures of the system to support the best effort of the workers to do their jobs.
3. It does not focus on failures of individual workers to do their jobs according to reasonable standards (which, for support personnel, are often defined in job descriptions). Deficiencies in the performance of an individual worker are handled administratively, by supervisors of support personnel and by the OR suite's professional leadership (the OR nurse manager and the chiefs of

clinical services, such as anesthesiology, general surgery, and orthopedics, whose physicians work in the ORs). Quality improvement is not aimed at improving performance of individual workers. It is not designed to identify and weed out "bad apples." Problem workers contribute relatively little to quality problems in the OR suite.

Administrative Structure Supporting Continuous Quality Improvement

The OR suite should have one person through whom all information relevant to quality of patient care flows. Even in large OR suites, this role is likely to be just one part of the quality coordinator's job description. The designated person should have a broad understanding of the way the OR suite functions and of the roles of all professional and support personnel in making things run. An RN often assumes the role of quality coordinator (or some equivalent title).

Quality improvement activities should involve substantial interaction among workers with various roles; the workers are responsible for the processes in which quality problems are likely to occur. They are best able to help identify systems problems and how to correct them. This analysis usually takes place in regular meetings of the quality improvement committee, to which the quality coordinator brings an agenda of items for analysis and discussion. The task list prepared at the end of such meetings might include collecting and plotting data to learn more about a given problem (see the discussion of plotting techniques in Conventional Continuous Quality Improvement Process: Pareto Diagrams and Statistical Process Control Charts) or implementing changes based on previous analysis and discussion.

Whether the quality coordinator or the OR director or nurse manager chairs the meeting depends on local preferences and traditions. However, the leader of the OR suite must be an active player in the OR suite's quality improvement program. That person must make it clear to everyone in the organization that the goal of quality improvement is not to identify and weed out problem personnel, but to identify and correct systems problems.

The multidisciplinary OR quality improvement program should be integrated with departmental quality improvement programs—principally nursing, anesthesiology, and surgery, but also such departments as pathology, radiology, housekeeping, and transportation—through representatives who are members of OR and departmental committees. Periodic joint meetings of the committees aid integration.

IDENTIFYING OPPORTUNITIES FOR SELF-IMPROVEMENT IN THE SYSTEM

Fear

Creating a work environment that is amenable to self-improvement is an essential role of OR leadership. Most workers, both professional and support, have been inculcated during their formative years with a deep-seated fear of being blamed if things go wrong: "If you don't do it right, I'll write you up." This threat is effective only as long as a written incident report is perceived by the organization's leadership to be a tool for identifying bad actors rather than bad systems.

Fear of being blamed when things go wrong should be targeted for extinction by the OR leadership. One of the most important of Deming's 14 points (see Table 6-1 on page 76) is "Drive out fear, so that everyone may work effectively for the company." Fear of adverse consequences after identifying problems (being blamed) is anathema to self-improvement in the OR suite.

Once a fearless environment is established, it is remarkable how freely opportunities for improvement are identified by the workers. "It's a systems problem" becomes a common assertion, and this statement is probably true more than 90% of the time. Much of the inservice training on quality improvement should be dedicated to helping the OR staff understand how systems problems contribute to poor quality. This educational process should be ongoing and never ending.

Conventional Continuous Quality Improvement Process: Pareto Diagrams and Statistical Process Control Charts

A 12-step approach to improving quality is detailed in Appendix 11-2 (page 165), with an example of how this process can be applied. Opportunities for improvement can often be identified by judicious plotting of data. Two particularly valuable graphical displays are Pareto diagrams and statistical process control charts.

Vilfredo Pareto was a nineteenth-century Italian economist and sociologist who in 1896 published a mathematical law describing distribution of wealth that has been widely interpreted as showing that 80% of a population's wealth is possessed by 20% of the population. A similar principle relevant to quality improvement was expounded by Willie Sutton when he was asked why he robbed banks: "That's where the money is!" Pareto diagrams are bar graphs showing frequency of various events and ordering them from highest to lowest frequency. These diagrams are used to identify "where the money is," so that analytic and remedial efforts can be efficiently directed. (See Figure A11-2B on page 167 for an example of a Pareto diagram.)

Statistical process control charts are plots of the frequency of events along a time line. They show hour-to-hour, day-to-day, week-to-week, month-to-month, or year-to-year variation in the frequency of events. Control charts help to identify whether an event (e.g., on-time start for first operation of the day, postoperative wound infection, or instrument pans requiring resterilization because of breaks in sterile packaging) is occurring significantly more or less frequently over time.

A certain amount of variation in the rate of events over time is normal. Expected random variation is sometimes called *common-cause variation*, and trends or periodic departures outside expected control limits are called *specific-cause variations*. Specific causes for the trends or departures should be sought out. Statistical process control charts are usually used to determine whether processes are "in control" (i.e., whether the frequency of adverse events is stable—having variation constrained within specified control limits). Control charts can also be used to demonstrate trends over time, showing either deterioration or improvement in performance. The two statistical control charts in Appendix 11-2 (page 166 and page 168) illustrate a process that was in control before and after an intervention substantially reduced the frequency of an adverse event.

INFORMED CONSENT

Informed consent is an imperative of medical ethics. The doctrine stems from the principle of self-determination or autonomy, which is defined as the right of individuals to make decisions for themselves based on their personal values. Acceptance of this ethical principle is sufficiently universal that adherence to the requirement for informed consent is embodied in laws enforced by many governmental jurisdictions and in standards generated by many voluntary standards-writing organizations. Hospitals and other health care organizations usually have specific policies regarding informed consent based largely on externally imposed laws and standards.

Informed consent is considered by many health care providers (and by most hospital attorneys) to be primarily a legal doctrine. It is a legal doctrine, but only to the extent that the law reflects the ethical standards of society. When ethical and legal considerations appear to be in conflict, the ethical consideration should be given preference. That is, if a course of action is in the best interest of the patient, but some would deem that action not to be in strict compliance with the law, the decision on what should be done should be weighted strongly in favor of what is best for the patient (Case Study 11-1).

OR personnel must clearly understand the policies regarding informed consent in their particular health care organizations and should be generally familiar with the laws and standards on which the policies are based. An important part of an OR manager's job is to make certain that appropriate policies governing informed consent are followed in the OR suite. The OR manager should be an arbiter and a definitive source of knowledge in matters involving informed consent. When indicated, legal counsel should be consulted.

Consent Forms

Whether informed consent is documented with a written form or with a note entered into the medical record by a physician is based on local legal requirements and tradition. Some authorities advocate use of detailed written consent forms in which as many adverse outcomes as can be contemplated are listed and described. Others advocate that a physician simply record in the medical record that the risks of the procedure have been explained to the patient along with alternative forms of therapy and their attendant risks, and that the patient consents to the planned procedure. The JCAHO standards are not specific: "Anesthesia options and risks are discussed with the patient and family prior to administration" (TX.2.2);

CASE STUDY 11-1. Legal Informed Consent at Community Medical Center

Eight-year-old Jeremy was brought by his father to CMC because of high fever and vomiting. Acute appendicitis was diagnosed, and the child was scheduled for an appendectomy. After the surgeon obtained the father's written consent for the procedure, a nurse in the PHU noticed that the father's surname was different from the patient's. When inquiries were made, the parent turned out to be Jeremy's stepfather, who had not yet adopted his wife's child from a previous marriage. The patient's mother, who had legal custody of Jeremy, was on a safari in Africa and was unavailable to give telephone consent.

To delay Jeremy's appendectomy until his mother could be located to give informed consent would clearly not be in the patient's best interests. Hence, the surgery should have proceeded in the absence of a legally ironclad informed consent. However, if the scenario had been, "Eight-year-old Jeremy was brought by his stepfather to CMC for bilateral tympanotomy and insertion of pressure equalizing tubes," with all other facts the same, would the prudent decision have been different? (In general, the more elective the surgical procedure, the more rigorous should be the efforts to obtain legally sound informed consent.)

"Before obtaining informed consent, the risks, benefits, and potential complications associated with procedures are discussed with the patient and family" (TX.5.2); "Alternative options are considered" (TX.5.2.1).*

Written consent forms usually have space for the patient and the physician to sign and date the document. The patient's signature signifies that the patient understands the risks and alternatives and has consented to the procedure. The physician's signature signifies that the physician has explained the risks and alternatives to the patient. Sometimes space is allowed for the signature of a witness. Unless specifically indicated on the consent form, the meaning of a witness's signature is ambiguous—it may mean that the witness observed the patient's signature, or it may mean that the witness observed the explanation given by the physician, questioning by the patient, and signing by the patient and physician. It is advisable for a written consent form to state explicitly what all signatures signify, including those of the patient and the physician.

Ensuring that the patient has signed an appropriate consent for the surgical operation has always

been a joint responsibility of the surgical team (surgeon, anesthesiologist, and circulating nurse). Increasing emphasis has been placed on ensuring that the correct side of the body (e.g., right leg vs. left leg) is identified not only on the consent form, but also in the OR just before surgery commences. Most policies designed to eliminate wrong-side surgery require that OR personnel verify the correct site of surgery with the patient and ensure that the patient's statement is consistent with the written consent. A more rigorous approach requires that some type of indelible mark be made on the body at the site of surgery by the surgeon before induction of anesthesia so that the patient can participate in this positive means of identification. The mark should be visible after the surgical field has been prepped and draped.

Consent for Surgical and Anesthetic Procedures

The surgeon and the anesthesiologist are responsible for obtaining consent for the surgical and anesthesia procedures, respectively. Ideally, informed consent for the surgical procedure should be obtained when the decision to perform the procedure is made jointly by surgeon and patient. Some hospitals discharge their legal responsibility to patients regarding informed consent by having a written policy stating that scheduling an operation by a surgeon

---

*Comprehensive Accreditation Manual for Hospitals: The Official Handbook. Oakbrook Terrace, IL: Joint Commission on Accreditation of Healthcare Organizations, 1999.

(or the surgeon's agent) constitutes assurance by the surgeon that appropriate informed consent has been obtained for the scheduled operation.

Consent for Blood or Blood Products

Until the late 1990s, standards for informed consent were for the most part silent on the issue of administration of blood and blood products. One exception to this silence has been the long-standing recognition by hospitals that some patients express the desire not to be given any blood or blood products (see Denial of Permission to Administer Blood or Blood Products). The JCAHO requires that hospitals meet the following standard for accreditation: "Discussions with the patient and family about the need for, risk of, and alternatives to blood transfusion when blood or blood components may be needed are considered" (TX.5.2.2).

Hence, a consent form for procedures performed in the OR suite must contain explicit language dealing with consent for the administration of blood or blood products, if such administration is likely to be required during the surgical procedure to which the patient is consenting.

The surgeon is usually responsible for obtaining consent for blood transfusion, because surgeons are in the best position to be able to predict whether blood transfusion may be required by the nature of the surgery. Similarly, the surgeon should determine whether autologous blood donation is indicated and discuss the indications with the patient. Even though the anesthesiologist usually administers blood or blood products during surgical operations, the surgeon is the logical person not only to obtain consent for blood transfusion, but also to arrange for autologous* or directed donation,[†] which must often be planned weeks ahead of the operation in which the blood will be transfused.

Autologous blood refers to the patient's own blood. When autologous blood transfusion is contemplated, the patient donates blood at prescribed intervals (e.g., every 2 weeks), and the blood is frozen until the patient needs it.

[†]*Directed donation* is the donation of blood by a relative or acquaintance of the patient who has a blood type compatible with the patient's. The blood is then reserved for transfusion to the patient, if needed.

Denial of Permission to Administer Blood or Blood Products

Some patients do not want to receive any blood or blood products. This restriction is often handled by having the patient sign a special form designed expressly for the purpose of declaring that the patient does not consent to receive blood therapy and understands and accepts the potential adverse consequences of this denial of permission. A generic form used for this purpose appears in Appendix 11-3 (page 169).

An additional problem sometimes arises when a patient specifies that no blood or blood products are to be administered and the surgical procedure carries a relatively high probability of considerable blood loss (e.g., repair of an abdominal aortic aneurysm). Some nurses or anesthesiologists may have personal ethical concerns that a conflict may arise between commitment to the patient's desire and preventing the patient's death. If OR personnel think that making such a commitment to a patient is unethical, those personnel should not be required to participate in the operation, especially if it is electively scheduled.

Do Not Resuscitate

Automatically discontinuing do-not-resuscitate (DNR) orders when a patient came to the OR suite for a surgical procedure was once a virtually universal practice in the United States. The reasoning behind this tradition was that patients consented to DNR status because they did not wish to be resuscitated from cardiopulmonary arrest resulting from fatal disease. However, consent for DNR rarely included a directive regarding resuscitation from a condition precipitated by medical care in the OR, such as sudden and unexpected blood loss or temporary overdose of anesthetic. Hence, it was previously concluded that DNR orders were, de facto, invalid in the OR, and therefore they were discontinued.

Principles of medical ethics have, however, matured on this issue. The American Society of Anesthesiologists in 1993 developed and adopted *Ethical Guidelines for the Anesthesia Care of Patients with Do-Not-Resuscitate Orders or Other Directives That Limit Treatment* (Appendix 11-4, page 170), and in

---

CASE STUDY 11-2. "Do Not Resuscitate" during Emergency Surgery at Community Medical Center

A woman with preterminal liver disease is rushed to the OR suite at CMC in the middle of the night for control of gastrointestinal bleeding, and the patient is in a confused state of mind because of her liver disease and recent bouts of hypovolemia and hypoxemia. The patient had signed a DNR directive stating that she does not want to receive cardiopulmonary resuscitation or other extraordinary treatment, such as mechanical ventilation or kidney dialysis, to prolong her life. No family member is available with whom to consult. Should the patient's previously declared desire not to be resuscitated be honored in the OR?

This question is complicated, because the surgery itself might be considered a violation of the advance directive. Beyond that, the decision about whether to perform cardiopulmonary resuscitation during the operation might reasonably be based on the surgeon's and anesthesiologist's judgment about whether the precipitating event is most likely a result of the patient's disease or of the anesthetic or surgical intervention. In the former situation, resuscitation should be withheld according to the DNR directive.

1995 AORN developed and adopted the position statement *Perioperative Care of Patients with Do-Not-Resuscitate (DNR) Orders* (Appendix 11-5, page 172). These and similar ethical guidelines may impose a substantial burden on OR personnel because of ambiguities associated with a DNR order (Case Study 11-2).

To avoid procedural problems in the OR associated with nonspecific DNR orders, either the surgeon or the anesthesiologist should revisit the issue of DNR with the patient as part of preparation for surgery. The difference between cardiopulmonary arrest caused by the patient's fatal disease and cardiopulmonary arrest caused by temporary and often easily reversible complications of the anesthetic or operation should be explained and the DNR order amended to include or exclude specific interventions that are likely to be part of the anesthetic or operative procedures, such as tracheal intubation, mechanical ventilation, and invasive monitoring. The OR leadership might want to put in place a policy requiring review and revision, if necessary, of all DNR orders before patients with such orders are brought to the OR suite for surgery.

Here again, ethical issues may arise in the minds of some OR personnel who consider it unethical to withhold resuscitative measures in the OR. When feasible, these concerns should be dealt with by substituting personnel who are in agreement with the appropriateness of decisions that have been made regarding withholding resuscitation.

Emergency Surgery with Lack of Consent

Operations must sometimes be performed expeditiously to save the life, limb, or vital organs of patients. When circumstances preclude obtaining appropriate informed consent, a surgeon's note in the chart, stating that the patient's welfare demands the surgical intervention, is generally accepted to be sufficient.* Circumstances vary in different jurisdictions, however, and advice of counsel is always warranted when any doubt exists.

Informed Consent under the Influence of Hypnotic Drugs

Prudent anesthesiologists ensure that appropriate consent for the surgical procedure is in the medical record before administering any sedative or hypnotic drugs during the immediate preoperative period. (In some jurisdictions, anesthesiologists are held accountable for ensuring that a proper consent is present.) If consent has not been obtained before the

---

*The intent of TX.5.2 through TX.5.2.2, the JCAHO's standards for informed consent in the *CAMH*, states, "Patients [should] receive adequate information to participate in care decisions and provide informed consent. *If the patient's condition does not allow for such interaction, appropriate documentation is provided in the medical record.*" (Italics added for emphasis.)

CASE STUDY 11-3. Informed Consent from a Sedated Patient at Freestanding Surgical Center

A nurse in the preoperative unit of FSC informed an anesthesiologist by telephone that the next patient scheduled for the OR in which he was working had an admission blood pressure of 195/105 mm Hg. The patient, who had no history of hypertension, was very anxious about her impending vein stripping. The anesthesiologist gave the nurse a verbal order for an intravenous dose of midazolam for sedation, which brought the patient's blood pressure down to 165/95 mm Hg. It was subsequently discovered that the patient had not yet given written consent for the operation. When the surgeon and anesthesiologist went to the bedside, they decided that the anesthesiologist should administer flumazenil to counteract the sedative effects of the midazolam before the patient signed the consent form.

The operation went well. However, the patient subsequently had persistent pain in her legs at the site of surgery and filed a malpractice suit against the surgeon, the anesthesiologist, and the surgical center. The patient asserted that she had not been informed that persistent pain was a possible consequence of the vein stripping and that, if she had been so informed, she would not have consented to the procedure. She further alleged that her consent for the operation had been obtained improperly while she was under the influence of a sedative drug.

Although the patient would not likely be awarded damages for her alleged adverse outcome under normal circumstances, would uncertainty about whether the consent had been legally obtained be likely to tilt the legal balance in favor of the plaintiff? Because of the elective nature of the surgery, would postponing the operation in the absence of legally sound consent have been more prudent, even though postponement would have inconvenienced the patient?

---

patient has been sedated, or if the surgeon decides at the last minute to modify the surgical plan, questions arise about whether a patient can legally or ethically give informed consent after having received sedative or hypnotic drugs.

No absolute answer to this question exists, because circumstances vary greatly from case to case. Risk-averse health care organizations are likely to require postponement of elective operations for which appropriate consent was not obtained before the patient was sedated. Emergency operations can usually be justified by a surgeon's note in the chart stating that the surgery is necessary to prevent patient harm. Whatever approach is contemplated, seeking counsel from the health care organization's attorney before proceeding with an operation for which appropriate informed consent has not been obtained is always advisable. If a decision is made to delay the operation to provide time for the patient to metabolize the drug, a physician should document justification for the length of the delay relative to the pharmacokinetic characteristics of the hypnotic drug involved. (See Case Study 11-3.)

FURTHER READING

ASA Standards, Guidelines and Statements, October 1998. Park Ridge, IL: American Society of Anesthesiologists, 1998.
Comprehensive Accreditation Manual for Hospitals: The Official Handbook. Oakbrook Terrace, IL: Joint Commission on Accreditation of Healthcare Organizations, 1999.
National Fire Protection Association. Life Safety Code: NFPA 101-1997. Quincy, MA: National Fire Protection Association, 1997.
National Fire Protection Association. National Electrical Code: NFPA 70-1996. Quincy, MA: National Fire Protection Association, 1996.
National Fire Protection Association. Standard for Health Care Facilities: NFPA 99. Quincy, MA: National Fire Protection Association, 1996.
Quality of Care: Selections from The New England Journal of Medicine. Waltham, MA: The New England Journal of Medicine, 1997.
Questions and Answers about Transfusion Practices (3rd ed). Park Ridge, IL: American Society of Anesthesiologists, 1998.
Standards, Recommended Practices, and Guidelines. Denver: Association of Operating Room Nurses, 1999.

Appendix 11-1
Sample Evacuation Plan

FIRE EVACUATION PLAN: OPERATING ROOM SUITE

1. Your main responsibility is life safety, not fire fighting or combating other adverse elements.
2. The person identifying the fire
   a. Should rescue anyone in immediate danger
   b. Should report the fire by
      (1) Activating the fire alarm pull station
      (2) Notifying the nurse-in-charge or anesthesiologist-in-charge, who will call security (telephone extension), giving the location and nature of the fire
   c. Should confine fire and smoke by closing all doors in the area
   d. Should extinguish the fire with a fire extinguisher or by smothering if the fire is small and contained (e.g., in a wastebasket) and if this can be done without danger to self or others (A clear exit should be maintained behind anyone attempting to extinguish a fire.)
3. The nurse-in-charge or anesthesiologist-in-charge
   a. Establishes a command post at the operating room control desk
   b. Turns off oxygen and nitrous oxide supply to selected operating rooms after notifying personnel in those rooms
   c. Makes decisions about whether to evacuate patients from involved areas
   d. If evacuation is necessary, establishes a remote command post at the receiving site
   e. Seeks consultation from the hospital's chief safety officer or fire marshall and from the fire chief after fire department personnel arrive
4. Evacuation procedures
   a. Horizontal evacuation
      (1) Horizontal evacuation should be used if possible.
      (2) Depending on the size of the fire, other patients in the block of operating rooms in which the fire is occurring may be moved laterally into another block. Blocks are separated by 1-hour fire wall barriers.
      (3) Patients should be moved beyond the double fire doors, if possible. If necessary, horizontal evacuation can be carried out beyond the 2-hour fire wall barriers between the main operating rooms and the personnel area (e.g., locker rooms, lounge).
      (4) Anesthetized patients should be evacuated by the surgical team performing the case, taking with them any equipment required to support the patient, such as an anesthesia machine and monitors. Additional personnel may be asked to help as needed. (The destination location should have electrical outlets to permit continued electronic monitoring and use of an anesthesia machine that has electrical controls.)
      (5) After evacuation has been completed, the oxygen and nitrous oxide lines to each operating room that has been evacuated should be turned off at the direction of the nurse-in-charge or the anesthesiologist-in-charge.

b. Vertical evacuation
   (1) Vertical evacuation should be carried out only if a safe location cannot be reached through lateral movement.
   (2) Patients should be carried up stairs via designated exit routes. (Elevators should not be used unless specifically designated by the local chief safety officer or fire marshall or a representative of the fire department.)

c. Notes
   (1) The primary concern is patient and staff safety.
   (2) Ambulatory patients should be moved first. An appropriate number of staff should accompany this group. They may immediately be vertically evacuated if safe and convenient.
   (3) If evacuation is necessary, patient charts should be moved to the receiving site.

Appendix 11-2
Continuous Quality Improvement: An Example*

Steps in the continuous quality improvement process:

1. Identify the problem to be addressed and the team to work on it.
2. Define relevant terms.
3. Delineate potential causes of the problem.
4. Identify data to be collected.
5. Collect data, including contributions of various potential causes of the problem.
6. Construct a control chart to characterize the baseline state and to identify outliers (outside 2 SD) that might require specific corrective action.
7. Construct a Pareto diagram to identify the most influential causes of the problem.
8. Analyze the most influential causes of the problem, recognizing that the causes are more likely to be related to faulty processes than to poor individual performance by individuals.
9. Carry out corrective action.
10. Collect another set of data after corrective action is taken.
11. Construct a control chart showing the situation after the corrective action was taken.
12. Continue periodic monitoring.

*Reprinted from American Society of Anesthesiologists. Quality improvement and peer review in anesthesiology. Manual for Anesthesia Department Organization and Management. Park Ridge, IL: American Society of Anesthesiologists, 1997. (Reprinted with permission of the American Society of Anesthesiologists, 520 N Northwest Highway, Park Ridge, IL 60068-2573.)

Example

1. Problem: Late starting times for the first case of the day
2. Definition of a late start: Patient entering the OR after 7:35 AM for a 7:30 AM procedure
3. Potential causes (sometimes depicted in a cause and effect or "fishbone" diagram):
   a. Processes, policies, and traditions
      (1) Number of transport personnel available
      (2) Starting time of transport personnel
      (3) Number of nurses in the preanesthesia holding unit
      (4) Starting time of the preanesthesia and OR nurses
      (5) Time allotted for preparing patients in the preanesthesia holding unit
      (6) Time ambulatory patients are scheduled to arrive at the hospital
      (7) Traditional arrival time of anesthesiologists
      (8) Traditional arrival time of surgeons
      (9) Location at which regional blocks are performed and invasive lines are inserted
   b. People
      (1) Anesthesiologists
      (2) Surgeons
      (3) Nurses
      (4) Patients
      (5) Transport personnel
   c. Equipment and space
      (1) Number of transport stretchers
      (2) Size of the preanesthesia holding unit
      (3) Availability of monitoring equipment in the preanesthesia holding unit

4. Data to be collected:
   a. Number of patients scheduled for a 7:30 AM operation who enter the OR after 7:35 AM
   b. Number of ORs scheduled for 7:30 AM operations that day
   c. Cause(s) for the late start (more than one factor may contribute to any given late start)
5. Baseline data:

Date	Number of ORs Starting Late	Number of ORs in Use	Percentage of ORs Starting Late
Feb. 1	3	12	25
Feb. 2	4	12	33
Feb. 3	2	10	20
Feb. 4	2	12	17
Feb. 5	2	11	18
Feb. 8	3	12	25
Feb. 9	4	12	33
Feb. 10	2	10	20
Feb. 11	4	12	33
Feb. 12	2	11	18
Feb. 15	3	12	25
Feb. 16	2	12	17
Feb. 17	2	10	20
Feb. 18	4	12	33
Feb. 19	3	11	27
Feb. 22	3	12	25
Feb. 23	3	12	25
Feb. 24	3	10	30
Feb. 25	4	12	33
Feb. 26	3	11	27
Mean percentage of cases starting late			**25**

6. The graph in Figure A11-2A illustrates the baseline data before intervention. Note that, on average, approximately 25% of the patients scheduled for 7:30 AM operations entered the OR after 7:35 AM. No special-cause variability was present, because all the data fell inside the control limits. Therefore, the variability was all common-cause and the process was in control. However, the mean percentage of late-starting cases (25%) provided substantial room for improvement.
7. The Pareto diagram (Figure A11-2B) displays causes of delays; it is useful for identifying problems on which to focus. Note that the total of the percentages represented by the bars is greater than 100% because two or more causes contributed to some of the late starts. Problems associated with the performance of the transport personnel and anesthesiologists were the principal causes of the late-starting cases, but analysis showed that the problems were caused by faulty processes and not by poor individual performance.
8. Analysis of the most influential causes of the problem:
   a. Transportation
      (1) Most of the late-starting cases were caused, at least in part, by failure of patients to reach the preanesthesia holding unit in time to be appropriately prepared for anesthesia and surgery.

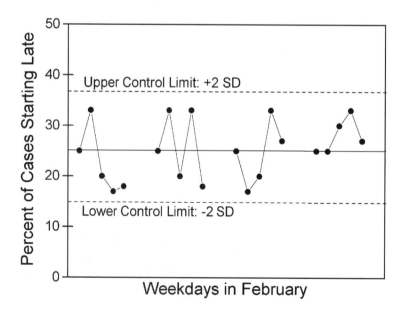

Figure A11-2A. "Before interventions" statistical control chart. On average, approximately 25% of the patients scheduled for 7:30 AM operations entered the operating room after 7:35 AM. All the data fall inside the control limits, showing that all the variability is common-cause, with no special-cause variability.

Figure A11-2B. Pareto diagram. Most of the late starts were caused by problems associated with performance of the transport personnel or the anesthesiologists.

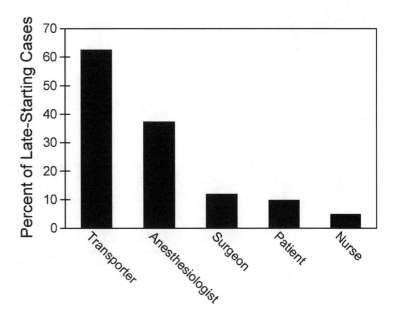

(2) Not enough transport personnel were available to move patients to the preanesthesia holding unit at a reasonable time.

(3) The available transport personnel could start earlier, but this would cause problems with preparing patients for surgery on the inpatient units.

b. Anesthesiologists

(1) A moderately large percentage of late-starting cases were caused by delays in performing regional blocks and inserting invasive monitoring lines in the preanesthesia holding unit.

(2) Electronic monitoring devices are used to monitor patients for regional blocks and insertion of invasive monitoring lines.

(3) Anesthesiologists often had to wait for an available electronic monitoring device.

(4) The OR nurses preferred that the patients not be taken into the ORs before 7:30 AM.

9. Corrective action:

a. Additional transport personnel were made available to the ORs first thing in the morning.

b. Two additional electronic monitoring devices were purchased for the preanesthesia holding unit.

10. Data after corrective action:

Date	Number of ORs Starting Late	Number of ORs in Use	Percentage of ORs Starting Late
April 5	2	12	17
April 6	3	12	25
April 7	1	10	10
April 8	0	12	0
April 9	1	11	9
April 12	2	12	17
April 13	2	12	17
April 14	0	10	0
April 15	1	12	8
April 16	2	11	18
April 19	2	12	17
April 20	1	12	8
April 21	2	10	20
April 22	3	12	25
April 23	2	11	18
April 26	1	12	8
April 27	3	12	25
April 28	2	10	20
April 29	2	12	17
April 30	2	11	18
Mean percentage of cases starting late			**15**

Figure A11-2C. "After interventions" statistical control chart. Compared with the baseline control chart, the average percentage of late-starting cases has been reduced from approximately 25% to approximately 15%. The process is still in control, with all common-cause and no special-cause variability.

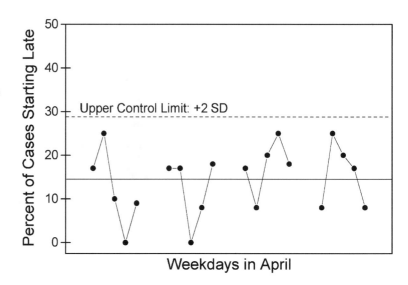

11. The graph in Figure A11-2C illustrates the control chart after corrective action had been taken. Note that the process is still in control, with no special-cause variability producing data outside the control limits. Compared to the baseline control chart, however, the average percentage of late-starting cases has been reduced from approximately 25% to approximately 15%, a substantial improvement.

Appendix 11-3

Sample Form: Refusal
of Treatment or Procedure

I refuse to consent to the following treatment or procedure:

_____

_____

I fully understand that such treatment or procedure may be needed and that, if it is needed, my refusal of such treatment or procedure may seriously imperil my life or health (or that of _____, who is a minor* or an incompetent patient for whom I have legal responsibility).

The risks and medical consequences attendant to my refusal have been fully explained to me by the physician treating me (him/her), and I understand and accept full responsibility for these and all other risks.

I hereby release Community Medical Center, its employees and former employees, and all physicians who were involved in any way with my care from, and waive against the forenamed parties, all actual or potential liability, claims, or actions relating in any way to my refusal of such treatment or procedure.

_____   _____   _____AM/PM
Signature of Patient   Date   Time

_____   _____   _____AM/PM
Signature of Person Authorized to   Date   Time
Consent for Patient if a Minor* or
Incompetent

_____
Relationship to Patient

_____   _____   _____AM/PM
Witness to Signing of This Form   Date   Time

_____
*Medical center counsel must be consulted if the refusal is on behalf of a child.

Appendix 11-4

Ethical Guidelines for Anesthesia Care: Do Not Resuscitate

ETHICAL GUIDELINES FOR THE
ANESTHESIA CARE OF PATIENTS WITH
DO-NOT-RESUSCITATE ORDERS OR OTHER
DIRECTIVES THAT LIMIT TREATMENT

(Approved by House of Delegates of the American Society of Anesthesiologists on October 13, 1993)*
These guidelines apply to competent patients and also to incompetent patients who have previously expressed their preferences.

I. Given the diversity of published opinions and cultures within our society, an essential element of preoperative preparation and perioperative care for patients with Do-Not-Resuscitate (DNR) orders or other directives that limit treatment is communication among involved parties. It is necessary to document relevant aspects of this communication.

II. Policies automatically suspending DNR orders or other directives that limit treatment prior to procedures involving anesthetic care may not sufficiently address a patient's rights to self-determination in a responsible and ethical manner. Such policies, if they exist, should be reviewed and revised, as necessary, to reflect the content of these guidelines.

III. Prior to procedures requiring anesthetic care, any changes in existing directives that limit treatment should be documented in the medical record. These include absolute injunctions as desired by the patient (or the patient's legal representative). When appropriate, the items that should be considered are:

A. Blood product transfusion
B. Tracheal intubation or instrumentation
C. Chest compressions and direct cardiac massage
D. Defibrillation
E. Cardiac pacing, internal or external
F. Invasive monitoring
G. Postoperative ventilatory support
H. Vasoactive drug administration

IV. When relevant, the anesthesiologist should describe and discuss the appropriate use of therapeutic modalities to correct deviations of hemodynamic and respiratory variables predictably resulting from anesthetic agents and techniques.

V. Additional issues that may be relevant to discuss are perioperative placement of naso/orogastric tubes or urinary catheters, administration of antibiotics, establishment of intravenous access, maintenance of intravascular volume with nonblood products and treatment with supplemental oxygen.

VI. It is important to discuss and document whether there are to be any exceptions to the injunction(s) against intervention should there occur a specific recognized complication of the surgery or anesthesia.

VII. Concurrence on these issues by the primary physician (if not the surgeon of record), the surgeon and the anesthesiologist is desirable. If possible, these physicians should meet together with the patient (or the patient's legal

*Reprinted from Ethical Guidelines for the Anesthesia Care of Patients with Do-Not-Resuscitate Orders or Other Directives That Limit Treatment. ASA Directory of Members 1997. Park Ridge, IL: American Society of Anesthesiologists, 1997; 400–401. (Reprinted with permission of the American Society of Anesthesiologists, 520 N Northwest Highway, Park Ridge, IL 60068-2573.)

representative) when these issues are discussed. This duty of the patient's physicians is deemed to be of such importance that it should not be delegated. Other members of the health care team who are (or will be) directly involved with the patient's care during the planned procedure should, if feasible, be included in this process.

VIII. Should conflicts arise, the following resolution processes are recommended:

A. When an anesthesiologist finds the patient's or surgeon's limitations of intervention decisions to be irreconcilable with his or her own moral views, then the anesthesiologist should withdraw in a nonjudgmental fashion, providing an alternative for care in a timely fashion.

B. When an anesthesiologist finds the patient's or surgeon's limitation of intervention decisions to be in conflict with generally accepted standards of care, ethical practice or institutional policies, then the anesthesiologist should voice such concerns and present the situation to the appropriate institutional body.

C. If these alternatives are not feasible within the time frame necessary to prevent further morbidity or suffering, then in accordance with the American Medical Association's Principles of Medical Ethics, care should proceed with reasonable adherence to the patient's directives, being mindful of the patient's goals and values.

IX. A representative from the hospital's anesthesiology service should establish a liaison with surgical and nursing services for presentation, discussion and procedural application of these guidelines. Hospital staff should be made aware of the proceedings of these discussions and the motivations for them.

X. Modification of these guidelines may be appropriate when they conflict with local standards or policies, and in those emergency situations involving incompetent patients whose intentions have not been previously expressed.

Appendix 11-5

Ethical Guidelines for Nursing Care: Do Not Resuscitate

PERIOPERATIVE CARE OF PATIENTS WITH
DO-NOT-RESUSCITATE ORDERS

(Position Statement: Association of Operating
Room Nurses)*

Preamble

Nurses have a responsibility to uphold the rights
of patients.[1] A patient with a do-not-resuscitate
(DNR) order may require surgical procedures and
anesthesia management. These procedures often
are for palliative care, to relieve pain or distress,
to facilitate care, or to improve the patient's quality of life. A DNR order should not mean that all
treatment is stopped and the need for medical and
nursing care is eliminated, but rather that the
patient has made certain choices about end-of-life
decisions.[2] A patient's rights do not stop at the
entrance to the operating room.[3] Automatically
suspending a DNR order during surgery under-
mines a patient's right to self-determination.[4]
Development of a policy related to DNR orders in
the operating room is supported by the Patient
Self-Determination Act,[5] the Joint Commission
on Accreditation of Healthcare Organizations
(JCAHO), the "ANA code for nurses with inter-
pretative statements—explications for perioperative nursing,"[6] and *A Patient's Bill of Rights*.[7]

*Reprinted with permission from Association of Operating
Room Nurses. Standards, Recommended Practices, and
Guidelines. Denver: Association of Operating Room Nurses,
1998; 102–103. (Copyright © AORN, Inc., 2170 South
Parker Road, Suite 300, Denver, CO 80231.)

Position Statement

Required reconsideration of DNR decisions with
patients is an integral component of the care of
patients undergoing surgery.[8] Required reconsideration of DNR decisions ensures that the risks
and benefits of anesthesia and surgery are discussed by health care providers and patients or
patients' surrogate decision makers before surgery.

Guidelines

Patient autonomy must be respected as the professional responsibility of the health care team.[9] The
patient's physicians are responsible for discussing and
documenting issues with the patient and/or family to
determine whether the DNR order is to be maintained
or completely or partially suspended during anesthesia
and surgery. The discussion needs to describe potential
resuscitation efforts during surgery and whether withholding resuscitation compromises the patient's basic
objectives for surgery.[10] Discussion involved with the
required reconsideration should include

- the goals of the surgical treatment,
- the possibility of resuscitative measures,
- a description of what these measures include, and
- possible outcomes with and without resuscitation.

If the patient has chosen to suspend the DNR order
during the intraoperative period, it should be documented when the DNR order is to be reinstated.

Preoperatively, communication among the health
care team, the patient, and the patient's family about
DNR decisions must occur. Adequate information
must be given so the surgical team supports the
patient's or the patient's surrogate's right to participate in the health care decision.[11] A method of com-

munication needs to be developed so that all health care team members are informed of the patient's decision. Following the discussion, the decision and plan must be clearly documented and communicated to all health care providers potentially involved in the perioperative care of the patient. Throughout the process, the patient has the right to modify any decision, and this also must be communicated to all involved health care providers. Patient situations that may require further ethical deliberation before surgical intervention may benefit from consultation with the hospital's ethics advisory committee.

The perioperative nurse, as a patient advocate, has a moral responsibility to the patient.[12] If the perioperative nurse has a moral objection to the patient's decision, he or she should be allowed to make a reasonable effort to find another nurse willing to provide care to the patient. If another nurse is not available, the patient's decision will be upheld, recognizing that there are times when a patient's wishes take precedence in a clinical situation.

Operational Definitions

The following are operational definitions of terms used in the statement.

Do-not-resuscitate (DNR) order. A specific directive, written by a physician, mandating that cardiopulmonary resuscitation should not be performed.[13]

Do-not-resuscitate (DNR) decision. The patient's or surrogate's directives regarding end-of-life choices.

Required reconsideration. An event that allows a patient or surrogate to participate in decisions about the use of cardiopulmonary resuscitation and that offers caregivers an opportunity to explain the significance of cardiac arrest and resuscitation in the perioperative setting.[14]

Health care team. Nurses, physicians, and all others involved in clinical disciplines.[15]

NOTES

1. S Igoe, S Cascella, K Stockdale, "Ethics in the OR: DNR and patient autonomy," *Nursing Management* 24 (September 1993) 112A, 112D, 112H.
2. JM Reeder, "Do-not-resuscitate orders in the operating room," *AORN Journal* 57 (April 1993) 947–951.
3. SJ Youngner, HF Cascorbi, JM Shuck, "DNR in the operating room: Not really a paradox," *Journal of the American Medical Association* 266 (November 1991) 2433–2434.
4. Igoe, Cascella, Stockdale, "Ethics in the OR: DNR and patient autonomy," 112A, 112D, 112H.
5. *Patient Self-Determination Act,* Public Law 101-508, *Federal Register* 57 (March 6, 1992).
6. "ANA code for nurses with interpretive statements—explications for perioperative nursing," in *AORN Standards and Recommended Practices* (Denver: Association of Operating Room Nurses, Inc., 1994) 39–56.
7. American Hospital Association, *A Patient's Bill of Rights,* second ed. (Chicago: American Hospital Association, 1994).
8. CB Cohen, PJ Cohen, "Required reconsideration of 'do-not-resuscitate' orders in the operating room and certain other treatment settings," *Law, Medicine & Health Care* 20 (Winter 1992) 354–363.
9. Igoe, Cascella, Stockdale, "Ethics in the OR: DNR and patient autonomy," 112A, 112D, 112H.
10. P Patterson, "Suspension of DNR orders in the OR being questioned," *OR Manager* 8 (February 1992) 1, 5–8.
11. Reeder, "Do-not-resuscitate orders in the operating room," 947–951.
12. MJ Keffer, HL Keffer, "The do-not-resuscitate order: Moral responsibilities of the perioperative nurse," *AORN Journal* 54 (March 1994) 641–650.
13. Cohen, Cohen, "Required reconsideration of 'do-not-resuscitate' orders in the operating room and certain other treatment settings," 354–363.
14. Ibid.
15. JL Levenson, L Pettrey, "Controversial decisions regarding treatment and DNR: An algorithmic guide for the uncertain in decision-making ethics (GUIDE)," *American Journal of Critical Care* 3 (March 1994).

SUGGESTED READING

American College of Surgeons. "Statement of the American College of Surgeons on Advance Directives by Patients: 'Do Not Resuscitate' in the Operating Room." *ACS Bulletin* 79 (September 1994) 29.

American Nurses Association Center for Human Rights Task Force. *Compendium of Position Statements on the Nurse's Role in End-of-Life Decisions.* Washington, DC: American Nurses Association, 1993.

American Society of Anesthesiologists. "Ethical guidelines for the anesthesia care of patients with do-not-resuscitate orders or other directives that limit care." In *ASA Standards, Guidelines, and Statements.* Park Ridge, Ill: American Society of Anesthesiologists, 1993.

Keffer, MJ; Keffer, HL. "Do-not-resuscitate in the operating room: Moral obligation of anesthesiologists." *Anesthesia and Analgesia* 74 (June 1992) 901–905.

Tomlinson, T; Brody, H. "Futility and the ethics of resuscitation." *Journal of the American Medical Association* 264 (September 1990) 1276–1280.

Walker, RM. "DNR in the OR: Resuscitation as an operative risk." *Journal of the American Medical Association* 266 (November 1991) 2407–2412.

Submitted: 3/95
Adopted: 3/6/95
House of Delegates,
Atlanta, Georgia
Sunset review: 3/2000

Chapter 12

Design and Construction

An expert is someone who knows some of the worst mistakes that can be made in his subject, and how to avoid them.

—*Werner Heisenberg (1901–1976)*

The structure of a building strongly influences the efficiency with which the functions it supports can be carried out. Effective design is particularly critical in OR suites, where efficient flow of patients, personnel, and materials is of utmost importance. OR designs, however, are frequently flawed. Even if they serve the needs of a health care organization reasonably well when they are initially built, changes in institutional function often require that the structure be modified. Consequently, we must consider not only how to do it right the first time—design—but also how to make it right at a later date—redesign.

All construction undertaken by a health care organization should be dictated by the organization's strategic plan. Therefore, before embarking on the planning for any contemplated construction, the strategic plan* should be reviewed to ensure that the planned construction is consistent with it. Likewise, the organization's master facility plan[†] should be reviewed for consistency of the contemplated construction with the master plan.

---

*The strategic plan describes the mission, the vision, and the goals and objectives of the health care organization, along with a set of strategies to accomplish the goals and objectives.
[†]The master facility plan describes the facilities required to carry out the strategic plan.

PLANNING TEAM

The design or redesign planning process should follow some well-established conventions. The owner of a building bears ultimate responsibility for all renovation or primary construction projects. For a health care organization, the term *owner* usually translates to *board of directors*, whether the organization is for-profit or not-for-profit. The board usually delegates responsibility for construction projects to a project manager.

Project Manager

The project manager, also referred to as the *owner's representative*, shepherds the design and construction from selection of the architect through final acceptance from the contractors. The project manager must be given full authority to represent the owner in all aspects of the project. The principal responsibilities of the project manager are listed in Table 12-1.

Health care organizations, especially large ones, often have a planning or facilities office that designates a project manager for construction undertaken by the organization. Such project managers have experience with and knowledge of the organization as an important asset. Smaller organizations without planning offices may designate an employee to be project manager on an ad hoc basis. Although this

Table 12-1. Duties of the Project Manager

Represents the owner in all phases of the project
Is responsible for project documentation
    Correspondence
    Meeting minutes
    Plans
Is the primary contact person for
    Owners
    Architects
    Contractors
    Regulatory agencies
    All those engaged in the planning process
Facilitates the flow of information among the above parties
Is responsible for obtaining cost estimates
Is responsible for contract administration
Is responsible for change orders
    Receives requests
    Negotiates with requesters
    Communicates approved changes to the architects
Is responsible for ensuring that the project proceeds according to the established time line
Is responsible for ensuring that the project proceeds according to the established budget
Is responsible for honoring pay requests from the architect, consultants, and contractors

practice appears to be cost effective, in the long run it may cost the health care organization more money. Employees of the organization often have political baggage encumbering them (e.g., people inside and outside the organization to whom they owe favors); an owner's representative who is devoid of such encumbrances can much more effectively constrain costs of the project. Project managers who are independent contractors may represent money well spent during a complex construction or renovation project, because a substantial amount of money can be saved by choosing vendors according to strict criteria and by keeping the project on schedule.

After the project manager has been selected and is on board, the next major task is to select the lead architect for the project. For an institution-wide construction project, choosing an architect is often carried out by a committee composed of one or more members of the board of directors, the CEO of the health care organization, and the project manager. For renovation of an OR suite, the OR manager, a representative of the health care organization, and the project manager are appropriate persons to select the architect. A set of selection criteria is developed

and the criteria prioritized. (Table 12-2 shows a typical set of architect selection criteria.) When a list of candidates possessing the essential criteria has been prepared, the contending firms should be evaluated by (1) communicating with the architects' previous clients, (2) evaluating ongoing or recently completed projects by reviewing descriptive material and visiting sites, (3) interviewing the architects in their own offices, and (4) discussing the project with the candidates at the site of proposed construction.

Another valuable consultant with whom organizations lacking full-time project offices may wish to contract (often through the project manager) is a professional cost estimator. Such an expert, who usually works directly for the project manager, can be brought into the process at any time. General contractors and architects are able to make cost estimates only when the planning process has progressed to a point at which line items can be costed out. In contrast, cost estimators have access to databases that permit them to provide reasonably sophisticated cost appraisals for projects that are defined relatively vaguely (e.g., "a freestanding four-OR ASC with supporting facilities"). Cost estimators, who often have had formal training and may even have attained advanced degrees in their field, tend to be cost-effective consultants who can be called on at each step in the planning process that requires cost estimates.

Primary Planners

The persons best qualified to make major design decisions for a facility are those who have had substantial experience working in similar facilities.

Table 12-2. Criteria for Selecting an Architect

Experience on similar health care projects of sizes similar to the project being planned
Record of repeat business with other clients
Special capabilities and/or facilities
Extent of professional services offered
Financial stability and capability
Types of staff and support personnel available
Experience and capability of consulting engineers normally used or of staff engineers
Previous performance on estimating costs of projects

Source: Adapted from C Laubach and T Ritter. Managing Hospital Design and Construction Programs. Agoura Hills, CA: Center for Management Programs, 1996; 26,28.

Intuition (and some architects) might suggest that an architect is better qualified than the users. However, reflection (and some architects) might argue instead that the major responsibility for planning should be in the hands of local experts. In this planning scenario, the architect acts as facilitator, guiding clinicians through the planning process and interjecting technical details when appropriate. An effective architect convinces the organizational planners that they—the future users—are themselves experts at OR design because they are experts in OR function. As noted earlier, structure and function are tightly linked.

When a Socratic forum is used to analyze an existing OR design, seasoned physicians and nurses with considerable OR experience can identify elements of design that, in their experience, work and those that do not. Effective OR designs are usually based on the collective experience of a group of veteran workers who understand very well how an OR suite should function and what structural factors are needed to make it function most efficiently. Of course, the architect's expertise is necessary to consolidate the collective wisdom of the organizational planners, to constrain their impractical impulses, to provide a wider range of design ideas from other institutions, and to add the elements of design that only an architect is qualified to supply.

The core planning group representing the institution is usually made up of selected OR nurses, surgeons, anesthesiologists, and OR management personnel—often just one representative of each group. At certain stages in the process, the planning group should request input from representatives of nonprofessional and professional support services, such as housekeeping, transportation, pharmacy, radiology, pathology, and laboratory medicine. The project manager is an ever-present entity, always representing the interests of the owner.

The architect, besides being a facilitator for the medical personnel, acts as coordinator for engineering consultants whose knowledge is essential to optimal design. (In some scenarios, the project manager assumes responsibility for coordinating consultants.) Specialists in fields such as structural engineering; electrical design; and heating, ventilation, and air conditioning are often consulted. Consultants in fields such as communication may also be asked to join the design team at certain stages in the planning process.

PLANNING AND DESIGN PROCESS

Once the architect and the in-house design teams are identified, the planning group systematically moves through the planning and design process. Facility planning and design begins with laying down broad concepts and progressively moves toward a final set of construction blueprints. Three major steps are involved: (1) facility plan, (2) functional program, and (3) design. The planning and design process is like developing and assembling a jigsaw puzzle made up of hundreds of pieces, each supporting necessary functions. First the individual pieces are free-formed (bubble diagrams—the facility plan); then they are given size and shape (space allocation—the functional program); and eventually they are fit together in a meaningful pattern (design) (Table 12-3).

The facility plan defines the functional needs of the organization. This plan is usually developed in interactive sessions involving the architect and the organizational planners. During these sessions, the architect-facilitator traditionally conducts a brainstorming session in which the organizational planners identify the functions that must be accommodated in the space being planned. The architect often displays these concepts on an erasable marker board, asking probing questions to help the group systematically refine the organization's needs. A scribe should be appointed to thoroughly document all of the ideas generated during each meeting. The functions and structures can be displayed in a bubble diagram (Figure 12-1). Bubbles of various sizes are sometimes

Table 12-3. Steps in the Planning and Design Process

Facility plan
    Definition of needs
    Bubble diagrams (which may include flow)
Functional program
    Space allocation (schematic documents)
    Floor loads
    Electrical supply, lighting
    Plumbing
Design
    Concept (schematic documents)
    Design and development (design documents)
    Working drawings (construction documents)

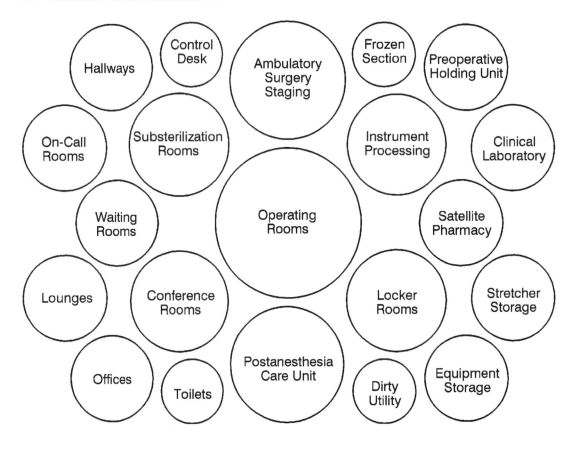

Figure 12-1. Bubble diagram illustrating the major functional and structural components of a project.

used to show the approximate size of the space needed for each function. Special bubble diagrams are sometimes prepared that have arrows showing flows of patients, personnel, and material.

The next step is to give more definition to functional and structural components (e.g., rooms, hallways, and stairwells) by assigning specific shapes and sizes to them. The outcome of this process is called the *functional program*. The initial step in this process is taken by the architect, who is an expert in the amounts of space typically needed to carry out specific functions and in how different types of spaces most effectively fit together. Also included in the functional program are such considerations as floor loads, plumbing, electrical capabilities, and lighting. Organizational representatives usually have one or more opportunities to recommend modifications to the architect's proposed functional program. Again, the project manager is

ever present as an expert representative of the interests of the owner (board of directors).

The design phase is divided into three stages: (1) concept, (2) design and development, and (3) working drawings. The output of the concept stage is schematic drawings, which are simple line drawings that show the overall layout of the job, room sizes, minimum room layout, and basic information about plumbing and electrical supply. The output of design and development is design plans that include complete room layouts and exact locations of plumbing fixtures and electrical switches and outlets. Finally, the output of the working-drawing stage is comprehensive construction drawings that include detailed specifications from which the contractor will build the structure.

Space configuration, which takes place during "concept" and "design and development," is governed by two considerations: (1) general principles on the efficient use of space and (2) flow of people and materials within the space and into and out of adjacent spaces. The architect identifies methods for efficiently using space. Efficient flow patterns are identified by a combination of the experience of the organizational planners (future users of the space) and the expertise of the architect.

Three flows are considered: flow of patients, flow of personnel, and flow of material (Table 12-4). In some areas, the flows of patients and personnel overlap, and in other areas they do not. Personnel work in all areas occupied by patients, but certain spaces in the OR suite are occupied only by personnel (e.g., staff lounges, locker rooms, offices). Good design usually separates spaces used exclusively by the staff from those used by the patients. Space occupied by personnel is further subdivided into staff areas, "clean" space where no sterile procedures are performed, and space where sterile procedures are carried out. Flow patterns reflect these separations. Personnel are usually expected to be dressed in scrub clothes when occupying clean space but not necessarily when in staff areas. They are further required to wear masks when entering space in which sterile procedures are carried out.

In general, the flow of material should be as innocuous as possible. Equipment, instruments, supplies, and waste may be transported into and out of ORs through the same corridors used by patients and personnel. The origins and destinations of material, however, are often different from those of patients and of personnel. Wherever possible, flow of material should be isolated from flow of patients and personnel. (For example, waste should not leave the OR suite on elevators used by patients.) With appropriate design, even when waste must travel in the same hallways as patients and personnel, the distances in which this overlap occurs can usually be minimized.

Early in the design process, those participating in the planning and design project have an opportunity to challenge and recommend modification of decisions that have been made. As the process progresses, however, the cost of making changes increases dramatically, because complexity of the construction project progressively increases with time. As a result, any change made late in the process has greater impact. All modifications necessarily result in changes to other components of the plan, because overall constraints of space and overall cost must be adhered to. These constraints can be relaxed only to the extent permitted by the limited resources allocated to the project.

Cost considerations mandate use of the "freeze." A freeze is an arbitrary but essential cessation of further changes by any representatives of the owner. The first of two freezes is imposed after agreement on concept in the design phase. Agreement on the concept, as noted previously, is reached through an iterative process during meetings involving the institutional planners, the architect, and the project manager. When agreement has been reached on concept, the owner is asked to approve, which involves the owner's representative (usually the project manager) signing and dating the plans to document approval. The architect then proceeds to the design and development stage.

After delivery of the initial design plans, further meetings take place so that the institutional planners can present their recommended modifications to the architect. After agreement on the design, the project director is again expected to sign off. This second freeze effectively ends the owner's direct participation in the planning process. From that point forward, the project is in the hands of the architect and the contractor. (As noted previously, the cost of changes beyond this point becomes excessive.) Of course, close contact between the project manager and the architect, consultants, and contractor continues up to the time the completed project is turned over to the owner. The job of the institutional planners is effectively completed, however, when the design is frozen.

Table 12-4. Major Flows within the Operating Room Suite

Patient flow: Patients do not normally enter staff areas
    Clean areas
    Sterile areas
Personnel flow: Personnel enter all space occupied by patients
    Staff areas (e.g., lounges, locker rooms)
    Clean areas
    Sterile areas
Material flow: Material flow should minimally overlap patient flow

OPERATING ROOM SUITE

Overall configuration of the OR suite is determined largely by corridor style. Therefore, a decision should be made early in the design process about which of the many options for corridor style to use. This decision is governed by the owner's priorities with respect to efficiency of flow (patients, personnel, and material) and by theoretical considerations having to do with the desirability of separating "clean" from "dirty." Although completely separating the flow of waste from the flow of patients may be intuitively appealing, modern concepts of materials management substantially reduce the practical importance of this degree of isolation. Therefore, efficiencies in the flow of patients and personnel should primarily determine which corridor style will be used.

Two general corridor styles are used: circumferential (outer; Figure 12-2A) and central (inner; Figure 12-2B). Other styles are variants of these general types. The triple corridor (Figure 12-2C) is a combination of both. When circumferential corridors are used, support space is sometimes placed in a central area separating the ORs (Figure 12-2D). The "pod," or "cluster," design (Figure 12-2E) is a variant of the central corridor design.

The triple-corridor OR suite, shown in Figure 12-2C, was popularized by the U.S. Department of Defense in the 1940s. This design is based on the premise that patients, personnel, and clean material should flow into and out of ORs through the "clean" central corridor, and dirty material (instruments and red-bag waste generated during operations) should leave via the "dirty" outer corridor. Such segregation, although theoretically advantageous, represents highly inefficient use of space, because roughly three times as much space is dedicated to hallways as in the central corridor design. The case cart system is a satisfactory alternative to providing a separate hallway for transporting waste out of ORs. With the case cart system, large, enclosed, wheeled stainless steel carts are used to transport all of the instruments and supplies needed for an operation into the OR. At the end of the procedure, all dirty instruments and waste are loaded into the cart, the doors are closed, and the case cart is transported to a utility area for processing of the dirty instruments and disposal of the waste. (See the discussion of the case cart system on pages 123–124.)

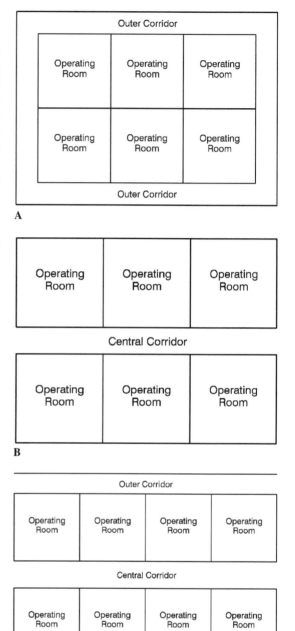

Figure 12-2. Corridor styles. **A.** Circumferential (outer) corridor. **B.** Central (inner) corridor. **C.** Triple corridor. **D.** Circumferential corridor with center core. **E.** Cluster design.

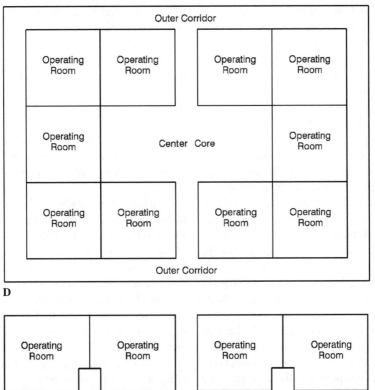

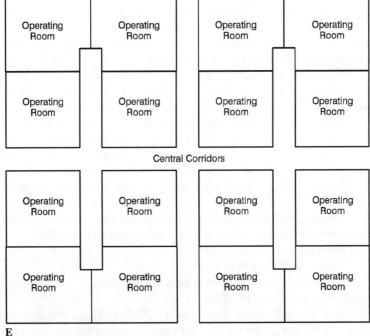

The average distance between ORs is considerably longer with circumferential corridors, which can be a negative feature when personnel (nurses or anesthesiologists) must cover two or more nonadjacent ORs. In addition, distances tend to be great between ORs and centralized patient-care locations (e.g., the PHU and the PACU).

A center core can be designed into OR suites that have circumferential corridors (see Figure 12-2D). The center core can accommodate either patient-care functions (e.g., preoperative holding, postanesthesia care, or both) or supply functions (e.g., storage or instrument processing). When the center core has been designed for storage or instrument processing, shelving on the center-core wall of each adjacent OR often opens through to the center core for ease of stocking, either routine or on demand. This design requires that the circulating nurse communicate with center-core personnel to request an item and then retrieve the item from a pass through.

Some hospitals have eliminated the need for center-core staff by making the center core "self-serve." To do this, a door is installed between each OR and the center-core space, and the center core is devoted entirely to storage. Circulating nurses can then directly obtain additional supplies or equipment during the progress of operations without involving other personnel. Instrument processing is moved to a nearby location, and instruments are transported to and from the ORs in case carts. A major bonus associated with a door that connects each OR to the center core is that it creates a shortcut between ORs on opposite sides of the center core. Without this route, personnel would have to travel a considerably longer circumferential route, rather than being able to cut through the center core.

The cluster design is generally preferred for larger OR suites. The version shown in Figure 12-2E combines four clusters of four ORs each, for a total of 16 ORs. In this design, the space at the end of the horizontal or vertical corridors can be allocated to functions such as case cart preparation (material flow), personnel locker rooms and lounges (personnel flow), and preoperative and postoperative patient care (patient flow). For example, in Figure 12-2E, the ASU, the (inpatient) PHU, and the PACU could be situated north of the vertical corridor. This setup would facilitate cross-functional use of space and personnel among the three units. (See Cross-Functional Use of Space on page 186.) Distance between the PACU and the ASU would be short. Personnel could enter and leave the ORs through locker rooms situated to the east or west, and material could flow to and from the south.

Storage and support areas are not shown in the figures displaying corridor styles. The role of the design team is to select specific locations for all of the functional space identified in the bubble diagram developed by the team early in the planning. Storage and support areas can be interspersed between the ORs or located on the periphery of the OR suite. Staff space (e.g., lounges and locker rooms) is usually located in the periphery, because it is not inte-

gral to the care of patients and therefore does not require close proximity for efficient function.

INDIVIDUAL OPERATING ROOMS

Shape

It is a general principle in architectural design that square rooms provide the most versatility and the most efficient use of space. This is particularly true for ORs.

The OR table is traditionally positioned parallel to the walls of the OR. Thus positioned, the table can be oriented in four different ways, with the head of the table pointing toward any of the four walls. Because the head of the OR table must be served by a gas supply for the anesthesia machine, which is located to the right of the patient's head, two of the walls are usually designated *head walls*. Furthermore, a sizable portion of one wall of the OR is usually allocated to shelving, which should be located to the side or at the foot of the OR table. (The two standard orientations of the OR table are illustrated in Figure 12-3.)

Of course, the OR table is not always positioned centrally as shown in the illustration. Orientation to one side or the other, toward the head or foot, or even in a diagonal direction is sometimes optimal. The position depends on the body part to which the surgeon needs access and on the need for positioning special equipment near the patient or within the surgeon's line of sight. Special configurations of the OR table and equipment are facilitated if the room is as nearly square as possible.

Location of Doors

Every OR has at least two doors, one an entrance for the patient and personnel, the other allowing personnel access to the substerile area. (A third may provide access to a storage room or to a center core, as described previously.) The main entrance should be located to facilitate the patient's arrival and departure on a stretcher. The path of the patient's arrival into the OR should not interfere with the scrub's simultaneously setting up the sterile table.

Because the anesthesia machine is positioned to the right of the patient's head (at least for the induc-

Figure 12-3. Two standard positions for an operating room table (drawn roughly to scale for a 20 ft × 20 ft room).

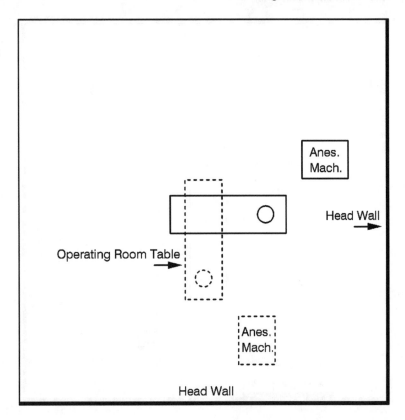

tion of anesthesia, although it is sometimes subsequently moved), the main entrance should not be located to the right of the head of the OR table. Similarly, having the main entrance to the right of the OR table's foot is not desirable, because anesthesia personnel entering the OR after the start of the operation have to maneuver past the sterile table to reach the anesthesia work station. The most desirable arrangement is to position the main entrance of the OR to the patient's left, either at the head (Figures 12-4A and 12-4C) or at the foot (Figures 12-4B and 12-4D).

The configurations depicted in Figures 12-4A through 12-4D work equally well when mirror images are used—that is, when the head wall is to the left rather than to the right, as shown. Locating one of the head walls adjacent to the main corridor of the OR suite is generally desirable, making the configurations shown in Figures 12-4A and 12-4B superior to those in Figures 12-4C and 12-4D. Having one head wall adjacent to the main corridor tends to minimize traffic from the door to the anesthesia workstation, whether the OR table is positioned parallel or perpendicular to the main OR corridor (running horizontally at the bottom in each figure). This not only reduces travel time but minimizes the possibility of contaminating the sterile field when entering or leaving the room.

Figures 12-4C and 12-4D show that having three doors in an OR is feasible. The trade-off is that less wall space is available for shelving. Additionally, having a third door may constrain positioning of the sterile table, which should not be near a doorway.

Size

ORs should be no smaller than 400 sq ft, making 20 ft × 20 ft nearly ideal dimensions. Rapid advances in endoscopic surgery have resulted in dramatic increases in the amount of equipment required for relatively straightforward operations. The same standard for size applies to ambulatory and inpatient surgery, because the amount of equipment needed for surgery performed in both settings is approximately the same.

Cardiac surgery requires an extracorporeal pump and, for minimally invasive thoracic operations,

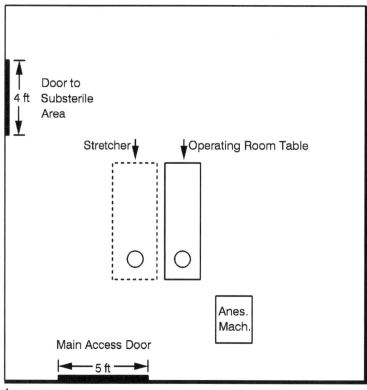

A

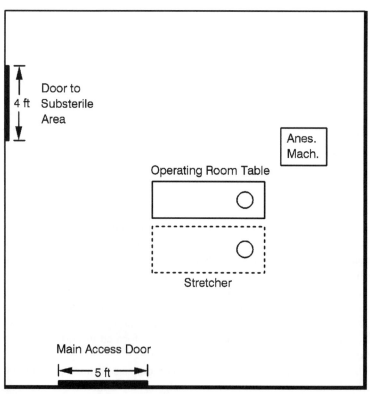

B

Figure 12-4. Positions of doors in the operating room (drawn roughly to scale for a 20 ft × 20 ft room). **A.** Preferred position of doors (orientation no. 1). **B.** Preferred position of doors (orientation no. 2). **C.** Alternative position of doors (orientation no. 3). **D.** Alternative position of doors (orientation no. 4).

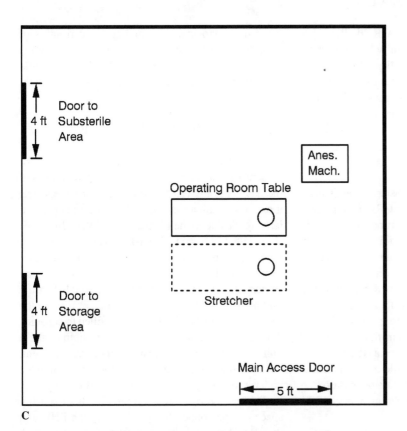

C

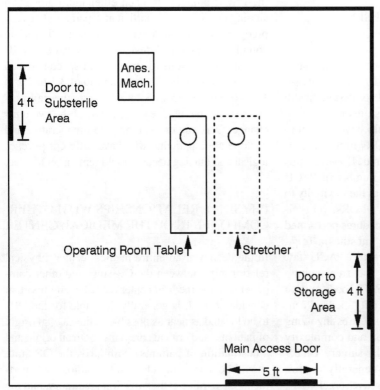

D

imaging equipment. Therefore, ORs dedicated to cardiothoracic surgery are generally larger, perhaps as large as 575–600 sq ft (roughly 24 ft × 24 ft). The particularly large sterile tables used for neurosurgery and transplantation surgery make larger ORs desirable for these specialties as well.

SUBSTERILE AREAS

In traditional OR design, one substerile area is interposed between and shared by two ORs. This arrangement has stood the test of time and is still recommended. In older methods for materials management, a washer-sterilizer between ORs was sometimes used for processing instruments between cases. This method is now generally considered too inefficient, except for those operations that have relatively modest instrument demands (e.g., fast-turnover cataract extractions). For selected instrument processing and for flash sterilizing instruments during operations, however, having a substerile area adjacent to every OR is essential. (See the discussion of flash sterilization under Instrument Sterilization on page 129.)

SIZE OF THE POSTANESTHESIA CARE UNIT

The number of beds that should be accommodated in the PACU depends largely on case mix. Historically, conventional wisdom (and some state health codes) dictated that small OR suites (e.g., those having three or four ORs) should have one more PACU bed than the number of ORs in which general anesthesia can be administered. However, this rule of thumb overestimates the number of PACU beds needed in an OR suite that has the flexibility to administer general anesthesia in all ORs, yet typically uses half of its ORs for procedures performed under regional block or local anesthesia (e.g., cataract extractions) that do not require PACU stay.

Small community hospitals and freestanding ASCs are likely to require fewer PACU beds relative to the number of ORs than university medical centers or large community hospitals. Cases involving sicker patients or greater duration and complexity (e.g., spine surgery, major vascular surgery, cancer surgery of the head and neck) generally require longer PACU stays than routine elective surgery (e.g., hernia repair, hysterectomy, diagnostic laparoscopy).

Either historical data or careful estimates of expected case mix should be used to determine the number of beds planned for the PACU. State regulations may dictate a minimum number of PACU beds.

CROSS-FUNCTIONAL USE OF SPACE

Certain space within the OR suite can be used for similar but distinct functions during different times of the day. Not only can this approach conserve space, it can also facilitate staffing. This concept is particularly applicable to the PHU and the PACU. In an OR suite with 12 ORs, at 7:30 AM 12 patients may be in the PHU but none in the PACU. During the remainder of the day, three to four patients may be awaiting surgery in the PHU, and at times, especially during mid-afternoon, there may be only one or two. At the same time, the PACU is likely to be filled to capacity. Allocating space to meet the needs of both of these units at their respective peak hours is not efficient, because both units (especially the PHU) will be underused during a considerable part of the day.

The preceding scenario lends itself to sharing space and personnel. Simply locating the PHU and the PACU adjacent to each other facilitates such sharing but provides insufficient separation between preoperative and postoperative patients. In a more complex yet practical design, electric sliding walls are used to adjust the distribution of space between the PHU and the PACU from a ratio of 3:1 to 2:2 to 1:3—or simply from 3:1 to 1:3—as the day progresses and the relative space needs of the two units change. One way or the other, the preoperative and postoperative patients, who have different psychological and nursing needs, should remain segregated.

PHYSICAL RELATIONSHIPS WITH OTHER COMPONENTS OF THE MEDICAL CENTER

In the design of an entire medical center, physical relationships between the OR suite and other components of the medical center represent an important consideration. It is generally desirable for the ORs to be located as near as possible to the ED (an origin of patients) and critical care units (both an origin and a destination of patients). Similarly, the OR suite should be reasonably close to the radiology department, the cardiac catheterization laboratory, and the blood bank. In smaller hospitals, locating the OR suite near the obstetric suite permits cesarean deliveries and other obstetric operations to be performed near the labor rooms. Larger hospitals often have dedicated ORs associated with the obstetric suite.

RENOVATION VERSUS
NEW CONSTRUCTION

Planning use of space for renovation is usually considerably more difficult than planning new construction, because constraints are imposed by existing structures. Additionally, renovation is often carried out because of a need to enlarge OR facilities to meet new requirements (e.g., additional ambulatory surgery), and non-OR functions may be displaced to make room for facilities that must be in close proximity to existing ORs.

Consideration should always be given to the possibility that replacing the existing OR suite with an entirely new suite may, in the long run, be more cost effective than patching up the structure that currently exists. This decision depends largely on how functional or dysfunctional the current OR suite is and how near it comes to meeting anticipated needs in its current configuration.

In the special case of enlarging the OR suite to accommodate increasing amounts of ambulatory surgery, one possibility is to build new ORs separate from the main OR suite expressly for surgery on ambulatory patients. This generally is not a good idea, because two smaller OR suites are invariably more expensive to operate than a single, larger suite. Flexibility of staffing (nursing, anesthesia, and support personnel) and flexibility of scheduling are lost with multiple sites because special equipment has to be kept in one location or the other. Flexibility can be preserved by hiring more staff and buying more equipment. The financial trade-off between these two options should be considered in making a decision about whether to tear down and add on or to build a second OR suite elsewhere.

FLEXIBILITY (AT A COST)

The degree to which flexibility should be designed into a new or renovated facility depends largely on the degree to which future needs can be predicted. For example, if a future need for additional ORs is fairly certain, then the plan under design should

include space for adding efficiently configured ORs. Space allocated for future ORs can be used temporarily for necessary functions such as storage. Then, when new ORs are needed, space-filling functions that do not require proximity to the OR suite can be relocated to accommodate the new ORs. The future location of displaced functions should be identified in the structure's master facility plan.

Flexible construction initially costs more than fixed-use construction, because expensive space is bought and, in the short term, used for storage. Therefore, flexibility should be designed into a plan only when future needs can be predicted with relative certainty. Otherwise, the increased cost of the flexible design may never be recovered.

BUILDING CODES AND
CERTIFICATE OF NEED

The architect should be an expert on relevant building codes. The project manager should also be knowledgeable about county and local building codes, approvals that are required before construction can begin, and inspections that are necessary during and after construction. Similarly, NFPA codes must be met. Although compliance with NFPA codes is voluntary, compliance with the standards in NFPA's Standard for Health Care Facilities (NFPA 99) is required by many insurance companies before they will write a fire insurance policy for a health care facility. (See Physical, Electrical, and Fire Safety on page 151 for a brief discussion of NFPA standards.)

Whether a CON is required depends on state law; some states require a CON, some do not. Well-informed health care administrators, project managers, and architects know whether a project requires a CON and, if one is needed, how and when to apply for it. The process of obtaining a CON can sometimes take many months, and it is unwise to progress very far along the planning process without obtaining state approval, if required.

SPECIAL CONSIDERATIONS IN THE
DESIGN OF AMBULATORY SURGERY
UNITS AND FREESTANDING
AMBULATORY SURGICAL CENTERS

In ASUs or freestanding ASCs, patients are admitted to a preoperative staging unit where nurses prepare them for surgery and where they wait until the OR is ready for them. Two design concepts are commonly used that have different effects on the flow of patients and on nursing staffing. The first is the "tidal," or "to-and-fro," design, which is based on the inpatient model (Figure 12-5A). In this design, the ASU functions the same way as an inpatient unit, in which patients are admitted to a bed that they occupy until discharge from the hospital. When patients leave an inpatient unit for diagnostic (e.g., radiology) and therapeutic (e.g., surgery) procedures, they return to the same beds (in the same rooms). In the tidal or to-and-fro design for ASUs and ASCs, the same concept applies; after discharge from the PACU, patients return to the unit to which they were admitted (although not necessarily to the same beds). They then undergo further recovery before discharge.

In the flow-through design for ASUs and ASCs (Figure 12-5B), patients are admitted to beds in a preoperative staging unit but do not return to that unit after surgery. Instead, on discharge from the PACU, they go to a lounge for further recovery until being discharged from the facility. In the overall design of the facility, a flow pattern is defined by locating the preoperative staging unit on one side of the OR space and the PACU and recovery lounge on the other side. The patients flow sequentially from the preoperative staging unit through the ORs to the PACU and from there to the recovery lounge. Freestanding ASCs are often designed so that the flow of patients is functionally circular, with the sequential units arranged in the general configuration shown in Figure 12-5B.

In the tidal model, the same cadre of nurses assumes preoperative and postoperative care of patients, whereas in the flow-through model a separate group of nurses cares for patients in the pre- and the postoperative areas. In the flow-through model, nurses staffing the recovery lounge usually also staff the PACU.

In neither of these models is it necessary for beds to remain empty while patients are in the OR. As soon as a bed in the preoperative staging unit is empty, another patient is placed in that bed. In practice, the "beds" in an ASU or ASC are stretchers.

When an ambulatory staging area must be located a considerable distance from the ORs, a PHU is sometimes used (Figure 12-5C). Such a unit is often designed into OR suites in inpatient facilities, because inpatients must be transported to the OR suite from nursing units that are usually a con-siderable distance from the ORs. With a PHU in place, patients can be brought to the OR suite early enough to avoid delay in entering the assigned OR once it is ready. Additionally, nurses sometimes start intravenous infusions and nursing assistants clip or shave hair at the surgical site while patients are in the PHU. Similarly, anesthesiologists sometimes insert epidural catheters or invasive monitors or perform peripheral nerve blocks in the PHU. In freestanding ASCs, where distances are usually short, the preoperative staging unit usually functions in the same way as the PHU in hospitals.

DESIGN OF OPERATING ROOM COMMUNICATION SYSTEMS

Communication within the OR suite is key to efficiency and patient safety. Personnel working in and managing ORs must communicate with each other within the OR suite and in adjacent support areas. They also must have links to the outside world, both within and outside the parent health care organization.

Control Desk

Traditionally, the OR control desk is the center of communication in the OR suite. This desk or work space, often behind a counter, is usually strategically located so that all patients entering or leaving ORs do so under direct observation by personnel at the control desk. When the primary method of communicating is an intercom, the central unit is located at the control desk. With more modern methods of communication, the control desk is the place where pages are initiated via computer and where personnel update the master computer displays of patient flow in real time.

Telephones and Intercoms

The standard telephone—which is present in every OR, as well as scattered throughout the OR suite—continues to be the primary method for communicating with the world outside the OR suite. The telephone should be widely used for communication within the OR suite as well. Speakerphones can be

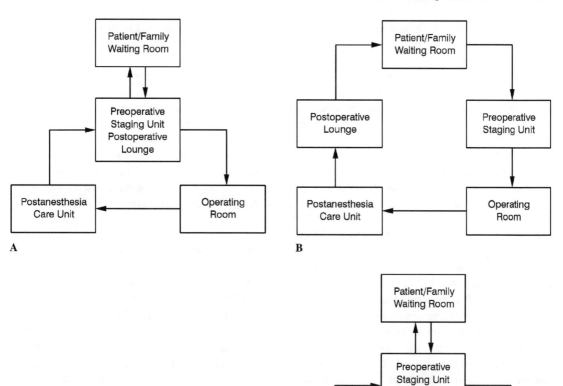

Figure 12-5. Patterns for flow in and out of ambulatory operating room suites. **A.** The tidal, or to-and-fro, design for ambulatory surgery units (ASUs) and freestanding ambulatory surgical centers (ASCs) is based on the inpatient model. **B.** The flow-through design for ASUs and ASCs generally provides more efficient patient flow than the tidal model. **C.** When the staging area of an ASU or ASC is a considerable distance from the operating rooms, a preoperative holding unit is used to minimize delays.

installed where hands-free use is desirable. One limitation of telephones is that even four-digit telephone numbers are hard to remember unless they are arranged in a familiar context. OR communications are substantially enhanced if telephone companies or the telecommunications divisions of large health care organizations can be convinced to assign meaningful telephone numbers. Thus, in an eight-room suite with ORs numbered 1 through 8, the local telephone numbers in the ORs should be something like 275-2221, 275-2222, . . . 275-2228. In an OR suite that has four-

digit OR numbers, the telephone numbers should be some access number followed by the four-digit OR number.

Intercoms based on the telephone may also be useful. The telephone intercom is particularly valuable if it is capable of sending an overhead page within the OR suite in the event of an emergency. (Such pages, however, should be used rarely.) Two advantages justify using the intercom feature of a digital telephone system rather than the core telephone system. First, intercom numbers might be easier to program in series that are easily remembered. Second, adding additional intercom numbers is likely to be less expensive than adding additional telephone numbers. Because calls cannot be made directly between ORs and locations outside the scope of the intercom system, intercoms should not be considered to be substitutes for conventional telephones.

Many ORs still use a nurse call intercom, which served OR communication well until better alternatives became available. The major drawback to the nurse call intercom is that it funnels all communication through a central location, usually the OR suite control desk. A few moments of reflection make the inefficiency associated with relaying messages through a central location apparent. Furthermore, sitting for a few minutes at a busy control desk that functions as a communications center will quickly convince an observer of the limitations associated with interposing the knowledge and vocabulary of even a well-trained clerk between two professional or technical medical personnel. It is difficult to justify using the nurse call intercom as a substitute for direct communication between two people by telephone or telephone-based intercom.

Pagers

Digital pagers are an effective method of communicating within the OR suite. Computer software is readily available to transmit digital messages from the OR control desk. Better paging programs permit entering into the computer the names and pager numbers of all personnel working in the OR suite. Hence, a clerk simply identifies on a menu the name of the person to be paged, types a brief message into the message box, and clicks "send" with a mouse. The software dials the paging system and transmits the message:

- To an OR technician: OR #3 needs a blood warmer.
- To an anesthesiologist: Patient Jones has arrived in the preoperative holding unit.
- To the nurse manager: Karen Epsom has called in sick.

Digital pagers are particularly useful for personnel who are unlikely to be in a given location when a message needs to be transmitted to them. For example, digital pagers are more valuable for the nurse manager than for circulating nurses, who spend most of their day in an OR near a telephone.

One major disadvantage of early paging technology was that it was unidirectional. Not only was the recipient of the message unable to respond to the message, but the sender received no confirmation that the message had arrived. Hence, acknowledgment, one of the most important components of effective communication, was absent from first-generation digital paging. Two-way messaging units are now available and should be used to close the loop for effective digital communication.

Computers, Intranets, and the Internet

Computers have several roles in OR communication. (See Table 10-2 on page 135 for a list of functions of an OR information system.) First, they can act as the front end of other communications devices, such as digital pagers. Second, they can be used to access the Internet or an intranet (see below) for reference information. Third, computers can be used for real-time tracking of OR activity (primarily patient flow).

Most people are familiar with the monitors in airports that track airline flights in real time. A similar method can be used to track patient flow through an OR suite. This requires that the fields in the ORDB pertaining to patient flow (e.g., "patient in PHU," "OR ready," "patient in OR," "patient in PACU") be updated when patients are transferred from one location to another and when other events occur. It also requires that large computer displays be located in strategic places in the OR suite (hallways, lounges, duty rooms) and that computer software to display the relevant fields in the database is available. Color coding can be used to make information on the display easier to read (e.g., black for a scheduled procedure waiting to be performed, yellow to designate that a patient has arrived in the PHU, green while a patient's operation is under way, red for a postponement, orange for an unscheduled, urgent procedure).

Physicians who do not spend most of their working day in the OR suite (e.g., surgeons, radiologists, and pathologists) should be able to access the computerized tracking system via modem, LAN, or the Internet (through a password-protected Web site). Telephone traffic to the control desk or to specific ORs is reduced, and, if the system is easy to use, surgeons and other physicians are likely to keep track of the status of their patients and therefore become more accessible as they anticipate the need for their presence in the OR suite.

The Internet or the health care organization's intranet can be a source of information for workers in the OR suite. Some health care organizations publish their policy and procedure manuals and other important public documents on the organization's intranet. Some even publish such documents on the Internet. To the extent that useful information is available through these sources, they become part of the communication system of the OR suite.

Overhead Page

Overhead paging is a much-overused method of communication in most hospitals and OR suites, perhaps because more effective or more easily used methods of communication are often unavailable. Health care organizations should minimize the use of overhead pages because of their substantial contribution to the noise and clutter of the health care environment. No other method of communication disturbs so many to communicate with so few (with apologies to Winston Churchill).

Appendix 1
Procedural Times Glossary*

PROCEDURAL TIMES GLOSSARY©

*Association of Anesthesia Clinical Directors
and Society for Technology in Anesthesia
National Database Committee*

1.   Procedural times
      For purposes of analyzing efficiency, each
      of the times defined below may be further
      classified by the subscripts S and A, for
      "Scheduled" and "Actual," respectively.
1.1. Patient in Facility (PIF) = Time patient
      arrives at health-care facility (applicable to
      Out-patient or Same Day Admission
      patients).
1.2. Patient Ready for Transport (PRT) = Time
      when all preparations required prior to
      transport (e.g., labs, consent, gowning) have
      been completed.
1.3. Patient Sent-for (PSF) = Time when trans-
      porting service is notified to deliver patient
      to the OR/PR [operating room/procedure
      room].
1.4. Patient Available (PA) = Time the patient
      arrives in the OR/PR pre-procedure area.
1.5. Room Set-up Start (RSS) = Time when per-
      sonnel begin setting-up, in the OR/PR, the
      supplies and equipment for the next case.
1.6. Anesthesia Start (AS) = Time when a mem-
      ber of the anesthesia team begins preparing
      the patient for an anesthetic.

1.7. Room Ready (RR) = Time when room is
      cleaned and supplies and equipment neces-
      sary for beginning of next case are present.
1.8. Patient In Room (PIR) = Time when patient
      enters the OR/PR.
1.9. Anesthesiologist, First Available (AFA) =
      Time of arrival in OR/PR of first anesthesi-
      ologist who is qualified to induce anesthe-
      sia in patient.
1.10. Procedure Physician, First Available (PPFA)
      = Time of arrival in OR/PR of first physi-
      cian/surgeon qualified to position and prep
      the patient.
1.11. Anesthesiologist of Record In (ARI) = Time
      of arrival in OR/PR of anesthesiologist of
      record.
1.12. Anesthesia Induction (AI) = Time when
      the anesthesiologist begins the administra-
      tion of agents intended to provide the level
      of anesthesia required for the scheduled
      procedure.
1.13. Anesthesia Ready (AR) = Time at which the
      patient has a sufficient level of anesthesia
      established to begin surgical preparation of
      the patient, and remaining anesthetic chores
      do not preclude positioning and prepping
      the patient.
1.14. Position/Prep Start (PS) = Time at which the
      nursing or surgical team begins positioning
      or prepping the patient for the procedure.
1.15. Prep-Completed (PC) = Time at which
      prepping and draping have been completed
      and patient is ready for the procedure or
      surgery to start.
1.16. Procedure Physician of Record In (PPRI)
      = Arrival time of physician/surgeon of
      record.

*Reprinted with permission from Association of Anesthesia
Clinical Directors. Procedural times glossary: glossary of
times used for scheduling and monitoring of diagnostic and
therapeutic procedures. Surgical Services Management
1997;3(9):11–15.

1.17. Procedure/Surgery Start Time (PST) = Time the procedure is begun (e.g., incision for a surgical procedure, insertion of scope for a diagnostic procedure, beginning of exam for an EUA [examination under anesthesia], shooting of x-ray for radiological procedure).

1.18. Procedure/Surgery Conclusion Begun (PCB) = Time when diagnostic or therapeutic maneuvers are completed and attempts are made by the physician or surgical team to end any noxious stimuli (e.g., beginning of wound closure, removal of bronchoscope).

1.19. Procedure Physician of Record Out (PPRO) = Time when physician/surgeon of record leaves the OR/PR.

1.20. Procedure/Surgery Finish (PF) = Time when all instrument and sponge counts are completed and verified as correct; all post-op radiological studies to be done in the OR/PR are completed; all dressings and drains are secured; and the physician/surgeons have completed all procedure related activities on the patient.

1.21. Patient Out of Room (POR) = Time at which patient leaves OR/PR.

1.22. Room Clean-up Start (RCS) = Time housekeeping or room personnel begin cleanup of OR/PR.

1.23. Arrival in PACU/ICU [post anesthesia care unit/intensive care unit] (APACU) = Time of patient arrival in PACU or ICU.

1.24. Anesthesia Finish (AF) = Time at which anesthesiologist turns over care of the patient to a post anesthesia care team (either PACU or ICU).

1.25. Room Clean-up Finished (RCF) = Time OR/PR is clean and ready for setup of supplies and equipment for the next case.

1.26. Ready-for-Discharge from Post Anesthesia Care Unit (RDPACU) = Time that patient is assessed to be ready for discharge from the PACU.

1.27. Discharge from Post Anesthesia Care Unit (DPACU) = Time patient is transported out of PACU.

1.28. Arrival in Same Day Surgery Recovery Unit (ASDSR) = Time of patient arrival in Same Day Surgery Recovery Unit.

1.29. Ready-for-Discharge from Same Day Surgery Recovery Unit (RDSDSR) = Time that patient is assessed to be ready for discharge from the Same Day Surgery Recovery Unit.

1.30. Discharge from Same Day Surgery Recovery Unit (DSDSR) = Time patient leaves SDSR unit (either to home or other facility).

2.   Procedural and scheduling definitions and time periods
(For purposes of analyzing efficiency, each of the time periods defined below may be further classified by the subscripts S and A, for "Scheduled" and "Actual," respectively.)

2.1. Anesthesia Preparation Time (APT) = Time from Anesthesia Start to Anesthesia Ready Time.

2.2. Average Case Length (ACL) = Total Hours divided by total number of cases performed within those hours.

2.3. Block Time (BT) = Hours of OR/PR time reserved for a given service or physician/surgeon. Within a defined cutoff period (e.g., 72 hours prior to day of surgery), this is time into which only the given service may schedule. (N.B., in some institutions, this is known as Available or Allocated Time.)

2.4. Case Time (CT) = Time from Room Set-up Start to Room Clean-up Finished.

2.5. Early Start Hours (ESH) = Hours of Case Time performed prior to the normal day's start time when it is not expected that the Patient Out of Room Time will be before the normal start time for that day.

2.6. Evening/Weekend/Holiday Hours (EWHH) = Hours of Case Time performed outside of Resource Hours.

2.7. In-own Block Hours (IBH) = Hours of Case Time performed during a Service's own Block Time. (N.B., for a case to be counted in IBH, it must begin during that given Service's Block Time.)

2.8. Open Time (OT) = Hours of OR/PR time not reserved for any particular Service, into which any Service or physician/surgeon may schedule according to the rules established by the given institution (N.B., in some institutions, this is known as Discretionary Time).

2.9. Outside-own Block Hours (OBH) = Hours of Case Time performed during Resource Hours but outside of the Service's Block Time.

2.10. Overrun Hours (OVRH) = Hours of Case Time completed after the scheduled closure time of the OR/PR (i.e., after the end of that day's Resource Hours).

2.11. Released Time (RT) = Hours of OR/PR time that are released from a service's Block Time and converted to Open Time (typically done when a service anticipates that it will be unable to use the block time due to meetings or vacation).

2.12. Resource Hours (RH) = Total number of hours scheduled to be available for performance of procedures (i.e., the sum of all available Block Time and Open Time). This is typically provided for on a weekly recurring basis, but may be analyzed on a daily, weekly, monthly, or annual basis.

2.13. Room Clean-up Time (RCT) = Time from Patient Out of Room to Room Clean-up Finished.

2.14. Room Close (RC) = Time at which the room should be empty and the assigned personnel free to be discharged.

2.15. Room Open (RO) = Time when appropriate staff are scheduled to be present and are expected to have the OR/PR available for patient occupancy.

2.16. Room Set-up Time (RST) = Time from Room Set-up Start to Room Ready.

2.17. Service = a group of physicians or surgeons that together perform a circumscribed set of operative or diagnostic procedures (e.g., Cardiothoracic Surgery, Interventional Radiology). Generally, any member of a service may schedule into that service's block time. Similarly, OR/PR time used by a given physician or surgeon is credited to his/her service's Total Hours.

2.18. Surgical Preparation Time (SPT) = Time from Position/Prep Start to Procedure/Surgery Start Time.

2.19. Start Time (ST) = Patient In Room Time.

2.20. Total Cases (TC) = Cumulative total of all cases done in a given time period. May be subdivided by Service or physician/surgeon.

2.21. Total Hours (TH) = Sum of all Case Times for a given period of time. TH = IBH + OBH + EWHH. May be subdivided by Service or individual physician/surgeon.

2.22. Turnover Time (TOT) = Time from prior Patient Out of Room to succeeding Patient In Room Time for sequentially scheduled cases.

3. Utilization and efficiency indices

3.1. Adjusted-Percent Service Utilization (ASU) = (IBH + OBH) ÷ BT × 100. This measures the percentage of time a Service utilizes their Block Time during Resource Hours. It is adjusted, compared to Raw Utilization, in that it gives a Service "credit" for the time necessary to set-up and clean-up a room, during which time a patient cannot be in the room. It may exceed 100% because of the inclusion of cases performed during Resource Hours that are Outside-own Block Hours.

3.2. Adjusted-Percent Utilized Resource Hours (AURH) = (TH − EWHH) ÷ RH × 100. This calculation provides the percentage of time that the OR/PRs are being prepared for a patient, are occupied by a patient, or are being cleaned after taking care of a patient during Resource Hours. It is adjusted, compared to Raw Utilization, in that it includes the time necessary to set-up and clean-up a room, during which time a patient can not be in the room.

3.3. Delays may be due to

3.3.1. Patient Issues
- Insurance problems
- Patient arrived late
- Patient ate/drank
- Abnormal lab values
- Surgery issues
- Complications arose

3.3.2. System Issues
- Test results unavailable
- Blood unavailable
- Patient not ready on floor
- Transport Delay
- Elevator Delay
- Previous case ran late
- Case bumped for emergency case
- Equipment unavailable
- Equipment malfunction
- X-rays unavailable
- X-ray technician unavailable
- Delay in receiving floor bed
- Insufficient post procedure care beds

- ICU delay
- Instrument problem

3.3.3. Practitioner issues
- Needs more workup (e.g., labs, consults)
- No consent
- Physician/Surgeon arrived late
- Anesthesiologist arrived late
- Physician/Surgeon unavailable
- Anesthesiologist unavailable
- Inaccurate posting
- Prolonged setup time

3.4. Early Start = When Patient In Room, Actual, is prior to Patient In Room, Scheduled.

3.4.1. With overlap—when a case starts early but prior to the Room Clean-up Finished, Actual, of the case originally scheduled to precede it (this occurs when either the preceding or following case is moved to a different OR/PR than originally scheduled).

3.4.2. Without overlap—when a case starts early but after the Room Clean-up Finished, Actual, of the case originally scheduled to precede it (this may occur because there is no preceding case or because the preceding case finishes earlier than scheduled).

3.5. Late Start = When Patient In Room, Actual, is after Patient In Room, Scheduled.

3.5.1. With no interference—when the Room Clean-up Finished, Actual, of the preceding case occurs before the Room Set-up Start, Scheduled, of the following case (i.e., the OR/PR is available prior to or at the time that preparation for the next case is supposed to begin).

3.5.2. With interference—when Room Clean-up Finished, Actual, of the preceding case occurs after the Room Set-up Start, Scheduled, of the following case (i.e., the OR/PR is not available at the time that preparation for the next case is supposed to begin, either because it is still occupied or because it has not been cleaned).

3.6. Overrun = When Room Clean-up Finished, Actual, for the last scheduled case of the day is later than Room Close. This may be caused by a late start, a Case Time, Actual, greater than Case Time, Scheduled, or a combination of late start and longer than scheduled Case Time.

3.7. Productivity Index (PI) = Percent of time per hour that a patient is in the OR/PR during the prime shift time (e.g., first 8 hours).

3.8. Raw Utilization (RU) = For the system as a whole, this is the percent of time that patients are in the room during Resource Hours (see Adjusted-Percent Utilized Resource Hours). For an individual service, this is the percent of its Block Time during which a service has a patient in the OR/PR (see Adjusted-Percent Service Utilization).

3.9. Room Gap = Time OR/PRs are vacant during Resource Hours

3.9.1. Empty Room (or Late Start) Gap (LSG)
Planned—When Patient In Room, Scheduled, is later than Room Open.
Unplanned—When Patient In Room, Actual, is later than Room Open.

3.9.2. Between Case Gaps (BCG)
Planned—When Patient In Room, Scheduled, is later than the Room Clean-up Finished, Actual, of the preceding case.
Unplanned—When Patient In Room, Actual, is later than the Room Clean-up Finished, Actual, of the preceding case.

3.9.3. End of Schedule Gaps (ESG)
Planned—When Room Clean-up Finished, Scheduled, occurs before Room Close.
Unplanned—When Room Clean-up Finished, Actual, occurs before Room Close.

3.9.4. Total Gap Hours (TGH) = LSG + BCG + ESG.

4. Patient categories

4.1. In-house (IH)—Patient admitted to and residing in the hospital prior to scheduled surgery/procedure.

4.2. Outpatient (OP)—Patient who is coming in on the day of surgery/procedure and is expected to return home following the procedure.

4.3. Same Day Admit (SDA)—Patient who is coming in on the day of surgery/procedure and will be admitted to the hospital following the procedure.

4.4. Overnight Recovery (ONR)—Patient who comes in on the day of surgery/procedure but requires overnight recovery prior to returning home. These patients are never admitted to the hospital as inpatients, but may remain in the recovery facility for 12–23 hours post surgery/procedure.

Appendix 2
Standards-Setting Organizations

ACCREDITATION ASSOCIATION FOR AMBULATORY HEALTH CARE (AAAHC)

Mission: "The AAAHC is a leader in ambulatory health care accreditation and serves as an advocate for the provision and documentation of high quality health services in ambulatory health care organizations. This is accomplished through the development of standards and through its survey and accreditation programs."*

Address: 9933 Lawler Ave., Suite 460
Skokie, IL 60077-3708

Telephone: (847) 676-9610

Fax: (847) 676-9628

Web Site: <http://www.aaahc.org>

AMERICAN ASSOCIATION FOR ACCREDITATION OF AMBULATORY SURGERY FACILITIES (AAAASF)

Mission: "To promote the highest standards in the delivery of ambulatory surgical care and to promote the common interests of those engaged in the delivery of such care. To maintain and improve the quality of surgical ambulatory care through the development, administration, and supervision of a voluntary program for the accreditation of surgical ambulatory care facilities. To develop and adopt criteria for the evaluation and accreditation of the facilities. To collect and analyze research data in order to develop new educational programs to improve the delivery of ambulatory surgical care."†

Address: 1202 Allanson Rd.
Mundelein, IL 60060

Telephone: (888) 545-5222

Fax: (847) 566-4580

Web Site: <http://www.aaaasf.org>

AMERICAN SOCIETY OF ANESTHESIOLOGISTS (ASA)

Mission: "The American Society of Anesthesiologists is a nonprofit association of reputable Doctors of Medicine or Osteopathy engaged in the practice of or otherwise especially interested in anesthesiology. As provided in the Bylaws, the Society holds to the following purposes:
"To advance the science and art of anesthsiology, and
"To stimulate interest and promote progress in the scientific, cultural and economic aspects of the specialty of anesthesiology."‡

---

*Source: <http://www.aaahc.org/pros/index.html>

†Source: Personal communication with AAAASF.
‡Source: Statement of Policy (Approved by House of Delegates on November 8, 1950 and last amended on October 19, 1994).

Address: 520 N. Northwest Highway
        Park Ridge, IL 60068-2573

Telephone: (847) 825-5586

Fax: (847) 825-1692

E-mail: mail@asahq.org

Web Site: <http://www.asahq.org>

ASSOCIATION FOR THE ADVANCEMENT OF MEDICAL INSTRUMENTATION (AAMI)

Mission: "The Association for the Advancement of Medical Instrumentation (AAMI), founded in 1967, is a unique alliance of nearly 7,000 members united by the common goal of increasing the understanding and beneficial use of medical instrumentation.

"AAMI is the primary source of consensus and timely information on medical instrumentation and technology, and is the primary resource for the industry, professions, and government for national and international standards.

"AAMI provides multidisciplinary leadership and programs that enhance the ability of the professions, health care institutions, and industry to understand, develop, manage, and use medical instrumentation and related technologies safely and effectively.

"AAMI helps members contain costs, keep informed of new technology and policy developments, add value in health care organizations, improve professional skills, and enhance patient care. . . .

"AAMI fulfills its mission through continuing education conferences, certification of health care technical specialists, and the publication of technical documents, periodicals, books, software."*

Address: 3330 Washington Blvd.
        Arlington, VA 22201-4598

Telephone: (703) 525-4890

Fax: (703) 525-1424

Web Site: <http://www.aami.org>

---

*Source: <http://www.aami.org/about/index.html>

ASSOCIATION OF PERIOPERATIVE REGISTERED NURSES (AORN)

Mission: "AORN is the professional organization of perioperative registered nurses whose mission is to promote quality patient care by providing its members with education, standards, services, and representation.

"AORN represents more than 43,000 registered nurses who facilitate the management, teaching, and practice of perioperative nursing, or who are enrolled in nursing education or engaged in perioperative research. AORN's members come from over 340 chapters across the US and in Puerto Rico."[†]

Address: 2170 South Parker Rd., Suite 300
        Denver, CO 80231-5711

Telephone: (303) 755-6300
        (800) 755-2676

Fax: (303) 750-2927 (Office of Executive Director)

Web Site: <http://www.aorn.org>

ECRI

Mission: "ECRI, an international nonprofit health services research agency and a Collaborating Center of the World Health Organization, is widely recognized as the world's leading independent organization committed to improving the safety, efficacy, and cost-effectiveness of healthcare technology."[‡]

Address: 5200 Butler Pike
        Plymouth Meeting, PA 19462-1298

Telephone: (610) 825-6000

Fax: (610) 834-1275

E-mail: info@ecri.org

Web Site: <http://www.ecri.org>

[†]Source: <http://www.aorn.org/abtaorn/index.htm>
[‡]Source: <http://www.ecri.org>

U.S. FOOD AND DRUG ADMINISTRATION (FDA)

Mission: "The American people expect and rely on a safe and wholesome food supply, and access to safe and effective drugs and medical devices. To meet those expectations, FDA inspects and oversees almost 95,000 establishments that produce:

- $487 billion worth of food
- $107 billion worth of drugs—prescription and over-the-counter—and biologics
- $350 billion worth of medical devices and radiation-emitting products
- $3 billion worth of animal drugs and medicated feed
- $39 billion worth of cosmetics and toiletries.

"In addition to overseeing the production of safe foods and the manufacture of safe and effective drugs and medical devices, the FDA has responsibility for:

- protecting the rights and safety of patients in the clinical trials of investigational medical products
- reviewing and approving in a timely manner the safety and efficacy of new drugs, biologics, medical devices, and animal drugs
- monitoring the safety and effectiveness of new medical products after they are marketed and acting on the information collected.

"As the nation's oldest consumer protection agency, FDA is also responsible for seeing that the public has access to truthful and non-misleading product information by

- monitoring the promotional activities of drug and device manufacturers
- regulating the labeling of all packaged foods.

"The FDA's public health mission also encompasses efforts to assure:

- the safety of the nation's blood supply
- the safety of all imported FDA-regulated products."[*]

---

*Source: <http://www.fda.gov/opacom/backgrounders/mission.html>

Address: U.S. Food and Drug Administration (HFE-88)
5600 Fishers Lane
Rockville, MD 20857

Telephone: (800) 532-4440
(301) 827-4420

Fax: (301) 443-9767

E-mail: execsec@oc.fda.gov

Web Site: <http://www.fda.gov>

HEALTH LEVEL SEVEN (HL7)

Mission: "The mission of HL7 is to provide standards for the exchange, management and integration of data that support clinical patient care and the management, delivery and evaluation of healthcare services. Specifically, to create flexible, cost effective approaches, standards, guidelines, methodologies, and related services for interoperability between healthcare information systems.

"These efforts enable effective, efficient communication between the constituents of the healthcare community as represented by our membership, which consists of an international community of healthcare organizations, vendors, developers of healthcare information systems, consultants and systems integrators, and related public and private healthcare services agencies.

"The mission of HL7 encompasses the complete 'life cycle' of a standards specification: development, adoption, market recognition, utilization and adherence. The HL7 specifications are unified by shared reference models of the healthcare and technical domains."[†]

Address: Health Level Seven, Inc.
3300 Washtenaw Ave., Suite 227
Ann Arbor, MI 48104-4250

Telephone: (734) 677-7777

Fax: (734) 677-6622

[†]Source: <http://www.hl7.org>

E-mail: hq@hl7.org

Web Site: <http://www.hl7.org>

JOINT COMMISSION ON ACCREDITATION OF HEALTHCARE ORGANIZATIONS (JCAHO)

Mission: "The mission of the Joint Commission on Accreditation of Healthcare Organizations is to improve the quality of care provided to the public through the provision of health care accreditation and related services that support performance improvement in health care organizations."*

Address: One Renaissance Blvd.
Oakbrook Terrace, IL 60181

Telephone: (630) 916-5600

Fax: (630) 792-5005

Web Site: <http://www.jcaho.org>

NATIONAL COMMITTEE FOR QUALITY ASSURANCE (NCQA)

Mission: "NCQA's mission is to provide information that enables purchasers and consumers of managed health care to distinguish among plans based on quality, thereby allowing them to make more informed health care purchasing decisions. This encourages plans to compete based on quality and value, rather than on price and provider network. Our efforts are organized around two activities, accreditation and performance measurement, which are complementary strategies for producing information to guide choice."†

Address: 2000 L St., NW, Suite 500
Washington, DC 20036

Telephone: (202) 955-5697

Fax: (202) 955-3599

Web Site: <http://www.ncqa.org>

NATIONAL FIRE PROTECTION ASSOCIATION (NFPA)

Mission: "The National Fire Protection Association is an international, nonprofit, membership organization founded in 1896 to protect people, their property and the environment from destructive fire. In more than 100 years of advocacy, NFPA has established its role as the leading worldwide advisor on the topics of fire safety and protection.

"More than 66,000 strong, NFPA's diverse membership represents nearly 100 nations and includes representatives from fire service, government, architecture, engineering, health care, education, insurance, transportation, manufacturing, and research industries.

"NFPA is the publisher of more than 300 codes and standards that comprise the National Fire Code covering life safety, electrical installations, and all areas of fire safety. In some way, virtually every building, process, service, design, and installation in society today is affected by codes and standards developed through NFPA's system.

"NFPA is the most comprehensive and authoritative source of information about fire problems, fire safety, and fire education."‡

Address: 1 Batterymarch Park
Quincy, MA 02269-9101

Telephone: (617) 770-3000

Fax: (617) 770-0700

Web Site: <http://www.nfpa.org>

OCCUPATIONAL SAFETY & HEALTH ADMINISTRATION (OSHA)

Mission: "The mission of the Occupational Safety & Health Administration (OSHA) is to save lives, prevent injuries and protect the health of America's workers. To accomplish this, federal and state governments must work in partnership

*Source: <http://www.jcaho.org/about_jc/jcinfo.htm>
†Source: <http://www.ncqa.org/pages/main/overview3.htm>
‡Source: <http://www.nfpa.org>

with the more than 100 million working men and women and their six and a half million employers who are covered by the Occupational Safety and Health Act of 1970."*

Address: OSHA
U.S. Department of Labor
200 Constitution Avenue, NW
Washington, DC 20210

Telephone: (202) 693-2000 (Office of the Assistant Secretary)

Fax: (202) 693-2106

Web Site: <http://www.osha.gov>

*Source: <http://www.osha.gov/oshinfo/mission.html>

Appendix 3
Table of Contents: Life Safety Code®*

National Fire Protection Association
NFPA 101-1997
Life Safety Code®†
Contents‡
(Relevant to Health Care Facilities)

---

*Portions reprinted with permission from NFPA 101-1997 Life Safety Code®. Copyright © 1997, National Fire Protection Association, Quincy, MA 02269.
†*Life Safety Code*® and *101*® are registered trademarks of the National Fire Protection Association.
‡Chapters 8–11 and 14–31 are not listed because they are not relevant to health care facilities.

Appendix 4
Table of Contents:
National Electrical Code®*

National Fire Protection Association
NFPA 70-1996
National Electrical Code®†
Contents

Appendix 5

Table of Contents: Standard for Health Care Facilities* (NFPA 99)

National Fire Protection Association
NFPA 99
Standard for Health Care Facilities
Contents

*Reprinted with permission from NFPA 99, Health Care Facilities. Copyright © 1996, National Fire Protection Association, Quincy, MA 02269.

Appendix 6

Table of Contents: Standards, Recommended Practices, and Guidelines*

Association of Operating Room Nurses
Standards, Recommended Practices, and Guidelines
Table of Contents

---

*Reprinted with permission from Association of Operating Room Nurses. Standards, Recommended Practices, and Guidelines. Denver: Association of Operating Room Nurses, 1998; i-ii. Copyright © AORN, Inc., 2170 South Parker Road, Suite 300, Denver, CO 80231.
†Indicates items newly revised in 1997 or published here for the first time.

Index

Note: Page numbers followed by *f* indicate figures; page numbers followed by *t* indicate tables.